Essentials of

Esthetic Dentistry

Principles and Practice of Esthetic Dentistry

Volume One

Essentials of

Esthetic Dentistry

Principles and Practice of Esthetic Dentistry

Volume One

Edited by

Nairn H. F. Wilson CBE DSc (*h.c.*) FDS FFD FFGDP FCDSHK FACD FADM FHEA FKC

Professor of Dentistry, King's College London Dental Institute,
London, UK

Series Editor

Brian J. Millar BDS FDSRCS PhD FHEA

Professor of Blended Learning in Dentistry;
Consultant in Restorative Dentistry; Specialist Practitioner, King's College London Dental Institute,
London, UK

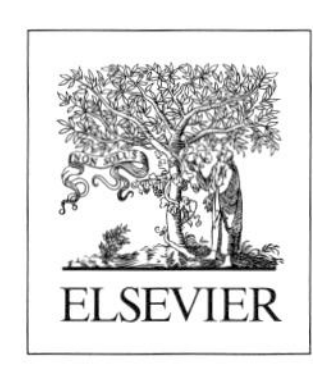

Edinburgh London New York Oxford Philadelphia St Louis Sydney Toronto 2015

ELSEVIER

ISBN 9780723455585
Reprinted 2015

Notices

Knowledge and best practice in this field are constantly changing. As new research and experience broaden our understanding, changes in research methods, professional practices, or medical treatment may become necessary.

Practitioners and researchers must always rely on their own experience and knowledge in evaluating and using any information, methods, compounds, or experiments described herein. In using such information or methods they should be mindful of their own safety and the safety of others, including parties for whom they have a professional responsibility.

With respect to any drug or pharmaceutical products identified, readers are advised to check the most current information provided (i) on procedures featured or (ii) by the manufacturer of each product to be administered, to verify the recommended dose or formula, the method and duration of administration, and contraindications. It is the responsibility of practitioners, relying on their own experience and knowledge of their patients, to make diagnoses, to determine dosages and the best treatment for each individual patient, and to take all appropriate safety precautions.

To the fullest extent of the law, neither the Publisher nor the authors, contributors, or editors, assume any liability for any injury and/or damage to persons or property as a matter of products liability, negligence or otherwise, or from any use or operation of any methods, products, instructions, or ideas contained in the material herein.

Printed in China

For Elsevier:
Content Strategist: Alison Taylor
Content Development Specialist: Clive Hewat
Project Manager: Anne Collett
Designer/Design Direction: Miles Hitchen
Illustrator: AEGIS Media

CONTENTS

CONTRIBUTORS

Subir Banerji BDS MClinDent
Programme Director MSc, Aesthetic Dentistry; Senior Clinical Teacher, Unit of Distance Learning
King's College London Dental Institute
Guy's Hospital
London, UK

Iain Chapple BDS FDSRCPS PhD FDSRCS CCST (Rest Dent)
Professor of Periodontology
University of Birmingham,
Birmingham, UK

Richard J. Foxton BDS PhD MFDS RCS (Ed) ISFE (Rest Dent) FHEA
Senior Clinical Lecturer/Honorary Specialist RegistrarDental Institute, King's College London
London, UK

Christopher C. K. Ho BDS(Hons) GradDipClinDent (Oral Implants) MClinDent (Pros)
Principal Dentist, CARE Dentistry; Visiting Clinical Teacher, Dental Institute, Kings College London
Sydney, Australia

Shamir B. Mehta BDS BSc MClinDent (Prosth) (Hons)
Clinical Senior Lecturer; General Dental Practitioner
Dental Institute, Kings College London
London, UK

Brian J. Millar BDS FDSRCS PhD FHEA
Professor of Blended Learning in Dentistry
Dental Institute, King's College London
London, UK

Jonathon Timothy Newton BA PhD CPsychol AFBPsS CSci
Professor of Psychology as Applied to Dentistry
Dental Institute, King's College London
London, UK

Amit Patel BDS MSc MClinDent MRD RSCEng FDS RCSEd
Specialist in Periodontics; Associate Specialist,
Birmingham Dental Hospital
Birmingham Community Health Trust
Birmingham, UK

Bill Sharpling MBA DipCDT RCS(Eng)
Director, London Dental Education Centre (LonDEC)
Senior Clinical Teacher, Dental Institute, King's College London
London, UK

Richard J. Simonsen BA BS DDS MS PhD (*h.c.*) FACD FICD FAAED
Dean and Professor of Dentistry
College of Dental Medicine, University of Sharjah
Sharjah, United Arab Emirates

Nairn H. F. Wilson CBE DSc (*h.c.*)) FDS FFD FFGDP FCDSHK FACD FADM FHEA FKC
Professor of Dentistry, King's College London Dental Institute
London, UK

David Winkler DDS
Owner, CastleView Dental
Windsor, UK

SERIES PREFACE

Esthetic dentistry is a complex subject. In many ways it requires different skills from those needed for disease-focussed clinical care. Yet in other ways esthetic dentistry is part of everyday dentistry. The team which has created this series shares the view that success in esthetic dentistry requires a broad range of additional skills. Dentistry can now offer improved shade matching through to smile design to reorganising the smile zone.

This first volume provides a wealth of useful, readily applicable information, and sets the scene for those wishing to develop further their practice of esthetic dentistry. The provision of esthetic dentistry requires a different philosophy in the dental clinic and the minds of the clinical team, a greater awareness of the aspirations of patients and a solid ethical footing. Also needed is an ability to carry out a detailed assessment of dental and psychological factors, offer methods to show the patient the available options and, in some cases, be able to offer a range of treatments.

An increasing concern to many clinicians is the amount of tooth reduction some would say destruction – carried out to enhance esthetics, while healthcare in general moves towards minimal intervention (MI). I believe patients should receive the best possible care, with the options not being limited by the clinician's skill (or lack of skills). Hence, the vision for this series.

The single biggest task the team faced in putting this series together was to create information for dentists across the world: recognising that there are differing views on esthetics, MI, essential understanding and skills, and patients with different attitudes and budgets. The specific challenge was creating a series of books which addresses these diverse opinions, ranging from the view that tooth reduction is acceptable and inevitable in producing beautiful smiles – thinking reflected in Volume 2 – to the view that such tooth reduction is abhorrent and unacceptable and the MI approach is preferable, as covered in Volume 3. I hope the series of books will satisfy both camps and enable practitioners at all levels to develop skills to practise esthetics, while respecting tooth tissue.

We intend this series to challenge your thinking and approach to the growing subject area of esthetic dentistry, particularly by showing different management of common clinical situations. We do not need to rely on a single formula to provide a smile make-over, promoting only one treatment modality where both the dentist and their patients are losing out; the patient losing valuable irreplaceable enamel as well as their future options.

This first book in the series will be of significant benefit to students and practitioners on subjects not taught in detail at the undergraduate level, but frequently learnt in a piecemeal way from short CPD courses, often giving a myopic view or single approach to dentistry. It is aimed at bringing together key elements of communication skills, understanding the patient with care and empathy and carrying out an assessment providing a foundation on which to base a treatment plan. Ethics are stressed and some of the simpler treatment options are covered in detail.

As the series progresses you can discover in greater depth the many clinical techniques to practise a range of effective procedures in esthetic dentistry.

Professor Brian Millar BDS, FDSRCS, PhD, FHEA

PREFACE

Esthetic dentistry is a global phenomenon that continues to grow and expand. To practise successful esthetic dentistry, practitioners must understand the art and science of the discipline and be up to date and competent in the use of modern materials and techniques. In addition, the successful practice of esthetic dentistry requires good communication skills, empathy with the esthetic concerns expressed by patients, and the ability to build a good rapport between the patient and the various members of the dental team.

Patients contemplating changes to their dental appearance, in particular their smile, wish to have their treatment provided by a practitioner they can trust, in an environment that they find reassuring and that gives them confidence. The present book, the first in a carefully planned series on the state of the art of esthetic dentistry, is an important foundation on which to build the knowledge and understanding required to practise effective, patient-pleasing, minimal intervention esthetic dentistry. If you do not know the difference between esthetic and cosmetic dentistry, need to know how to carry out a comprehensive examination and assessment of a patient seeking esthetic dental care, harbour uncertainties about the different approaches to enhancing dental attractiveness and about related ethical considerations, and have unanswered questions in respect to the application of contemporary materials and techniques in esthetic dentistry, then this book will be of great value to you.

The highly regarded international team of contributors to this book, who individually and collectively have considerable knowledge and expertise in the field of esthetic dentistry, have adhered strictly to the brief to deal, succinctly but comprehensively, with their allocated subject in a text that is engaging and pleasing to read. It has been a pleasure and an honour to edit and contribute to this book, which is intended to be of immediate practical relevance to students and practitioners alike – a book for everyone engaged in the modern practice of dentistry.

Being able to consistently provide high-quality esthetic dentistry that pleases patients, will survive the test of time and, as described in the introductory chapter to this book, makes others smile is very rewarding. Realising this goal requires good knowledge and understanding, meticulous investigation, planning and execution of all relevant procedures, strong team working and excellent patient relationships, as well as professionalism and clinical acumen in all aspects of esthetic dentistry. Whatever the level at which you presently practise esthetic dentistry, my fellow authors and I believe that this book will strengthen, enhance and hopefully expand the scope of your work. I have learnt a great deal in the process of editing this book, and am confident that all those who read and study its contents will share my experience. Your patients and practice will benefit greatly from you acquiring this book and becoming familiar with its contents.

Nairn Wilson CBE DSc (*h.c.*) FDS FFD FFGDP FCDSHK FACD FADM FHEA FKC

CHAPTER 1

Dental Esthetics: the Big Picture

DAVID WINKLER AND NAIRN WILSON

INTRODUCTION

Esthetic dentistry is here to stay. It is a widely held belief that individuals who are beautiful are happier, have more 'sex appeal', and are more confident, kind, friendly, popular, intelligent and successful than their less attractive peers. Who does not want to share some, if not all, of these perceived qualities? Having, or *acquiring*, an attractive smile (Fig. 1.1) can make an important contribution to realizing this goal.

Dentistry has changed dramatically over the past 30 years. Many have called it a revolution but this denotes sudden, monumental change. In contrast, it has been an evolutionary development, catalysed by various factors, including the following:

- Dentistry, as now practised by an increasing number of practitioners, has moved from being a needs-based service, focused on treating acute symptoms and mechanistic operative interventions to manage disease, to a consumer-driven, wants-based service, treating patients presenting with various wishes and expectations, typically to maintain and, wherever possible, enhance oral health using minimal intervention approaches.

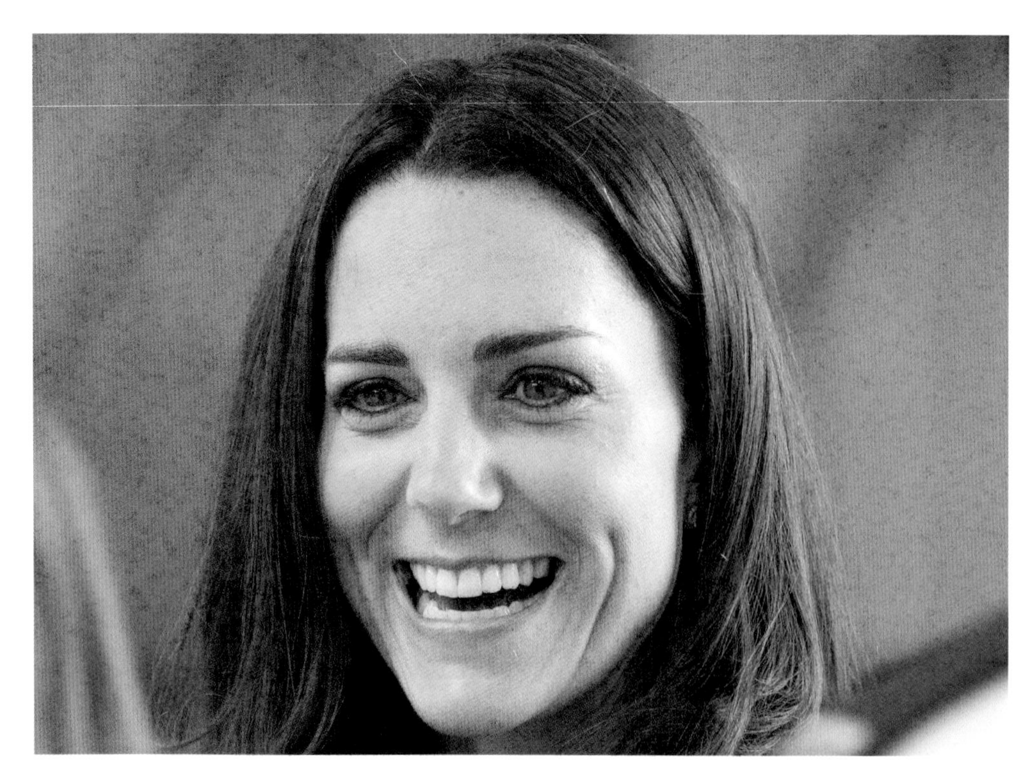

Fig. 1.1 An attractive smile. ***Photograph by Sarah Ivey-Pool, Getty Images Entertainment, Getty Images.***

- Patients have ready access to a wealth of information and are subject to media pressures in current society. This has increased the dental 'IQ' and awareness of most patients, who, as a consequence, are more questioning and have higher expectations.
- Dental attractiveness has increasingly become recognized as being part of looking youthful, vital and successful.
- Developments in tooth-coloured restorative systems and their application have created many new opportunities to enhance dental esthetics, increasingly using minimal intervention techniques as part of the drive to assist patients in having good-looking, functionally effective 'teeth for life'.

THE PATIENT'S CONCERNS

Although patients have access to information, it stems from the media and not the dental profession. This raises issues of unreasonable expectations, based on Photoshopped images in the press and elsewhere. Is what the patient is asking for really an achievable result? Do the media raise false expectations?

ESTHETICS *VERSUS* COSMETICS

What is the difference between esthetic and cosmetic dentistry? The terms 'cosmetic' and 'esthetic' dentistry ('esthetic' being used more widely on the international stage than the 'aesthetic' spelling) have been and continue to be employed interchangeably, causing much confusion in the profession and the population in general. The situation is compounded by the overlap between various esthetic and cosmetic treatments and by the fact that all esthetic and cosmetic procedures in medicine and surgery are considered to fall under the single umbrella of 'cosmetic practice'. In this introductory chapter of the first volume of a series of books on esthetic dentistry, it is important to discuss and clarify the use of the two terms.

There are many different and varying definitions of 'cosmetics' and 'esthetics'. What is the etymology of these two words?

As a noun, the word 'cosmetic' comes from Greek 'kosmetike', which is 'the art of dress and ornament'. As an adjective, 'cosmetic' derives from the Greek word 'kosmetikos', 'skilled in adornment or arrangement' or 'used or done superficially to make something look better, more attractive, or more impressive' (http://dictionary.reference.com; all websites accessed 14 February 2014). The word 'esthetic' comes from Greek 'aisthetikos', meaning 'sensitive and perceptive' (http://www.etymonline.com). The *Collins Concise English Dictionary* provides the following definitions for 'esthetic': 'relating to pure beauty rather than to other considerations' and 'relating to good taste or artistic' (http://www.collinsdictionary.com). The same source defines 'cosmetic' as 'having no other function than to beautify' and 'designed to cover up a greater flaw or deficiency; superficial'.

In essence, the way to differentiate between the terms 'cosmetics' and 'esthetics' is to consider esthetics as the theory and philosophy that explore beauty, while cosmetics refers to a preparation designed to beautify the body by direct application (http://www.thefreedictionary.com). Aristotle stated that esthetics is the art of imitating ideal objects.

KEY POINT SUMMARY

How important is it to understand the difference between cosmetics and esthetics?

Winkler and Orloff[1] describe the terms, as they pertain to the treatment of patients, as follows:

> *Cosmetic: This encompasses reversible procedures to attain a so-called optimal appearance that is sociological, cultural, geographic and time-dependent. Trends are time-dependent; what is acceptable and fashionable today can and will oftentimes be considered unacceptable and old-fashioned tomorrow.*
>
> *Esthetic: This demands tailoring and customisation to individual preference. It is a fluid and dynamic entity, but it is based on the patients' expectations, psychology and subjective criteria.*

Others, including Touyz,[2] have suggested that cosmetic dentistry, while improving appearance, does not strive to achieve enhanced function, whereas esthetic dentistry incorporates biological considerations and measures to achieve ideal form, function and appearance, with a view to long-term performance and survival.

These authors consider cosmetic dentistry to comprise measures designed primarily to enhance dental attractiveness, without necessarily improving function, whereas esthetic dentistry involves procedures on teeth and the associated soft tissues aimed at concurrently achieving ideal form, function and appearance. A useful distinction is considered to contrast a conformative approach to the enhancement of dental appearance (cosmetic dentistry), with a modifying or rehabilitative approach with changes in function (esthetic dentistry). In many cases, however, the measures and procedures undertaken comprise elements of both esthetic and cosmetic dentistry, resulting in the common but confusing interchangeable use of the terminology. If the measures and procedures involve any changes to function, then the treatment should be termed esthetic rather than cosmetic dentistry. As a consequence, most of the procedures undertaken to enhance dental attractiveness – with the exception, for example, of work such as bleaching that is limited to changing the shade of teeth, with no changes being made to form and function, including the replacement of any existing restorations and modifications to the adjacent soft tissues – should be classified as esthetic dentistry.

CLINICAL TIP

A decision often has to be made either to work with the status quo and achieve a compromised result, or to carry out a complete rehabilitation.

For the sake of completeness, two other terms also need to be considered: 'dental decoration' and 'dental mutilation'.

Dental decoration, including, for example, the bonding of a trinket or gemstone, possibly even a precious stone such as a diamond, typically to the labial surface of one or more upper anterior teeth (Fig. 1.2), may be considered to be a form of cosmetic dentistry. A dental decoration may be applied to cover a defect, such as

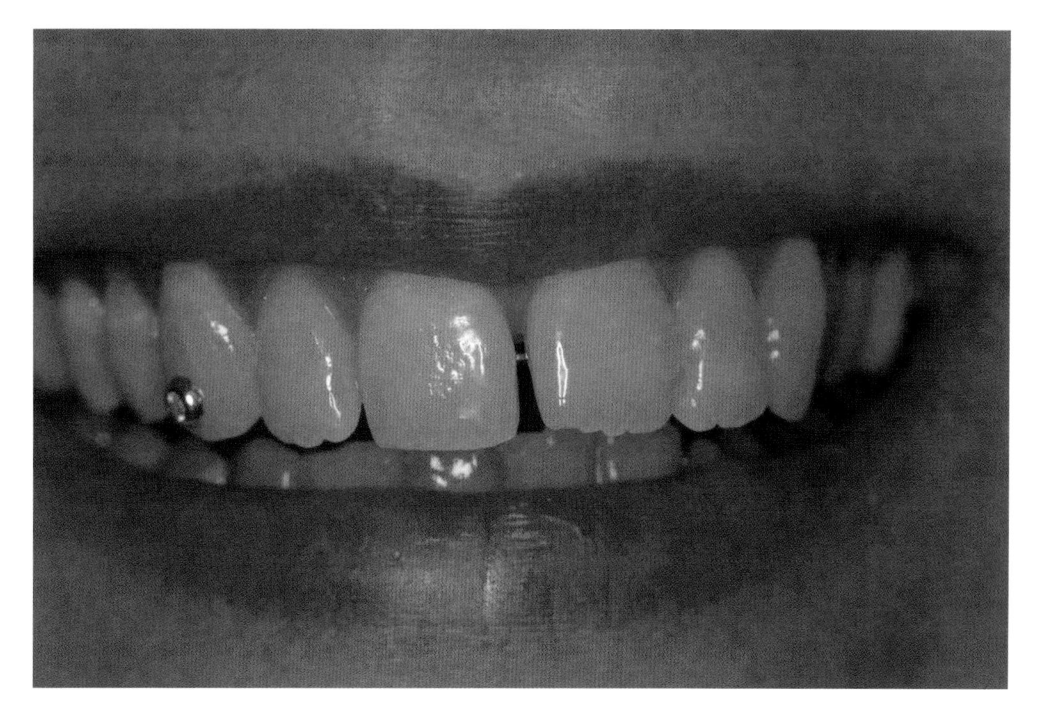

Fig. 1.2 An example of a dental decoration in a patient concerned about a midline diastema having opened up following the failure of an orthodontic retainer.

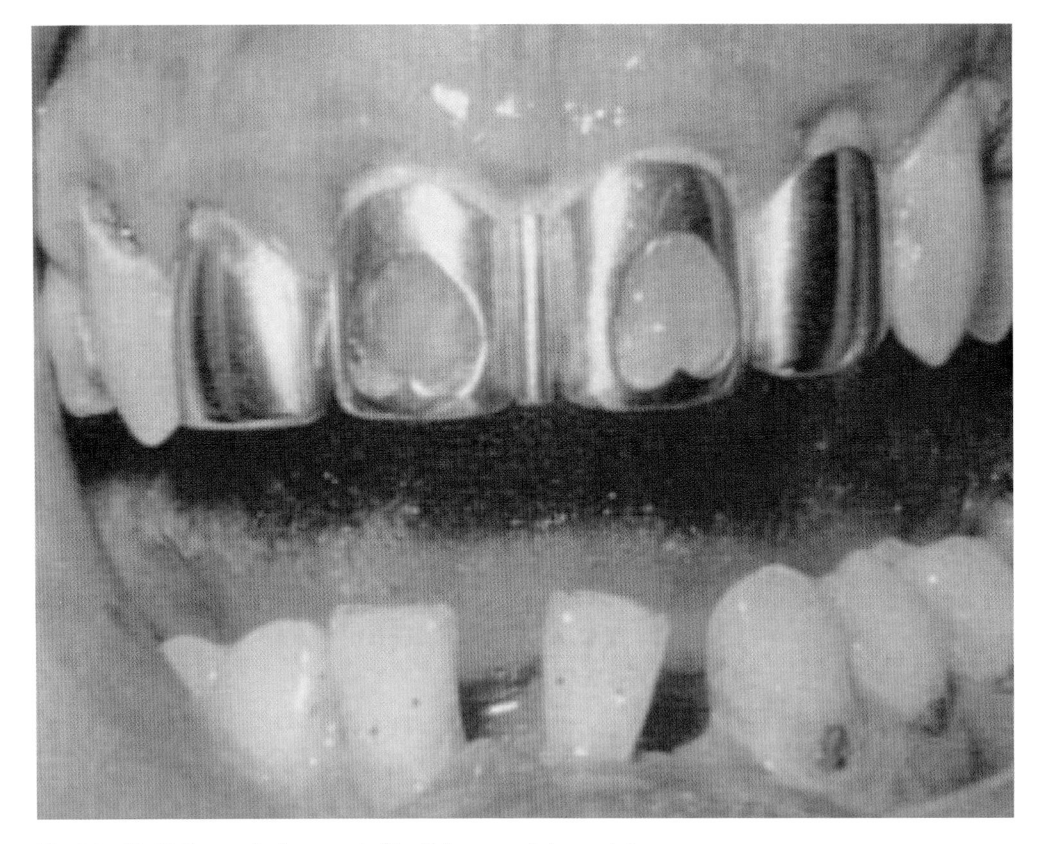

Fig. 1.3 Mutilation and adornment of teeth in present-day society.

a discrete area of hypocalcification in the labial surface of a maxillary anterior tooth, providing a means of minimal intervention to mask an unsightly feature.

Dental mutilation, as undertaken in some primitive societies, albeit to enhance dental attractiveness in the eyes of the participants and their family members, friends and acquaintances, cannot be considered to be part of esthetic and cosmetic dentistry, nor to have any relationship with them. Similarly, in present-day society, the mutilation and adornment of teeth (Fig. 1.3) is not considered to constitute either esthetic or cosmetic dentistry.

Other forms of 'body art' carried out in the mouth, such as tongue piercing (Fig. 1.4), which may have adverse dental consequences (Fig. 1.5), are not seen to fall within the scope of cosmetic dentistry, let alone esthetic dental practice.

ORIGINS OF ESTHETIC DENTISTRY

Pierre Fauchard, the Frenchman widely recognized to be the 'father of dentistry' and author of *Le Chirurgien dentiste, ou Traité des dents* – the book that has been

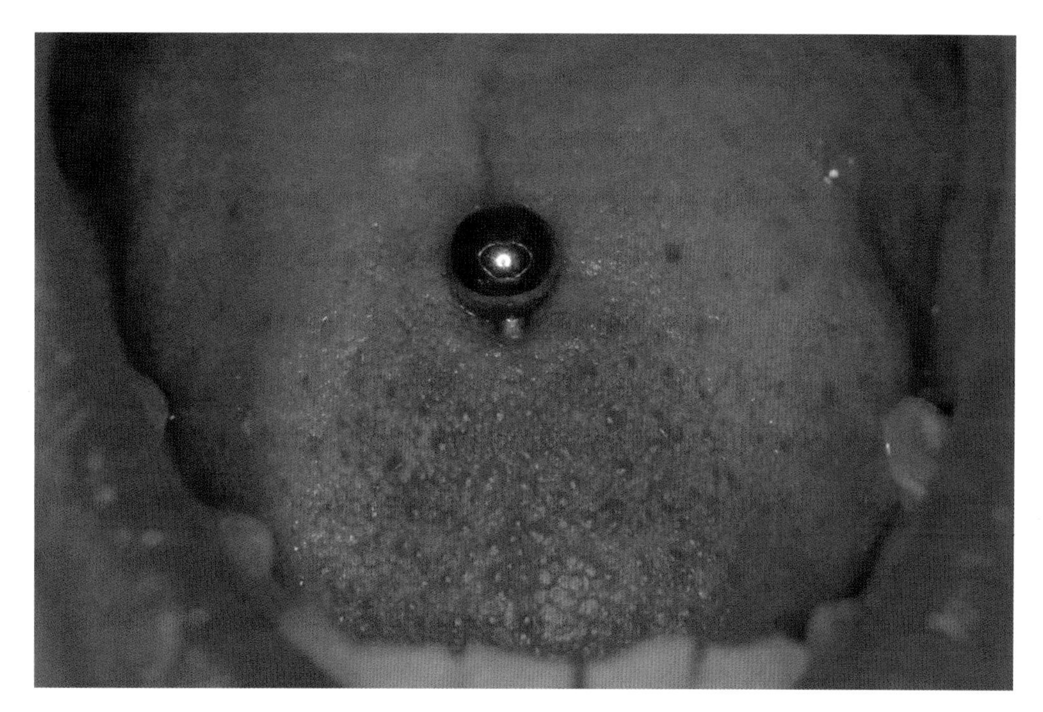

Fig. 1.4 **A tongue piercing.**

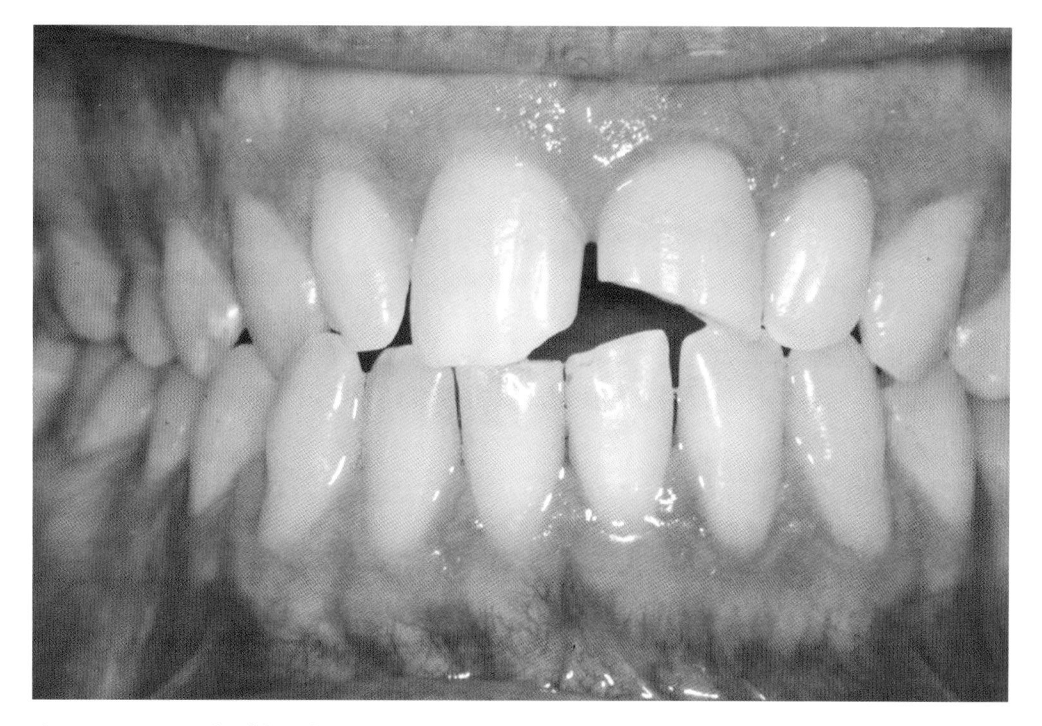

Fig. 1.5 **An example of dental trauma caused by a tongue piercing.**

claimed to have provided the foundations for the recognition of dentistry as a profession, should, it is suggested, be credited with the initial considerations of esthetic dentistry. Perhaps one of Fauchard's most notable contributions, in particular in the field of prosthetic dentistry, was his work on the colouring and enamelling of denture bases. His thoughts on colour and esthetics provided the foundations for subsequent developments in esthetic dentistry. Many of the ideals established and practised by Fauchard remain relevant today, nearly 250 years after their introduction.

Greene Vardiman Black, better known as G.V. Black – the father of dentistry as practised in the 20th century – was responsible for 'bringing dentistry into the modern world' and 'putting it on a solid scientific foundation'.[3] While best known for his cavity classification and work on dental amalgam, he made frequent references to esthetic considerations in his numerous publications and was working on the unsightly effects of fluorosis, including enamel mottling, at the time of his death in 1915. He is famously quoted as telling his students in 1896:

> *The day is surely coming ... when we will be engaged in practicing preventive, rather than reparative dentistry ... and will so understand the etiology and pathology of dental caries that we will be able to combat its destructive and unsightly effects by systematic medication.*

The first porcelain crown systems, which preceded early direct tooth-coloured filling materials, were developed in the 1880s by Drs M. Richmond and M. Logan. Although these crown systems were a technological breakthrough at the time, they required the radical removal of coronal tissue, with devitalization of the tooth to be restored, and were ill-fitting and lacking in esthetic qualities. Indeed, the completed crowns were typically considered to be unsightly.

Also in the 1890s there was the first known description of porcelain veneers, fixed in place with zinc phosphate cement. The esthetic qualities of these veneers, in common with the first porcelain crowns, were, at best, limited.

Subsequent to the invention of the electric furnace and the development of porcelains fusing at low temperatures, Charles Henry Land came up with a transformational innovation. Land's system for the provision of strong, esthetic porcelain jacket crowns was introduced in 1901. It revolutionized restorative dentistry at the time and is still used to this day, albeit in a greatly refined and modified form. For decayed and otherwise damaged anterior teeth, the alternative esthetic solution at the time was the use of silicate cements, which, in comparison to the tooth-coloured restorative systems of the present day, were crude and difficult to handle, and had limited shade-matching capabilities.

Between the early 1900s and the 1950s there were relatively few developments in esthetic dentistry, with the exception of advances in the esthetics of artificial teeth for dentures. Silicate cements were refined and marketed in a range of shades, and for the rich and famous, notably Hollywood film stars, various treatments became available that were the precursors to modern-day vital tooth bleaching, amongst other techniques. The primary purpose of dentistry of the time was the treatment of pain and disease, including the replacement of teeth lost mainly as a consequence of caries and periodontal disease.

In the 1950s and 1960s two major developments heralded a new era in esthetic dentistry: the introduction of enamel etching and bonding by Michael Buonocore in 1955, and the development of acrylic resins for use in dentistry. Relatively quickly thereafter, resin composite systems were introduced for the esthetic restoration of teeth. As an aside, it should be noted that Kramer and McLean published the first histological report on what is now termed a hybrid layer in 1952.[4] According to McLean, this layer (Fig. 1.6), formed by a material called Servitron, was not clinically relevant, as none of the restorative materials

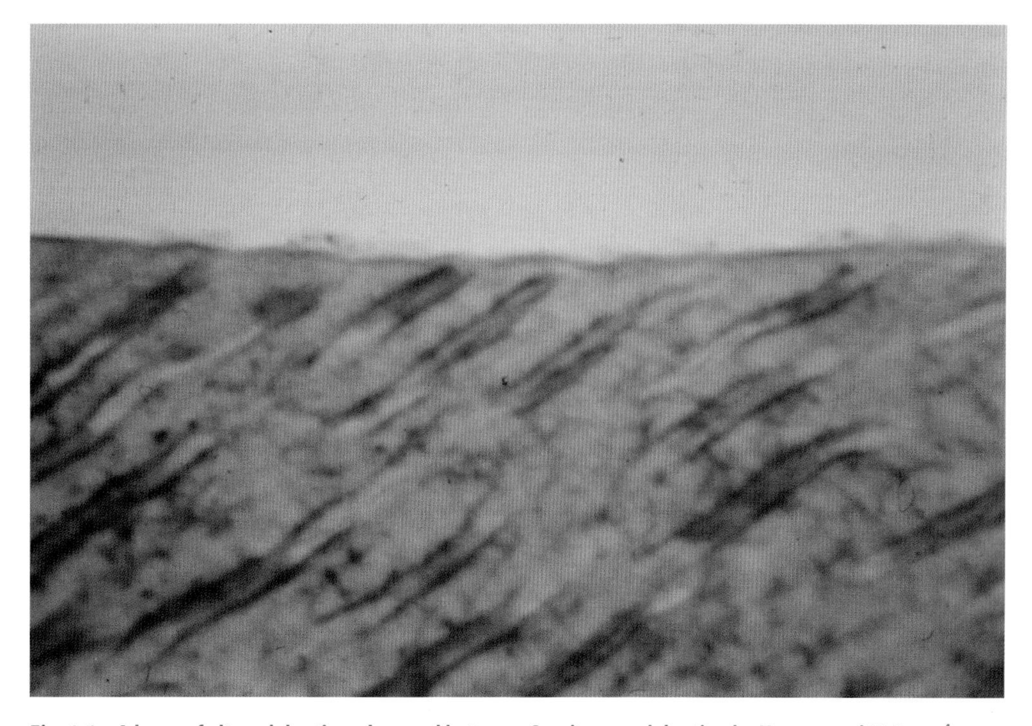

Fig. 1.6 A layer of altered dentine observed between Servitron and dentine by Kramer and McLean.[4]

available at the time was able to bond to the resin-impregnated dentine layer, making it vulnerable to breakdown in clinical service.

Stemming from the initial work on the bonding of restorative materials to remaining tooth tissues, rapid developments in tooth-coloured restorative systems, notably the visible light-cured resin composites, and concurrent innovations in dentals materials science, including developments in porcelain fused to metal systems, there were many new opportunities for the provision of esthetically pleasing restorative dentistry in the late 1970s and early 1980s. With the subsequent introduction of many other systems and techniques, including resin-bonded ceramic veneers and numerous other ceramic systems, dentine adhesives, innovations in osseointegration and implant dentistry, and new interests in colour science in dentistry, as well as growing patient interest and expectations in respect of dental appearance, esthetic dentistry, as we know it today, began to emerge and evolve. The profession now takes for granted a plethora of systems that may find application in the provision of esthetic dentistry, and remains anxious to see further developments and innovations that will facilitate easier, faster and better-quality esthetic dentistry, with increased patient acceptance and longevity.

THE SMILE

It was not until the 1980s and 1990s that attention turned to defining and describing the dental smile, as forms the basis of present-day esthetic dentistry. As in most, if not all, procedures in dentistry, success in the management of the dental smile involves careful assessment and diagnosis, the application of all relevant art and science, tempered by clinical experience and acumen, and the ability to communicate effectively with patients to understand their concerns and wishes fully. Although esthetically pleasing smiles include many common features and characteristics, no two smiles are the same. The wrong smile, albeit classical and ideal, in the wrong patient not only may look bizarre, but also may have adverse psychological and other effects on the patient. Conceiving, planning and providing the right, esthetically pleasing smile for a patient is the challenge and professional fulfilment of high-quality esthetic dentistry.

What's in a smile? There are many interactive components to an attractive smile: the head, neck and face in which it is set; facial structures and features; the nature, form, function and conditions of, in particular, the soft tissues of the lower third of the face, specifically the lips; the architecture and health of the gingival tissues; and last, but by no means least, the shapes, condition, shades, relationships and function of individual teeth and the dentition as a whole. The scientific and artistic principles that link all these features together are often collectively referred to as the principles of 'smile design'. The successful application of smile design in the practice of esthetic dentistry is not, however, limited to optimizing the health, appearance, relationship and function of the oral–facial tissues and structures; it also involves consideration of the attitudes, motivation, expectations and personality of the patient, and in some cases the attitudes and expectations of the patient's partner and family, and possibly even friends and acquaintances. Giving an individual a smile that is beautiful, makes the patient happy, and encourages others to smile, is what esthetic dentistry should aim to achieve.

THE GOLDEN PROPORTION

If we delve into the belief that dental esthetics is both an art and a science, then we have to ask the question: what is beauty? While the age-old adage that 'beauty is in the eye of the beholder' remains true, there is evidence that our perceptions of beauty are determined by a range of factors, including acquired, cultural and family values.

One of the earliest theories considered to underpin the science of beauty is that of the Golden Proportion – a ratio of 1 : 1.618 – attributed to Pythagoras in 530 BC. Luca Pacioli and Leonardo da Vinci are held responsible for introducing the concept of Golden Proportion into art. One of da Vinci's best-known drawings, the 'Vitruvian Man' (Fig. 1.7), is possibly the most famous example of its application. The man's height is equal to the combined length of his arms, which, together with the extended legs, touch the circumference of the surrounding circle. The ratio of the length of the sides of the square formed by the hands and feet to the radius of the circle is 1 : 1.618 – the Golden Proportion.

Biologists, botanists and other scientists have observed the Golden Proportion in many diverse natural forms,[5] including flowers, sea creatures such as the nautilus shell (Fig. 1.8) and starfish, and snowflakes. Natural structures that conform to the Golden Proportion, including faces and smiles, are invariably perceived to be esthetically pleasing.

R.E. Lombardi was one of the first to propose the use of the Golden Proportion in relation to dentistry.[6] He concluded that the form and arrangement of the teeth determine the esthetics of the smile, and smiles that display symmetry and Golden Proportion ratios are the most attractive. Ricketts developed Golden Proportion callipers to be used to evaluate and develop desirable ratios between the various elements of the face and dentition.[7] Present-day versions of these

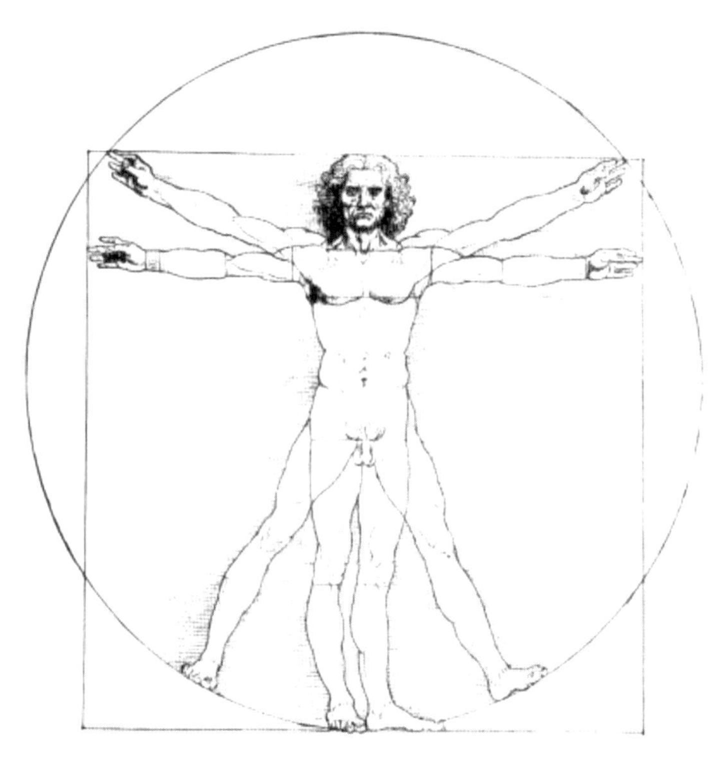

Fig. 1.7 The 'Vitruvian Man'.

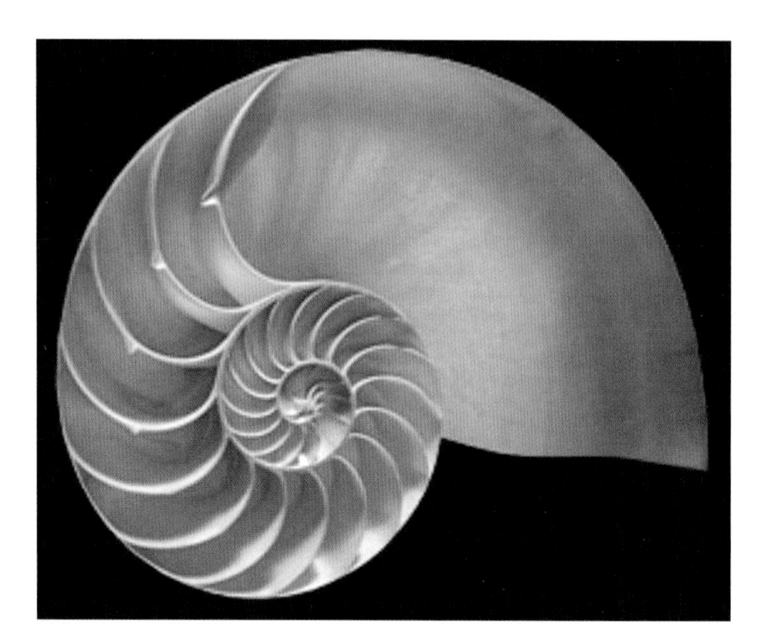

Fig. 1.8 Cross-section of a nautilus shell.

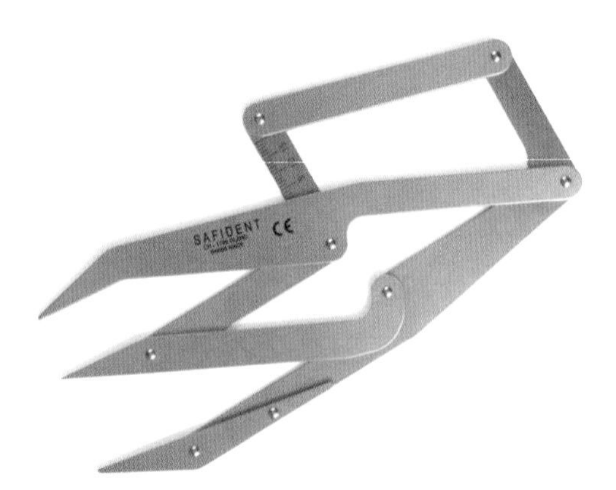

Fig. 1.9 Golden Proportion callipers.

callipers (Fig. 1.9) can find application in the contemporary practice of esthetic dentistry. It is widely accepted, however, that the use of Golden Proportion callipers provides a useful guide rather than constituting any form of objective measurement in the assessment and planning of esthetic appearance.

SYMMETRY

Symmetry is also important in perceptions of beauty; it suggests balance and the absence of discrepancies in growth and development. Can beauty exist without symmetry, let alone Golden Proportion dimensions? Edmund Burke, an 18th-century philosopher, highlighted the difference between classical beauty (that which has symmetry and obeys the Golden Proportion), and the sublime (art, a product of nature, or architecture that lacks symmetry and does not adhere to classical standards), indicating that the sublime may by no means be ugly, having its own esthetics and appeal. Many beautiful faces and attractive smiles may be found to lack symmetry and not to conform to the Golden Proportion, but faces and smiles that are symmetrical and do conform to the Golden Proportion tend to be more esthetically pleasing.

PHYSIOGNOMY

In Western and Eastern cultures there is a strong tendency to apply physiognomy judgement.[8] Physiognomy is the art of judging an individual's character or personality by the appearance of their face. In recreating damaged faces and smiles, with no pictures or other likenesses of the face to use as a reference, the art is to develop a face and a smile that are considered to match the character and personality of the patient. Such stereotyping can, however, lead to patient dissatisfaction, irrespective of the quality of the dental care provided. The patient, together with family, friends and colleagues, must identify and be comfortable with the appearance created. A smile can be judged to be, amongst other things, friendly, seductive, reassuring, young, old or fake. Planning and creating the smile that best suits the patient, let alone having certain patients agree and consent to the provision of what is considered by the clinician and possibly others to be the most appropriate smile, can be one of the greatest challenges in esthetic dentistry. Ultimately, the decision rests with the patient, but the clinician must ensure that he or she is cognizant of all the relevant information and possible consequences before reaching a decision.

ETHNIC AND CULTURAL CONSIDERATIONS

To be successful in the provision of esthetic dentistry to patients of various ethnicities and cultural backgrounds, it is important to understand and be sensitive to different ethnic and cultural esthetic values and perceptions of beauty.[9] Throughout the world, each culture has a different interpretation of a smile. What is attractive to patients of one culture or ethnic group may be unattractive, if not ugly, to others. As with physiognomy, stereotyping must be avoided. Such pitfalls may be best circumvented by spending time attempting to understand and appreciate what a patient really wants by way of treatment outcomes. Cases in which an individual wishes to change his or her dental appearance to look more like someone of a different ethnic or cultural group require special consideration and care.

'HOLLYWOOD SMILES'

In the Americas, a bright, white, wide, even, symmetrical smile is typically considered to signify wealth, vitality, health and success. In Europe, and increasingly in other parts of the world, more emphasis is placed on the natural smile, leading Europeans and others of similar inclination to classify the preferred smile in the Americas as the 'Hollywood smile'. It is interesting to note how the media represent both views: for example, Lisa Simpson being shown the *Big Book of British Smiles* by her orthodontist when being persuaded to go for the 'perfect smile', and remarks in newspapers and magazines in Europe about the artificiality and cloned appearance of the smile of celebrities who have obviously undergone extensive 'esthetic' dental treatment in the Americas.

Esthetic perceptions and values vary greatly within and between different cultures and societies. Perhaps this is best expressed by the Scottish philosopher Francis Hutcheson, who argued that beauty is 'unity in variety and variety in unity'. Over time, many, including those who have contributed to this book, would hope that natural beauty, rather than some artificial construct of esthetics, might prevail, with minimal intervention approaches being applied, where indicated clinically, to achieve long-lasting and esthetically pleasing smiles.

CONCLUDING REMARKS

Prior to embarking on a journey to understand and appreciate the many different aspects of dental esthetics better, you may wish to reflect on the explanations and definitions of esthetics and the following eloquent and apposite quotation attributed to St Francis of Assisi: 'He who works with his hands is a labourer; he who works with his hands and his head is a craftsman; he who works with his hands and his head and his heart is an artist.' In the context of clinical practice, this quotation could possibly be expanded by adding '... and he who works with his hands, head and heart in the best interests of his patients is a true clinical professional'.

Finally, in sojourning in the complex field of esthetic dentistry, it is best to remember, as stated in Sullivan's pervading law, that in all true manifestations of the head, heart and soul, 'form ever follows function'.[10]

REFERENCES

1. Winkler D, Orloff J. Ethics behind esthetics: Nordic Dentistry 2003 Yearbook. Berlin: Quintessence; 2003.

2. Touyz LZ. Cosmetic or esthetic dentistry? Quintessence Int 1999;30:227–33.

3. Ring ME. Dentistry: an illustrated history. New York: Abradale; 1985.

4. Kramer IRH, McLean JW. Alterations in the staining reaction of dentine resulting from a constituent of a new self-polymerising resin. Br Dent J 1952;93:150–3.

5. Huntley HE. The divine proportion. New York: Dover; 1970.

6. Lombardi RE. The principles of visual perception and their clinical application to dental esthetics. J Prosthet Dent 1973;29:358–82.

7. Ricketts RM. Divine proportion in facial esthetics. Clin Plast Surg 1982;9:401–22.

8. Hassin R, Trope Y. Facing faces: studies on the cognitive aspects of physiognomy. J Pers Soc Psychol 2000;78:837–52.

9. Wilson NHF, Scully C. Culturally sensitive oral healthcare. London: Quintessence; 2006.

10. Sullivan LH. The tall office building artistically considered. Lippincott's Magazine 1896;(March):403–9.

CHAPTER 2

Ethics Considerations in Esthetic Dentistry

RICHARD SIMONSEN

INTRODUCTION

> *The first time you compromise your ethics is always the hardest. After that it gets easier. (J.R. Ewing, Dallas)*

'It doesn't make a difference whether you are in business, or in politics, or in law [or in dentistry] – ethics is ethics, is ethics,' I still remember hearing Michael Josephson say in a National Public Radio broadcast some time in the 1990s. Josephson, the founder of the Joseph and Edna Institute of Ethics, and a frequent media commentator on ethics in the United States, was discussing ethics in the workplace. The understanding of ethics as it applies to dentistry is fundamental to the profession's vitality, and a vital cog in the continuance of the unwritten bond we have with the general public. The profession's autonomy is dependent on public trust – a trust that is now under challenge, particularly in the fields of esthetic and cosmetic dentistry.

WHAT IS ETHICS?

Ethics is the study of what is good and what is bad, what is right and what is wrong. One can wonder if ethics can be taught or if it is somehow an innate standard of moral behaviour, drilled into us (or not) from our early years by our families and members of the wider community. Growing up, it mortified me to hear of schoolmates who shoplifted for fun. Now, that did not necessarily make me a better person; it just made me believe I had better guidance from my parents. So, can we guide our dental students towards what is right and discourage them from taking advantage of vulnerable patients for personal gain? Can we hope that dental manufacturers will provide us with the best products for our patients, or will they compromise their ethical standards in order to garner the highest profits at our expense, to the detriment of their ultimate customer – the patient? Dare we believe that our colleagues will refuse to mislead the public with unethical advertising or will they use the medium dishonestly in the pursuit of financial reward? Will the truth become the preserve of a minority while trust in dental professionals continues its downward spiral?

One of our most prolific writers on dental ethics, David Chambers, editor of the *Journal of the American College of Dentists*, believes that individuals cannot be considered ethical in any meaningful sense unless they are part of a community:

> *By analogy, dentists who materially mislead patients during informed consent, who upgrade (dental) insurance claims, and who practice so close to the standard of care that mishaps are expected are all no longer professional. They are*

not poor dentists; they have stepped outside the community of dental practice. What makes their 'crime' so heinous is that they continue to hold themselves out as belonging to the profession, while they operate outside it. Unethical practitioners claim the advantages of being a professional, while simultaneously damaging the credit the public extends to all professionals. Unethical behavior means cheating in the game of building a community.[1]

CHEATING

Cheating is endemic in today's world. We are bombarded by major ethical breakdowns in journalism and politics, such as the 2012 phone-hacking scandal in the UK, as well as other, more minor, travesties. The pushing of the competitive envelope in the media phone-hacking cases eventually led to the closure of one of the UK's best-known newspapers – the *News of the World* – owned by Australian media giant Rupert Murdoch. At the time of writing, we are still awaiting the outcome of a number of criminal trials arising from the police investigations.

In recent years we have also seen journalists such as Jayson Blair resign from prestigious publications like the *New York Times* for making up stories. We have witnessed all kinds of fakery being pushed on the Internet. Some of our sports stars have been discredited, even Tour de France winners Floyd Landis and the once legendary Lance Armstrong, the latter eventually admitting to blood doping and the use of other illegal pharmaceutical supplements, subsequent to being stripped of his titles. 'Big Pharma' has paid a radio host for giving their drug marketing lectures, a fact he did not disclose to listeners of his show.[2] Our universities and colleges have seen cheating at all levels: by teachers under pressure to meet targets[3]; by a student who gained entry to one of the most highly regarded institutions in the world – Harvard – using fake documents[4]; and by the Dean of Admissions at another top-notch school – the Massachusetts Institute of Technology – who was forced to resign when she admitted to having fabricated her own educational credentials.[5]

RESEARCH SCANDALS

Perhaps some of the more serious instances of cheating in the healthcare world have involved the fudging of data, or their outright invention, in some of our scientific publications. A paper may not be exposed as flawed until it is withdrawn or retracted, too late in many cases to assuage the damage already done. Parents all over the world withheld vaccinations from their children based on the study of British medical researcher, Andrew Wakefield; in an article published in the prestigious *Lancet*, Wakefield claimed a possible link between the measles, mumps and rubella (MMR) vaccine and autism.[6] Study after study has failed to reproduce Wakefield's results and no correlation has been found between vaccination and autism. A General Medical Council inquiry found Wakefield guilty of serious professional misconduct on several charges relating to his research and struck him off. *The Lancet* retracted the paper. How many children are now living with a disability or even died as a result of Wakefield's actions?

Then there was the study conducted by the Norwegian, Jon Sudbö, who concluded that anti-inflammatory drugs reduce the risk of oral cancer; it emerged that his conclusions were based on fabricated data.[7]

Equally seriously, perhaps, the *Chronicle of Higher Education* reports that many images used in research studies are faked, including those appearing in one paper on the role of cell growth in diabetes.[8]

'BIG PHARMA' MISCONDUCT

In 2009, we saw the world's largest drug company, Pfizer, plead guilty in court to criminal charges that it broke the law in marketing the drug Bextra. It agreed to pay a record US$1.195 billion fine, plus a further $1 billion to settle civil claims relating to the marketing of Bextra and other medications.[9]

Pharmaceutical companies have vast sums of money riding on the outcome of clinical trials and there must be a real temptation to delay those that do not appear to be producing the desired results, to cherry-pick or massage data, and to send out 'stories' based on incomplete findings.

Big Pharma has also, on occasion, buried results that fail to show its products in the best light. Pharmaceutical companies have been known to sue to prevent researchers from presenting or publishing data not seen as favourable.

ETHICS AND LEGALITY

The examples above are but a grain of sand in the desert of alleged and proven fraud and cheating through which we are struggling today. When a cheating scandal hit several US dental schools in 2006 and later, in one situation involving half of the senior class of a large institution, it became difficult to see where it all would end. Harvard University has recently announced that over a hundred students have been investigated for cheating. Will our children grow up thinking that this is simply normal behaviour? As Chambers says, 'We have reached a critical mass of chronic low-grade cheating.'[10]

In his excellent book, *Profit with Honor*, Daniel Yankelovich notes that, 'Every viable society depends on ethical norms to guide and restrain conduct. For most forms of conduct, norms are far more important than legal constraints.' The law only sets minimal standards of conduct. Yankelovich continues, 'one can act legally and still not act ethically.'[11] Thus one can say that ethical standards become the moral rules that fill in the spaces between laws – laws that cannot completely determine societal behaviour.

CODES OF ETHICAL CONDUCT IN DENTISTRY

Most countries have ethical codes or standards of professional conduct for dental practice. These guidelines, such as the American Dental Association (ADA) *Principles of Ethics and Code of Professional Conduct*, outline the principles that an ethical practitioner of dentistry is expected to uphold.[12] The dental profession holds a special position of trust within society. In return, the profession makes a commitment that its members will adhere to high standards of ethical conduct. In essence, the ADA code is a written expression of the duties and obligations inherent in the implied contract between the dental profession and members of society. This implied contract supports the autonomy that is granted to the profession by the public.

The ADA code discusses five principles that underlie the duties of a dentist:

- patient autonomy
- non-maleficence
- beneficence
- justice
- veracity.[12]

These five principles are all intertwined. However, they are guidelines only, and in practice there is nothing that the ADA, or any other body not involved with issuing the licence to practise, can do in instances of violation, other than expelling a member from the organization.

PATIENT AUTONOMY

The dentist has a duty to respect the patient's right to self-determination and confidentiality. This duty has emerged from the days when healthcare professionals, including dentists, often exhibited a paternalistic attitude towards patients, who may have felt unable or unwilling to question the dentist about treatment and generally accepted what was proposed. The situation today is very different. Patients are better educated about dental health and expect, and in most cases receive, multiple options for treatment, laid out by the dentist in an open and honest discussion. There are, however, clear examples in the published literature of 'induced consent' rather than 'informed consent'.[13] By induced consent, I mean that the treatment 'chosen' is clearly what the dentist, rather than the patient, wanted, generally for economic motives. Guiding choice in this way, for any reason other than a genuine concern for the long-term interests of the patient, is in violation of the first principle of patient autonomy. As Ozar and Sokol put it, 'A dentist can make his/her explanation of alternative treatment options persuasive in any direction he/she chooses.'[14] Yet even when it comes to proper informed consent, where adequate information is provided, it has been shown that a high proportion of patients do not understand the consent process.[15] Thus the responsibility for selecting the appropriate treatment rests heavily on the shoulders of the dentist.

NON-MALEFICENCE

The second principle is non-maleficence – doing no harm. Dentists have a clear duty to heal, not harm, the patient – guarding the patient's welfare, recognizing the scope of their own skills and knowledge, and seeking advice or referring the patient to a specialist or another practitioner if the problem lies outside their area of expertise. If a patient is denied the appropriate information about, say, an elective esthetic procedure and consents to significant tooth structure removal to improve their 'smile' when another less invasive procedure would have sufficed, that patient has been harmed, particularly in the long term. As Bader and Shugars put it, 'An implicit, if not explicit, assumption covering any treatment is that the benefits of the treatment will, or at least are likely to, outweigh any negative consequences of the treatment ... in short, that treatment is better than no treatment.'[16]

BENEFICENCE

The third principle is one of beneficence – doing 'good.' Professionals have a duty to act for the benefit of others and to promote the patient's welfare. As a treating dentist, one should always consider whether the patient will be better off after treatment than if nothing had been done. One can appear to be 'doing good' by obtaining a short-term improvement in appearance via an elective esthetic treatment, for example, but if the result is significant reduction of tooth structure that later requires endodontic care and/or additional extensive restorative treatment, the patient has not been well served. The British author Martin Kelleher has written eloquently about this serious problem from the European perspective.[17–19]

Tongue-in-cheek, he invented the terms 'hyperenamelosis' to describe the imaginary condition of a patient with too much enamel (to justify the gross over-removal of enamel seen in many 'cosmetic' treatments) and 'porcelain deficiency disease' (to describe the imaginary condition of a patient who thus requires the brutal removal of natural enamel so that it can be replaced with porcelain). This phenomenon has been documented by me over the years.[20-24] It is hard to retain a sense of humour when viewing some of the more egregious examples of over-treatment that fill the pages of the dental literature.

JUSTICE

The fourth principle is justice or 'fairness'. Professionals have a duty to be fair in their discussions with patients and in their actions. If dentists do not put the patient's interests first, they are not fulfilling this obligation. This principle is most frequently violated in the form of advertising and treatment planning, where the dentist's willingness to push the ethical boundaries of propriety can lead to the promotion of short-term profit rather than long-term health.

VERACITY

The fifth and final principle is veracity or 'truthfulness', which applies to any communication between dentist and patient. Violations are most common in advertising and can be found en masse on dentists' websites. Dentists may attempt to promote unproven 'science', such as that of neuromuscular dentistry, which some are said to favour as a 'justification' for carrying out unnecessary full mouth reconstruction. Or they may argue against the use of amalgam for restorative dentistry, in an effort to persuade patients to have all their old amalgam alloy restorations replaced. Such statements are in direct violation of the ADA position statement on the use of dental amalgam. And while dental amalgam has lasted much longer than I incorrectly predicted in the early 1990s,[25] there is no justification for removing otherwise adequate amalgam restorations, other than in a very small minority of allergic patients.

ETHICS IN ESTHETIC DENTISTRY

In 1955, Michael Buonocore published the first article on the etching of enamel.[26] This historic report has formed the basis for tremendous changes in clinical practice: in particular, in preventive dentistry – for example, pit and fissure sealants (Fig. 2.1). In restorative dentistry, etching of enamel heralded the arrival of minimally invasive preparations, determined by the extent of caries and not by the principles of G.V. Black (Fig. 2.2). The introduction of an array of elective and minimally invasive procedures based on the etching of enamel changed esthetic

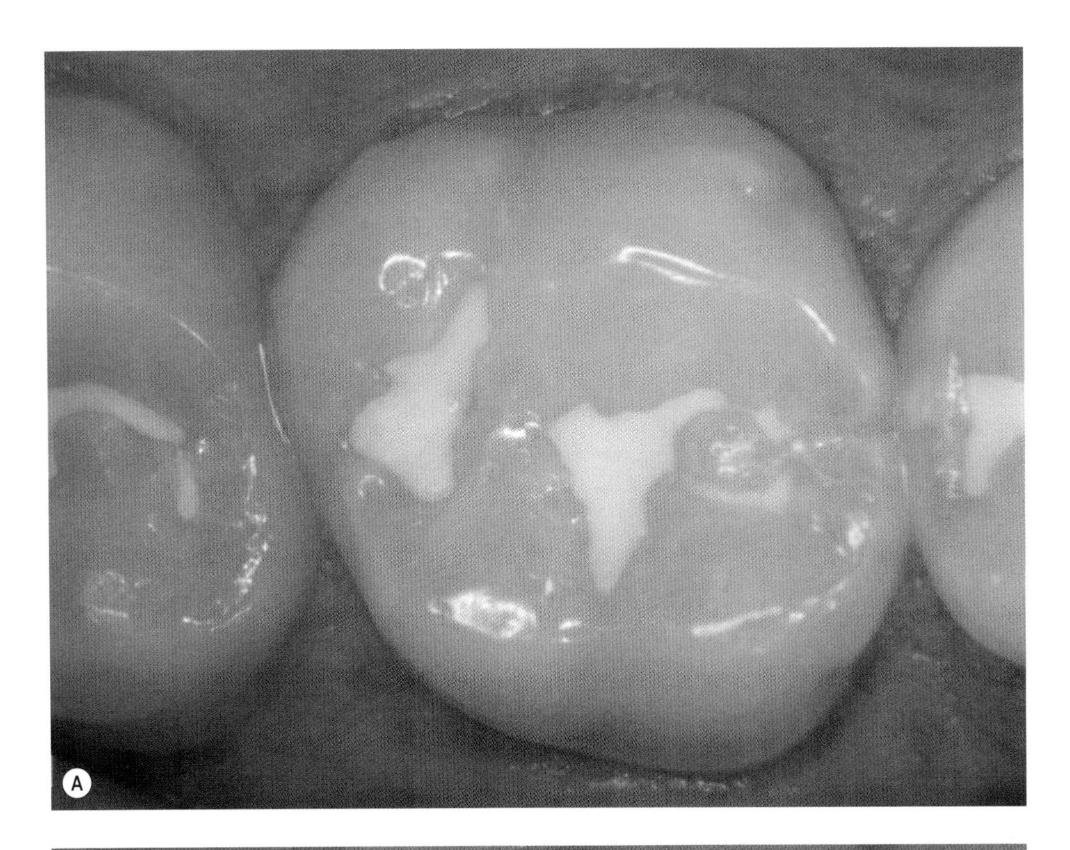

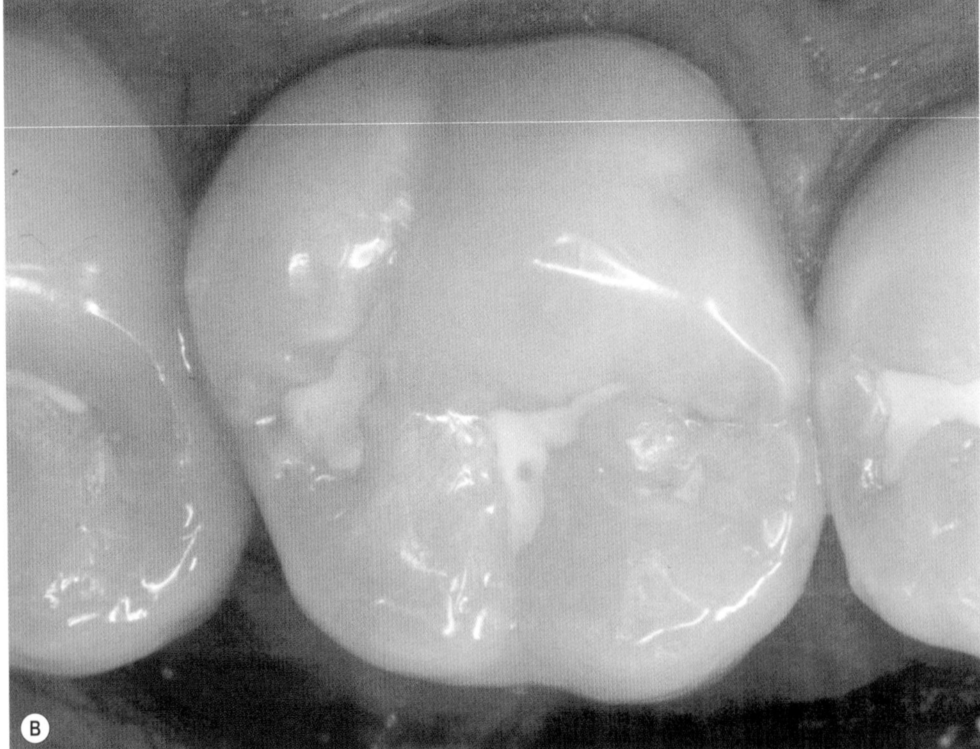

Fig. 2.1 Pit and fissure sealant. A. The sealant at 5 years old. B. The same sealant, now 15 years old.

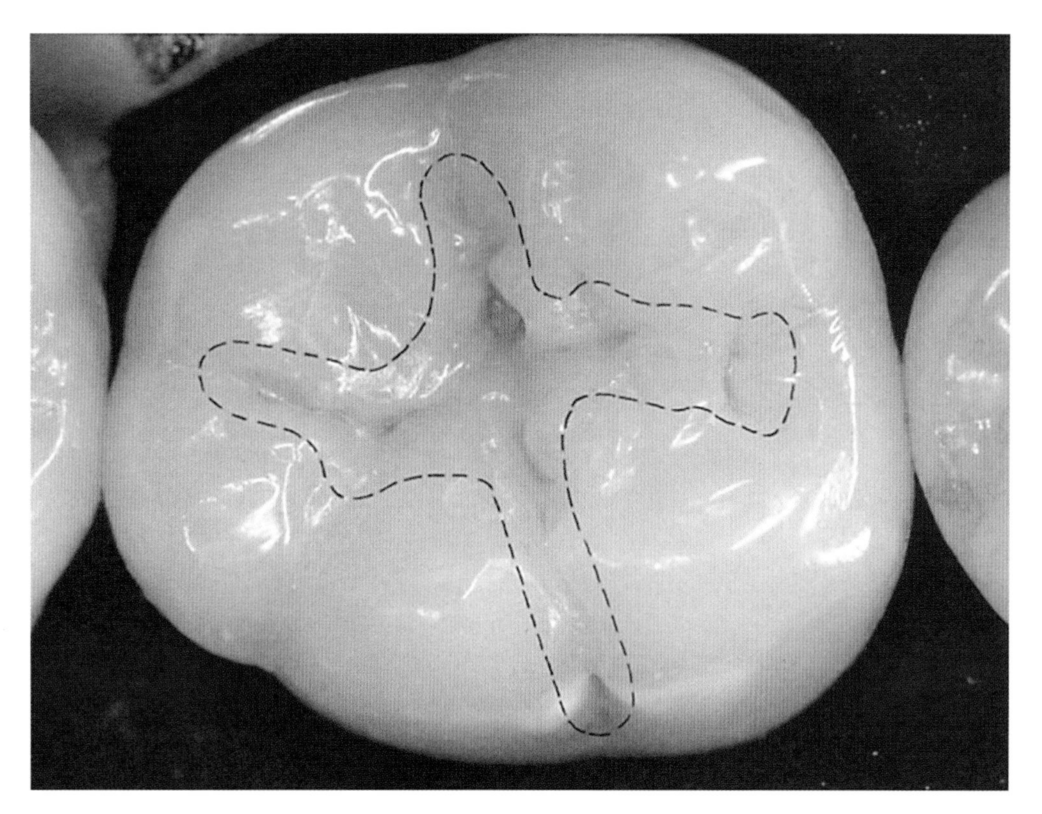

Fig. 2.2 Traditional Cavity Outline. It would be ethically inappropriate to carry out a conventional class I G.V. Black cavity preparation (outline form in dotted lines) on a molar with incipient caries in two confined areas such as this when a conservative preparation removing only the carious tooth structure can be used (Preventive Resin Restoration).

dentistry forever. Indeed, Buonocore's original research may be the key that opened the door to the modern practice of esthetic dentistry, as well as other clinical techniques that utilize the acid etch technique, especially, perhaps, in orthodontics.

With these changes have come opportunities. On the positive side, dentists now have the ability to provide conservative options to address a patient's esthetic concerns. For example, whereas it used to be necessary, just a few decades ago, to place a full crown (or, in the case of children, a basket crown) to repair a fractured central incisor, today a bonded composite resin can accomplish the same functional and esthetic task, while removing virtually no tooth structure (Fig. 2.3). On the negative side, there has been an upswing in over-treatment, pandering to some patients' vanity. Lured to the surgery by glossy media images of that super-smile, such individuals are easy prey for the minority of dentists who threaten the ethical standards of the rest of the profession. A minimally invasive treatment option may not be considered by the unethical dentist, or is quietly discouraged. Disputed approaches such as neuromuscular dentistry are sometimes part of the package, convincing some in the dental community and

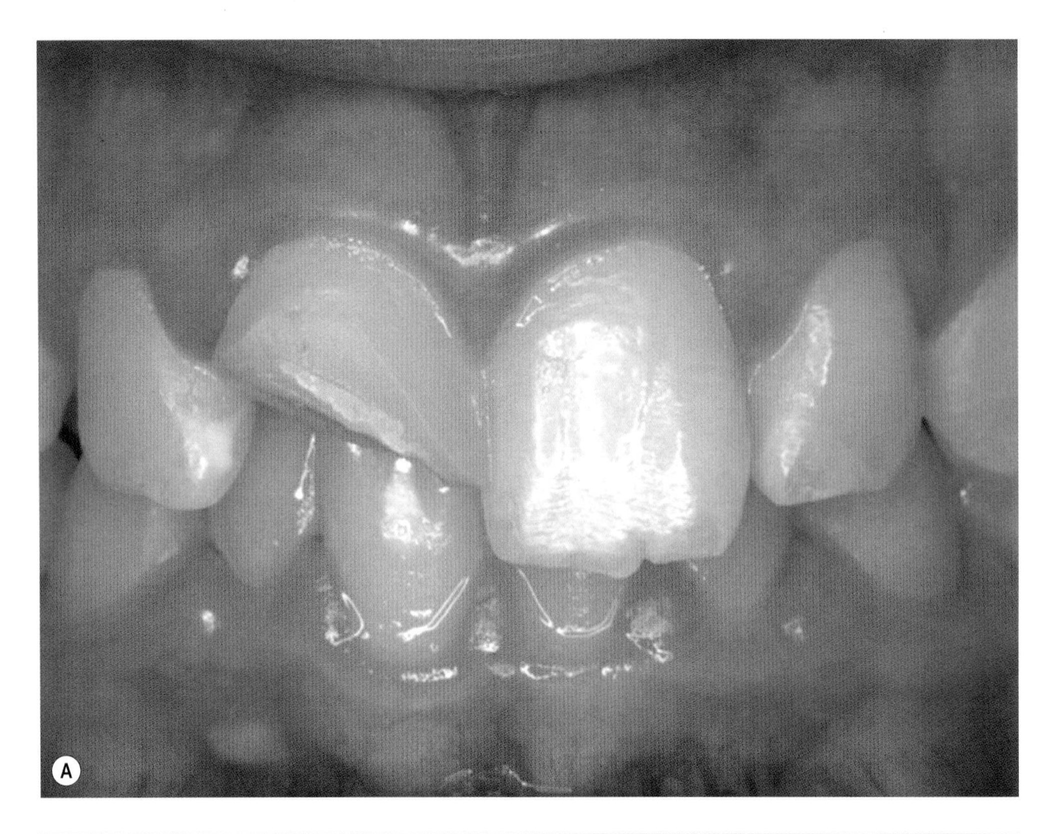

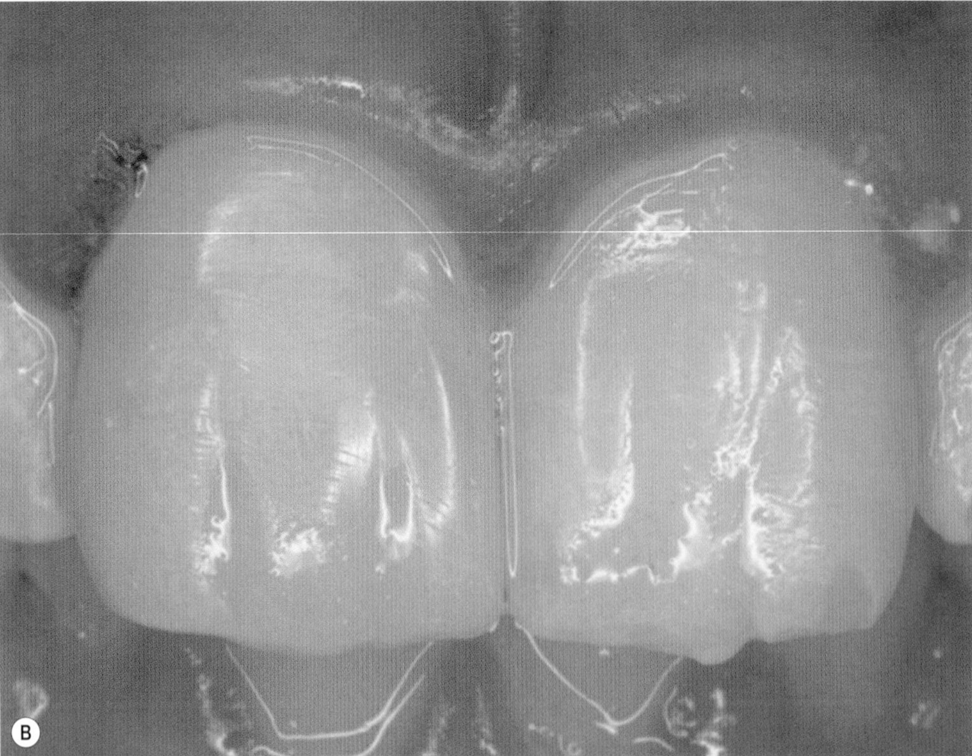

Fig. 2.3 The traumatic fracture of anterior teeth. A. This can be devastating to young patients and their parents. It is ethically appropriate to provide informed consent for all treatment options. B. The fracture can be quickly and conservatively treated with the acid-etch technique and composite resins. Conservation of tooth structure is ethically appropriate.

clusters of insecure patients that they need full mouth reconstruction – a cure without a disease. Greed and vanity can be powerful motivators.

OVER-TREATMENT

We must remember that the vast majority of dental practitioners serve the public in an ethical manner. Most enter the profession with a sense of wanting to help people, whether by relief of pain or correction of a life-affecting cosmetic concern. Some, however, violate their ethical obligations by pursuing the path to riches via unethical choices and taking advantage of their sometimes gullible patients in a most egregious manner.

Dentists are sometimes placed in an uncomfortable position. They have one foot in the world of healer and provider of care, and the other in the commercial world. While many hold salaried positions and have made no personal financial investment in the surgery or in costly equipment and supplies, others have put in large amounts of money and must cover these costs from the remuneration they receive from patients. Without a sufficient flow of income the practice would go bankrupt, and patients in the neighbourhood would lose their surgery. Running a dental practice like a business is, therefore, a necessary evil to some degree. Chambers notes:

> *Dental practice is inherently a profession only; it is a business in an accidental and derivative sense ... Quality in dentistry should be determined by what it means to practice oral health care and not by looking for good economic returns in pandering to the wants of a small segment of patients.*[27]

It must be clear that the ethical standards relating to a patient's treatment cannot take into account the business needs of the practitioner. Connected to this is how the dentist chooses to advertise the practice. Ethical standards governing health-care promotion are frequently violated by those who would take advantage of patients for financial gain. This leads to appearance being put before health, anecdote before evidence, and profit before public interest. Those who follow such a path are putting the autonomy of the dental profession at risk.

NEUROMUSCULAR DENTISTRY

Neuromuscular dentistry is an approach that is promoted by fringe elements of the profession and is often used, in my opinion, as a means to justify full-mouth reconstruction. Such actions make the evidence-based scientific community react with shock and dismay. One can certainly question the motives and ethics behind such treatment if it is used to lure patients who are unhappy with their appearance into undergoing extensive and invasive treatment at great financial and oral health cost.

No dental school of which I am aware teaches neuromuscular dentistry as part of the dental curriculum, let alone as a recommended treatment. No legitimate expert in oral pain, prosthodontics or temporomandibular joint science that I have ever asked for an opinion has indicated that there is any scientific method behind neuromuscular dentistry. A recent 600-page textbook on the subject of temporomandibular dysfunction gives it not a single line.[28] Other recent texts on temporomandibular disorder,[29] headache, oro-facial pain and bruxism,[30] and on oral rehabilitation,[31] equally lack any such reference. So, it really puzzles me how certain colleagues can base their work on this disputed practice.

However, the Las Vegas Institute (LVI), a for-profit, private continuing dental education centre, makes claims of 'changing lives' while placing neuromuscular dentistry at the core of its programme. It uses terms like 'graduates', 'alumni' and 'faculty', which invite comparisons with universities, and describes itself as a postgraduate institute, but the requirements for gaining a qualification are far fewer than those demanded by a university. The programme has been exported globally and dentists in many countries now claim affiliation. A significant proportion of the LVI programme is focused around how to increase office productivity. Thus neuromuscular dentistry is presented as a substantial source of income.

The institute also awards qualifications like LVIM (Mastership) and LVIF (Fellowship) that are only obtainable at LVI (unlike academic degrees such as MS or PhD that can be obtained world-wide at accredited universities). It describes itself and its mother organization as 'world-renowned', yet the majority of the full-time faculty listed on their website as of September 2014 seem to lack any recognized academic postgraduate qualifications beyond their primary dental degrees.[32] Nevertheless, they all have LVIM and LVIF titles, which seem to be aimed at gaining credibility with the public. As has been noted on their website over the years, 'It won't be long before "LVIM" after the name of a doctor will indicate superior skills and training to the public.' The motives appear clear – that the LVIF and LVIM titles should be treated as a badge of quality and expertise.

What would the ADA code say in such a case? 'The use of abbreviations to designate credentials shall be avoided when such use would lead the reasonable person to believe that the designation represents a quality assured professional qualification or academic degree, when such is not the case.'[12]

One could write a whole book on the over-treatment seen in the pages of dental magazines over the past years. It is unfortunate that the success of one very fine minimally invasive procedure, that of porcelain veneers, has been turned to the benefit of some clinicians in the name of esthetic dentistry. Done properly, porcelain veneers are highly successful in terms of retention and esthetics, but even minimally invasive porcelain veneers may be classed as over-treatment when they are placed in situations where simple bonding composite resin would suffice. Indeed, any treatment used where a less invasive option is available can be regarded as over-treatment.

One particularly troubling example illustrates this ethical minefield. It involves the treatment of a young lady (in her early twenties, judging from her photograph), whose only esthetic issue was a discoloured proximal-incisal (class IV) composite resin on her maxillary left central incisor. The rest of her teeth were impeccable and restoration-free. The dentist, who brazenly entitled the paper *Conservative Elective Porcelain Veneers*,[13] proceeded to cut into and treat no fewer than eight teeth for maxillary veneers from central incisors to first bicuspids. Each veneer, of course, adds to the cost of the procedure, removes enamel from a virgin tooth, and creates a restoration that will require constant follow-up and possible replacement in future decades. The author puts the onus on the young patient, saying:

> *After discussing the options of vital bleaching and direct bonding with composite resin or porcelain veneers, the patient opted for porcelain veneers because she [my italics] considered them the longest lasting, most durable, and most stain-resistant option. It was still possible, however, to maintain most of her natural tooth structure for the future by using stacked porcelain and performing minimal preparation of the specific teeth involved.*[13]

The purpose of the seven veneers that performed no useful function was presumably the result of the domino effect – wanting the neighbouring teeth to match the one tooth that did need treatment. Esthetic improvement using composite resin would have been minimally invasive and equally attractive, albeit lacking the longevity of porcelain.

So was this informed or induced consent? I do not know the details of the advice given to the patient, but I find it hard to believe that any normal human being, presented with the pros and cons, would choose the more invasive and much more costly option. It has been shown that, when offered an informed choice, two-thirds of patients select the non-invasive composite veneer over the mildly invasive porcelain veneer.[33] The only reason for choosing the veneers would be if they presented a significant esthetic benefit. If there is no such benefit, it is difficult to see any advantage, other than an economic one for the dentist. If that was the motivation, it would, of course, have been unethical.

ETHICS OF ADVERTISING IN DENTISTRY

Advertising serves a useful purpose for consumers, providing information about individual businesses that offer services the public may wish to purchase. One could argue that the more information is available to patients, the better prepared they will be to make what is, in reality, a purchasing decision about their health. So, why should they not have information about the training and skill level of the clinician they are considering using and which treatment option they should choose? Isn't that a part of informed consent? Certainly, the US legal system has recognized that advertising can play a large role in providing the information patients may need. The problem comes when advertising becomes deceptive or unfair, such that the consumer is faced with a false choice.

Ever since the US Federal Trade Commission (FTC) started to break down the self-imposed restrictions on advertising by dentists (brought in by the various State Boards of Dentistry), the role of advertising in the profession has been fraught with emotional and political issues. On one side, the State Boards (generally made up of a large majority of practising dentists) are trying to protect the interests of their constituency. On the other, the FTC and the courts aim to protect the public from the potential self-interested actions of some State Boards and some dentists, who may choose to walk the fine line between ethical and unethical advertising. The promotion of competition is also a goal of advertising and of the FTC, while the profession of dentistry prides itself on collegiality.

In an article called 'Ethics and Advertising,' Geoffrey Klempner wrote that three charges can be levelled against advertisers[34]:

- 'They sell us dreams; entice us into confusing dreams with reality.
- They pander to our desires for things that are bad for us.
- They manipulate us into wanting things that we don't really need.'

Would we wish any of these characteristics to be associated with our profession? I think the answer is very clearly, 'No!' However, at the peak of the esthetic revolution of the 1990s and 2000s, and even today, some of those charges might perhaps have been levelled against a certain segment of our community who employed exaggeration and hyperbole in an attempt to present themselves as experts and specialists in the area of esthetic dentistry (not, in fact, a recognized specialty).

The battle over advertising in the United States was fought and lost by its opponents when the FTC ruled that dentists should be allowed to advertise, providing the advertisement is not false or deceptive. State Boards then tried to regulate but found that the bar had been placed quite low. Advertisements are permitted that are self-aggrandising and unprofessional. They lure consumers by appealing to their vanity. Some manipulate patients by making them want something that they do not need, and that in many cases is harmful to their long-term oral health. Unprofessional? Yes. Unethical? Yes. Yet it's all still legal.

In the early days of dentistry, advertising took the form of harmless self-promotion on business cards and free 'give-aways' imprinted with the name of the practice or dentist. There followed a long period of essentially minimal advertising before we reached the point we are at today, most dentists carrying out some form of practice information delivery.

Examples of Victorian-era trade cards can be seen in Figures 2.4–2.9. These date from circa 1885–1895 and some depict claims that would be considered

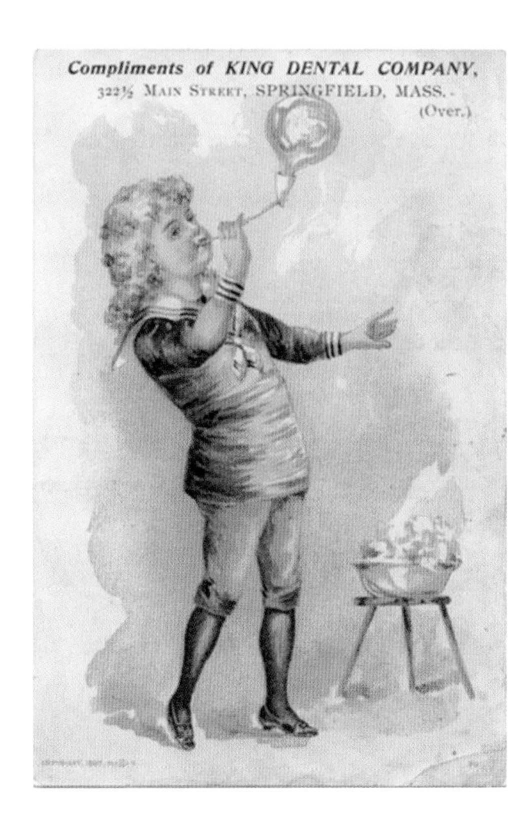

Fig. 2.4 Victorian-era advertising trade card. (Courtesy of Dr Theodore P. Croll, Doylestown, PA)

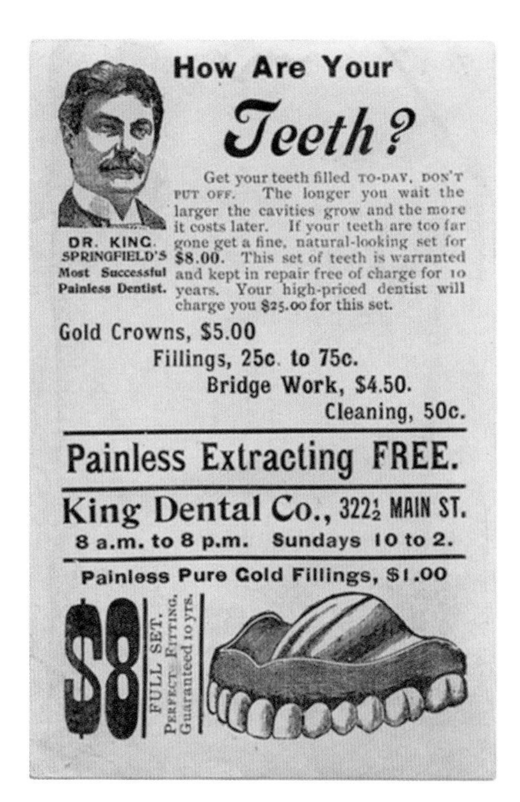

Fig. 2.5 Victorian-era advertising trade card. (Courtesy of Dr Theodore P. Croll, Doylestown, PA)

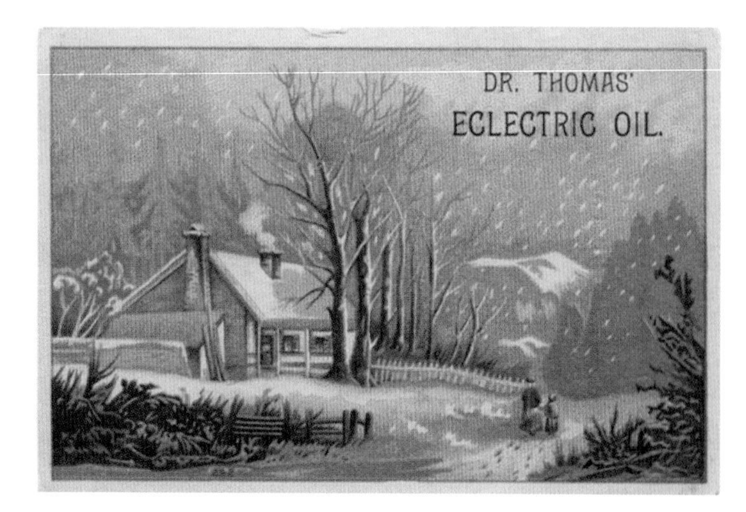

Fig. 2.6 Victorian-era advertising trade card. (Courtesy of Dr Theodore P. Croll, Doylestown, PA)

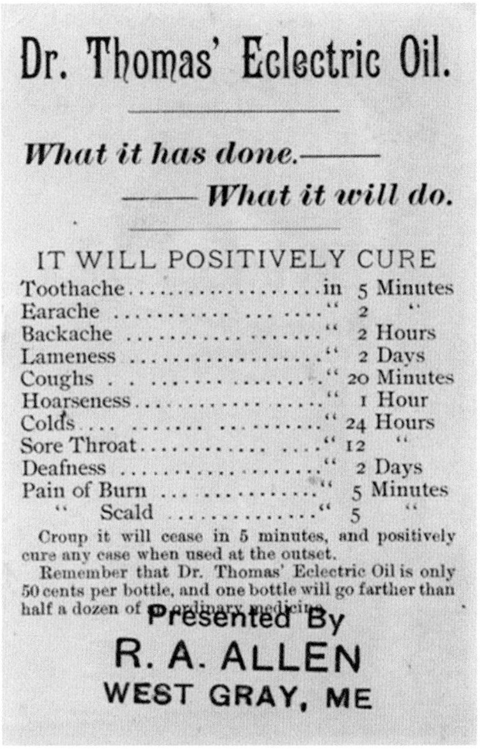

Dr. Thomas' Eclectric Oil.

What it has done.——

——What it will do.

IT WILL POSITIVELY CURE

Toothache ....in 5 Minutes
Earache .... " 2 "
Backache .... " 2 Hours
Lameness .... " 2 Days
Coughs .... " 20 Minutes
Hoarseness .... " 1 Hour
Colds .... " 24 Hours
Sore Throat .... " 12 "
Deafness .... " 2 Days
Pain of Burn .... " 5 Minutes
" Scald .... " 5 "

Croup it will cease in 5 minutes, and positively cure any case when used at the outset.
Remember that Dr. Thomas' Eclectric Oil is only 50 cents per bottle, and one bottle will go farther than half a dozen of ordinary medicine.

Presented By
R. A. ALLEN
WEST GRAY, ME

Fig. 2.7 Victorian-era advertising trade card. (Courtesy of Dr Theodore P. Croll, Doylestown, PA)

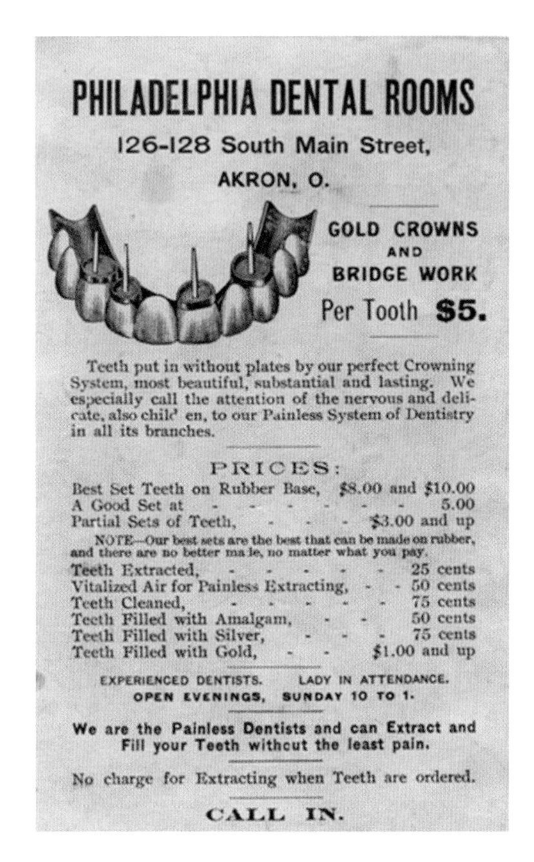

Fig. 2.8 Victorian-era advertising trade card. (Courtesy of Dr Theodore P. Croll, Doylestown, PA)

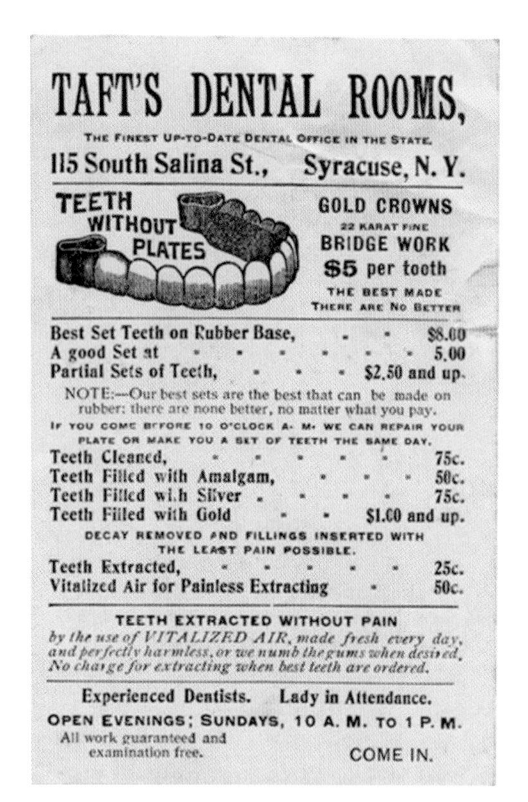

Fig. 2.9 Victorian-era advertising trade card. (Courtesy of Dr Theodore P. Croll, Doylestown, PA)

deceptive and unethical today, referring, for example, to a 'perfect crowning system' or 'painless dentistry'. Another card talks with apparent hope of 'painless extracting' while perhaps coming closer to the truth with 'Decay removed and fillings inserted with the least pain possible'. Apart from word of mouth, such cards were the only way to advertise one's services during this period.

While dentists no longer produce trade cards, I have seen advertisements for dentists in the present day that employ questionable professional standards, such as those printed on the back of grocery store receipts or on the sides of an advertising van (Fig. 2.10).

Today, the most popular form of advertising is surely a well-designed and well-managed website. Such a site, displaying truthful statements about the dentist and his/her team, with some educational materials also available, can be a very positive advertisement for dentist and practice. However, many exaggerate a dentist's credentials and are misleading and deceptive. It seems there is a blurring of the formerly sharp line between a profession and a trade, at least in terms of advertising standards, and this is especially noticeable in glossy magazines sporting advertisements for cosmetic dental 'spas' placed between those touting tummy tucks and tattoo artists. Is that really how we wish the public to visualize our profession?

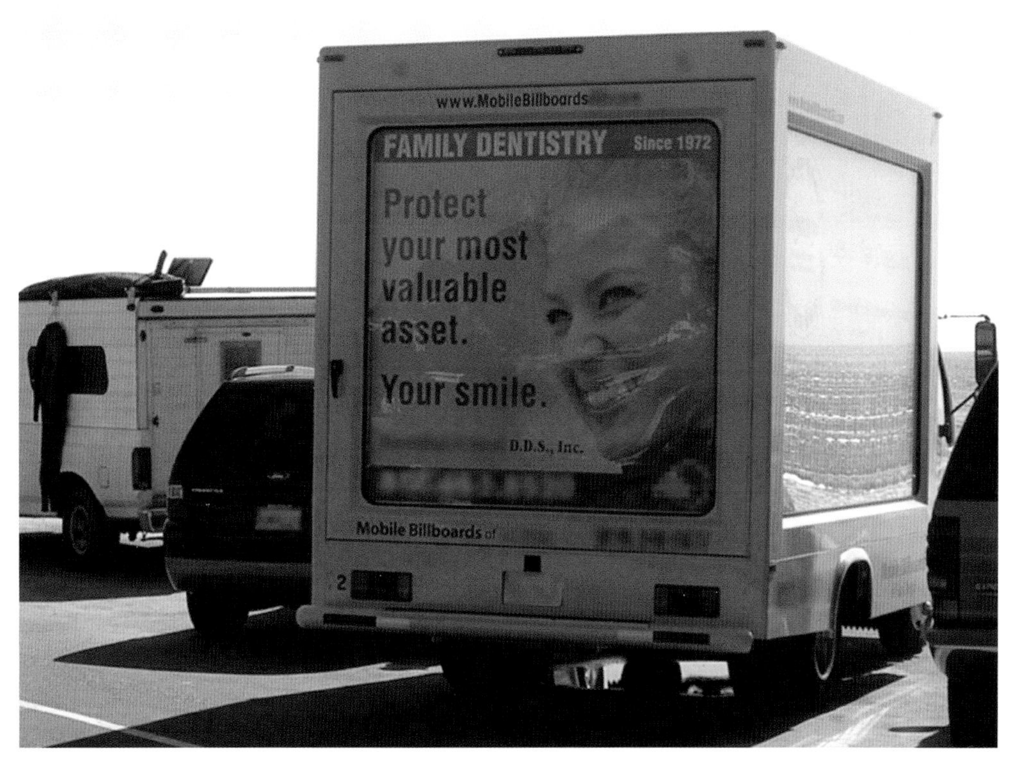

Fig. 2.10 Advertising van in the USA. Promoting a practice in this manner does nothing to enhance the image of the profession in the public mind.

TRUST

At the core of ethical advertising for the dental professional lie three issues, the first of which is trust. Trust is the most fundamental building block of any practice and should be the basis on which the relationship between dentist and patient rests. Without it, an adversarial relationship, such as that seen during the purchase of a car, for example, is set up and there can rarely be a truly happy outcome as each side tries to gain an advantage. The buyer wants the best possible car for the lowest possible price, while the seller is trying to pocket as much money as he or she can.

It is trust that enables the dentist to complete the best treatment plan for the patient, who, in turn, is happy to receive such treatment, trusting that it has been delivered with their best interests in mind. And yet the adversarial relationship is also creeping into dental practice, as many office managers and staff are trained to 'up-sell' additional treatments, or the patient tries to bargain for extra services to be included. This is the inevitable outcome of advertising (for example, 'free teeth whitening with examination') and has been going on since the early trade cards ('No charge for Extracting when Teeth are ordered' – see Fig. 2.8). It is unfortunate that the trust factor in the dentist–patient relationship appears to be under severe challenge today. This can only lead to an erosion of our professional autonomy.

MISLEADING CLAIMS

After trust comes the responsibility to refrain from making claims that can mislead – an extremely problematic area. Often the intent seems to be to mislead the patient (deceptive advertising) into believing that Dr X is better than any other dentist at a particular procedure or in a particular community (Fig. 2.11). This leads us into a grey area where the FTC would probably rule that it is acceptable to say that one is good, but not to draw comparisons with colleagues that are impossible to prove. Any attempt to claim superiority is fraught with collegial issues and is certainly unprofessional and, to my mind, unethical.

TITLES

The third core component of ethical advertising is to stay within one's area of professional competence and abilities, and not to imply that one is a specialist if not qualified to do so. Unfortunately, in a rush to follow the business principles that really should not be applied to a healthcare profession, many colleagues stray over this ethical boundary. The unsuspecting public is not familiar with the accredited specialty areas and it is easy to deceive by exaggeration. Calling

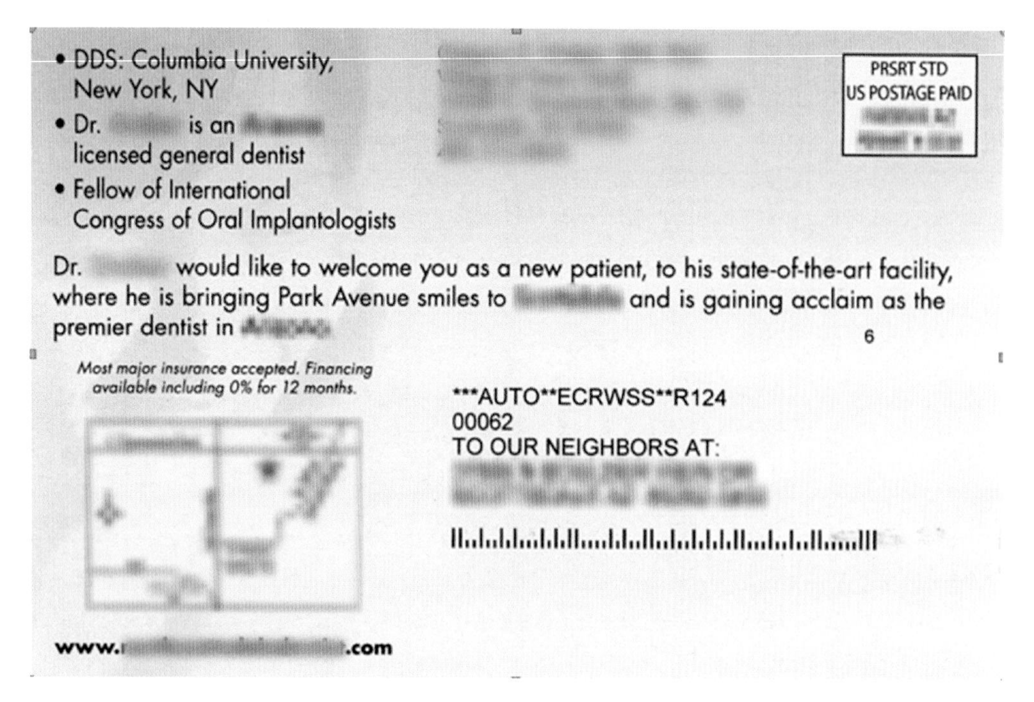

Fig. 2.11 Advertising card mailed to private homes in a US town, promoting the 'premier dentist in the state'. Saying one is better than one's colleagues is unprofessional and shows a lack of collegiality.

one's practice a '[YourTown] dental implants specialist's' or 'specialists' implant centre', especially when there is no such specialty and the dentists involved are not, therefore, implant specialists, seems to me deceptive. The key is to ask the question: Is a member of the general public likely to be misled into thinking that the dentist in question is a specialist in the area advertised? If so, the advertisement, in the form of the practice name, is, in my view, unethical.

BEING TRUTHFUL AND HONEST

The onus is on dentists to present their skills and qualifications truthfully and honestly, and not even to hint at any claim that might stray into questionable ethical territory. Subjective claims concerning the quality of the services provided or the relative quality of the treatment should be avoided. For example, many practices try to set themselves apart by claiming to provide 'advanced dentistry'. And one has only to search the Web to find general practitioners who call themselves the 'best cosmetic dentist'. How do we, or they, know they are the best? And what are your colleagues down the road, also general dentists, going to call their practice? While it may be true that the level and quality of care provided in any particular surgery is of a higher standard than that of others in the vicinity, how can that be proved without objective evidence?

In its policy on advertising, the American College of Dentists (ACD) puts the onus on the public to verify the claim, noting in a list of points that an advertisement is deceptive if it 'contain[s] a representation or implication regarding the quality of dental services which would suggest unique or general superiority to other practitioners which are not susceptible to reasonable verification by the public'.[35] The ADA code also makes itself quite clear when it declares:

> *In order to properly serve the public, dentists should represent themselves in a manner that contributes to the esteem of the profession. Dentists should not misrepresent their training and competence in any way that would be false or misleading in any material respect ... Although any dentist may advertise, no dentist shall advertise or solicit patients in any form of communication in a manner that is false or misleading in any material respect.*[12]

QUALIFICATIONS AND DEGREES

The use of letters after one's name that represent unearned or non-health degrees is another way in which we can potentially mislead the public. In the USA, dentists may use the title 'Doctor' or 'Dentist', or either of the commonly awarded degrees – DDS or DMD (but not, as is often seen, Doctor *and* the doctoral degree, as that is redundant) – plus any advanced degree such as MS or PhD, providing the degree in question has been awarded in a relevant healthcare subject. Thus MD is acceptable, but MA would only be acceptable if dentally or medically related. Similarly, a PhD in Oral Biology may be mentioned but not one in Theology. Similar rules exist elsewhere in the world. The reasons are obvious:

> *The use of a non-health degree in an announcement to the public may be a representation which is misleading because the public is likely to assume that any degree announced is related to the qualifications of the dentist as a practitioner.*[12]

It should almost go without saying that one must only utilize degrees professionally awarded in healthcare, in a healthcare practice, and not in diploma 'mills'. Some years ago, a regular contributor to the *Journal of the American Dental Association* listed a Master's degree after his name and dental degree on the title page. This MBA suddenly disappeared when its legitimacy was questioned but the publications continued. The degree had been purchased from a diploma mill and seems to have been used to bolster the author's qualifications and ego. It appears that the transgression, major as it was, was not serious enough for the journal to consider losing a potential source of a column.

THE AMERICAN COLLEGE OF DENTISTS

The ACD, a highly respected fellowship organization, has been at the forefront of promoting ethical standards in the profession. Its position on advertising is straightforward: while recognizing that advertising is legal, the ACD 'does not encourage or support advertising by dentists and feels that any form of advertising by dentists is demeaning to the profession, is not in the best interests of the profession, and is not in keeping with its perception of professionalism'.[36]

The College does, however, recognize that advertising is here to stay and, 'when properly done ... may help people to better understand the dental care available to them and how to obtain that care'. The ACD states that advertising should be designed to increase public confidence in the dental profession and in the individual practitioner, and should not be misleading or false in any way. In particular, advertising should avoid creating any false expectations for a favourable treatment outcome and should not primarily target a lay person's fears.

Advertising in dentistry has its good and bad points. On the plus side, dentists can get their message across, and patients can benefit from extra information concerning the dentist's education, training and interests. On the minus side, advertisements can make the profession look like all the trades that advertise in a non-professional manner. False, misleading or overtly deceptive advertising not only becomes a stain on the individual dentist, but also spreads to everyone else in the profession. Advertising should be professional, honest, informational and accurate, so as to convey the sense of a profession communicating its goals of service to the general public. Anything else chips away at the unwritten laws of trust and autonomy, hard earned by the generations of colleagues that went before us.

DENTAL PUBLISHING

While much has been noted about the dishonest and unethical researchers who fudge, manipulate or even invent data, there is also a trend that attempts to make pure hype and sales-oriented publications look and feel like scientific reports. Authors throw in a few references to make an article look scientific and format the report just like a peer-reviewed paper to disguise its real intent. Also, many papers in the trade magazines (I refuse to call them 'journals') are ghost-written by dental product manufacturing companies. 'Serial endorsers' are paid to add their names to a paper that they have not written or participated in, other than to approve the content.

Another source of dental advertising, particularly for esthetic dentistry and implant surgery, is airline magazines. Certain of the advertisements are sponsored by some of the most self-promotional dentists you will find anywhere. Each one appears to be the only 'cosmetic or esthetic dentist with real credentials'. Since there is no such specialty as cosmetic or esthetic dentistry, what are these 'real credentials'? Does this mean that everyone else has 'fake' ones? This sort of advertisement certainly implies that impossible scenario.

PLAGIARISM

Plagiarism and the stretching of one study into multiple publications are significant ethical problems in dental publishing today. Everyone is aware of the ease of plagiarizing articles from the Web. So much information is freely available and can be easily transferred to one's own documents. The intent may often be to modify and paraphrase, and mistakes are easy to make in such situations. But mistaken or purposeful copying is plagiarism and is unethical. Authors must pay special attention to quoting and referencing appropriately.

Double publishing is another serious ethical transgression. It is hard to plead a mistake when two virtually identical papers are prepared and submitted to two different journals – particularly when it is commonplace to have to sign a form stating that the work in question has not been published or submitted elsewhere. In the Spring of 1988, as Editor-in-Chief of *Quintessence International*, I became personally involved in a brazen example of double publishing. A colleague submitted essentially the same paper at about the same time to *Quintessence International* and to another journal, *Gerodontics*, and I was alerted to this fact by an observant reader. The senior author of both articles denied that the papers were virtually identical, claiming that the one in *Gerodontics* was directed at the older population. It was not difficult to see that the illustrations, data and bulk of the text were more or less the same.[37,38] What made the situation worse was that the lead author was a consultant to the company making the toothbrushes reviewed in the articles, so there was also a clear but undeclared conflict of interest. Both papers were retracted.

Other more serious issues in research conduct (such as the Wakefield MMR and autism study) have been discussed previously.

ETHICS IN THE DENTAL PRODUCT INDUSTRY

What are the ethics that lie behind the manufacturing and selling of dental products? Where do you draw the line when deciding whether to market a product that is going to be placed in the human body? (In the interests of full disclosure, I should note that from 1989 to 1999 I worked at 3M Dental Products Company – now 3M ESPE.)

There are a large number of companies making dental materials, ranging from divisions of international conglomerates to small family-owned businesses. US dental products from US-based manufacturers are sold all over the world, so can be said to have a global impact. The industry's record of material production for dental practice in recent decades is marked by some outstanding successes but also some stunning failures. Who can forget Artglass ('the first and only true polyglass'), which, in its early form, caused tremendous problems? 'Many dentists have been financially damaged by having to repair faulty and inadequate restorations through no fault of their own,' noted the *ADA News*.[39] Then there were the so-called 'condensable composites' – a disgraceful foray by manufacturers who competed prematurely to grab the amalgam market for composite resin by marketing materials that all failed quickly and miserably in their original versions. It was well known that these materials could not be 'condensable' in the sense that an amalgam was condensable (as liquids are not condensable), yet one advertisement boasted 'real condensability'. Another claimed, on its introduction in 1997, 'A full 5 mm depth of cure (go ahead, bulk fill)'. These dual virtues gave the product an unfair competitive advantage over others that did not make the same claim, and for 16 years the company continued to repeat the statement in its marketing materials. However, a recent study showed that the product had just 2.53 mm depth of cure, and in Knoop Hardness tests it emerged that, if placed as directed, the composite would not be fully cured at depth.[40]

This is a classic example of manufacturers (unethically) promoting the use of their material for purposes not supported by the evidence, and when the evidence indicates that the material will fail in a way that may not be detectable for some time due to inadequate polymerization of the deeper layers.

With appropriate controls, failures should rarely make it to the market. Adequate and proper testing should disclose the more obvious inadequacies and prevent the material from failing in the mouth, providing the manufacturers are willing to run the proper clinical trials prior to launch. Unfortunately, that is not always the case, and by default, our practices become the testbed for new materials. This is an unethical adaptation to competitive pressure. Many products therefore have a very short market life, being withdrawn and replaced with an amended version until the manufacturers get it right. Meanwhile, patients need restorations replaced and dentists suffer the embarrassment of explaining why it is necessary to replace work done just months before.

It is worth noting here the paradox of the professional standard that encourages dentists not to criticize each other's work to lay people. I was educated to believe that it is unethical to express criticisms of a patient's dental work to the individual concerned; instead, one should call the treating dentist and question the treatment. That is all very well and good the first time one sees inadequate or shoddy work, or obvious over-treatment. But I believe the dentist is obligated, by those same professional standards, to be the whistle blower in cases of repetitive maltreatment. Failing to do so would be unethical, in my opinion. If it is clear that the treatment is grossly inadequate and that the poor treatment was not affected by conditions outside the control of the treating dentist – such as a patient's failure to return for follow-up care, or a lack of cooperation precluding optimal treatment at the time of the appointment, the dentist needs to be informed that the case will be submitted for peer review. Turning a blind eye to over-treatment or inadequate care has the distinct potential to harm the patient, or subsequent patients who visit the treating dentist, and blatant mistreatment should be reported to collegial association peer-review boards or the regulatory body.

CONCLUDING REMARKS

What is a professional? According to McCullough, the concept of a profession may be described as the 'public, sanctioned promise that one will blunt one's own self-interest, and the guild interests of one's professional group, to protect and promote the best interest of those one serves in dentistry'. If we fail in this moral commitment, 'dentistry will revert to a trade, a way to do business and earn money.'[41]

With the advent of Buonocore's acid-etch technique[26] and the development of the first composite resins by Bowen,[42] an array of conservative, minimally invasive dental procedures was made possible.[43] As well as maintaining high standards of personal ethical behaviour, we must do as much as we individually are able to try to influence future generations of dentists, growing up surrounded by cheating and unethical behaviour, to be ethical healthcare professionals. We must encourage our younger colleagues to treat the bond that they have with their patients as ethically inviolable and to understand the boundaries between profit and patient care. Dentists must apply ethics to all dentally related healthcare issues and consider people's oral health as a part of their general wellbeing. As Jon Huntsman said, in the title of his fine book, '*Winners Never Cheat*'![44]

Going back to where I started this chapter – Michael Josephson's radio talk, I will exercise editorial licence and substitute the words 'dentistry/the profession' for 'business', and 'we/our' for 'they/their' from Josephson's original words: 'Probably no one in dentistry has the power to change everything in the profession, but we have the power to change something, and that's what our obligation is.'

REFERENCES

1. Chambers DW. Large ethics. J Am Coll Dent 2008;75:36–47.
2. Harris. Radio Host Has Drug Company Ties. New York Times, November 21, 2008.
3. <http://www.cbsnews.com/2100-18563_162-20077025.html>; [accessed 14 February 2014].
4. <http://www.huffingtonpost.com/2010/05/19/harvard-hoax-adam-wheeler_n_582451.html>; [accessed 14 February 2014].
5. Lewin. Dean at M.I.T. Resigns, Ending a 28-Year Lie. New York Times, April 27, 2007.
6. Wakefield AJ, Murch SH, Anthony A, et al. Ileal–lymphoid–nodular hyperplasia, non-specific colitis, and pervasive developmental disorder in children. Lancet 1998;351:637–41.
7. Wade. Cancer Study Was Made Up, Journal Says. New York Times, January 19, 2006.
8. Young JR. Journals find many images in research that are faked. Chron Higher Educ June 6, 2008;54(39).
9. <http://www.justice.gov/opa/pr/2009/September/09-civ-900.html>; [accessed 14 February 2014].

10. Chambers DW. Lying through your teeth. J Am Coll Dent 2004;71:7–13.
11. Yankelovich D. Profit with honor. New Haven: Yale University Press; 2006.
12. American Dental Association. Principles of Ethics and Code of Professional Conduct. <http://www.ada.org/194.aspx>; [accessed 14 February 2014].
13. Nash RW. Conservative elective porcelain veneers. Comp Cont Ed Dent 1999;20:888–97.
14. Ozar DT, Sokol DJ. Dental ethics at chairside: professional principles and practical applications. 2nd ed. Washington: Georgetown University Press; 2007.
15. Tahir MAM, Mason C, Hind V. Informed consent: optimism versus reality. Br Dent J 2002;193:221–4.
16. Bader JD, Shugars DA. Variation, treatment outcomes and practice guidelines in dental practice. J Dent Educ 1995;59:61–5.
17. Kelleher MGD. The 'daughter' test in aesthetic (esthetic) or cosmetic dentistry. Dent Update 2010;37:5–11.
18. Kelleher M. Ethical issues, dilemmas and controversies in 'cosmetic' or aesthetic dentistry. A personal opinion. Br Dent J 2012;21:365–7.
19. Kelleher M. Porcelain pornography. Faculty Dent J 2011;2:134–41.
20. Simonsen RJ. Greed and the gravy train: is this success? J Esthet Dent 1999;11:287–8.
21. Simonsen RJ. From needs to wants; from service to self-interest; from profession to trade: whatever happened to Hippocrates? Gen Dent 2001;49:232–4.
22. Simonsen RJ. Delusions of grandeur or what the public doesn't know about shortcuts. J Esthet Restor Dent 2005;17:69–71.
23. Simonsen RJ. Commerce versus care: troubling trends in the ethics of restorative dentistry. Dent Clin N Am 2007;51:281–7.
24. Simonsen RJ. Overtreatment? You bet it is! J Esthet Restor Dent 2007;19:235–6.
25. Simonsen RJ. The death of amalgam. Quintessence Int 1991;22:173.
26. Buonocore MG. A simple method of increasing the adhesion of acrylic filling materials to enamel surfaces. J Dent Res 1955;34:849–53.
27. Chambers DW. Concerning the current high demand for snake oil. J Am Coll Dent 2004;71:2–3.
28. Laskin DM, Greene CS, Hylander WL. TMDs: an evidence-based approach to diagnosis and treatment. Chicago: Quintessence; 2006.
29. Wright EF. Manual of temporomandibular disorders. Ames, IA: Wiley–Blackwell; 2010.
30. Selvaratnam P, Niere K, Zuluaga M. Headache, orofacial pain and bruxism. Edinburgh: Churchill Livingstone/Elsevier; 2009.
31. Klineberg I, Kingston D. Oral rehabilitation: a case-based approach. Ames, IA: Wiley–Blackwell; 2012.

32. <http://www.lviglobal.com/full-time-faculty>; [accessed 14 February 2014].

33. Nalbandian S, Millar BJ. The effect of veneers on cosmetic improvement. Br Dent J 2009;207:72–3.

34. <http://klempner.freeshell.org/articles/advertising.html>; [accessed 14 February 2014].

35. <http://acd.org/policy1.htm>; [accessed 14 February 2014].

36. <http://www.acd.org/policy1.htm>; [accessed 14 February 2014].

37. Silverstone LM, Featherstone MJ. A scanning electron microscope study of the end rounding of bristles in eight toothbrush types. Quintessence Int 1988;19:87–107.

38. Silverstone LM, Featherstone MJ. Examination of the end rounding pattern of toothbrush bristles using scanning electron microscopy: a comparison of eight toothbrush bristle types. Gerodontics 1988;4:45–62.

39. Berthold M. Dentists sue Heraeus Kulzer. ADA News October 21, 2002;33(19):14.

40. Tiba A, Zeller GG, Estrich C, et al. A laboratory evaluation of bulk-fill versus traditional multi-increment-fill resin-based composites. ADA Professional Product Review 2013;13–26.

41. McCullough LB. Ethics in dental medicine: a framework for moral responsibility in dental practice. J Dent Educ 1985;49:219–24.

42. Bowen RL. Dental filling material comprising vinyl silica and a binder consisting of the reaction product of bisphenol and glycidyl methacrylate. Washington, DC: Commissioner of Patents and Trademarks, US Patent No. 3,066,112; Nov. 1962.

43. Simonsen RJ. Clinical applications of the acid-etch technique. Chicago: Quintessence; 1978.

44. Huntsman JM. Winners never cheat – even in difficult times. Upper Saddle River: N.J. Pearson Prentice-Hall; 2011.

Additional reading

Chambers DW. In, Journal of the American College of Dentists. All issues.

Rule JT, Veatch RM. Ethical questions in dentistry. 2nd ed. Chicago: Quintessence; 2004.

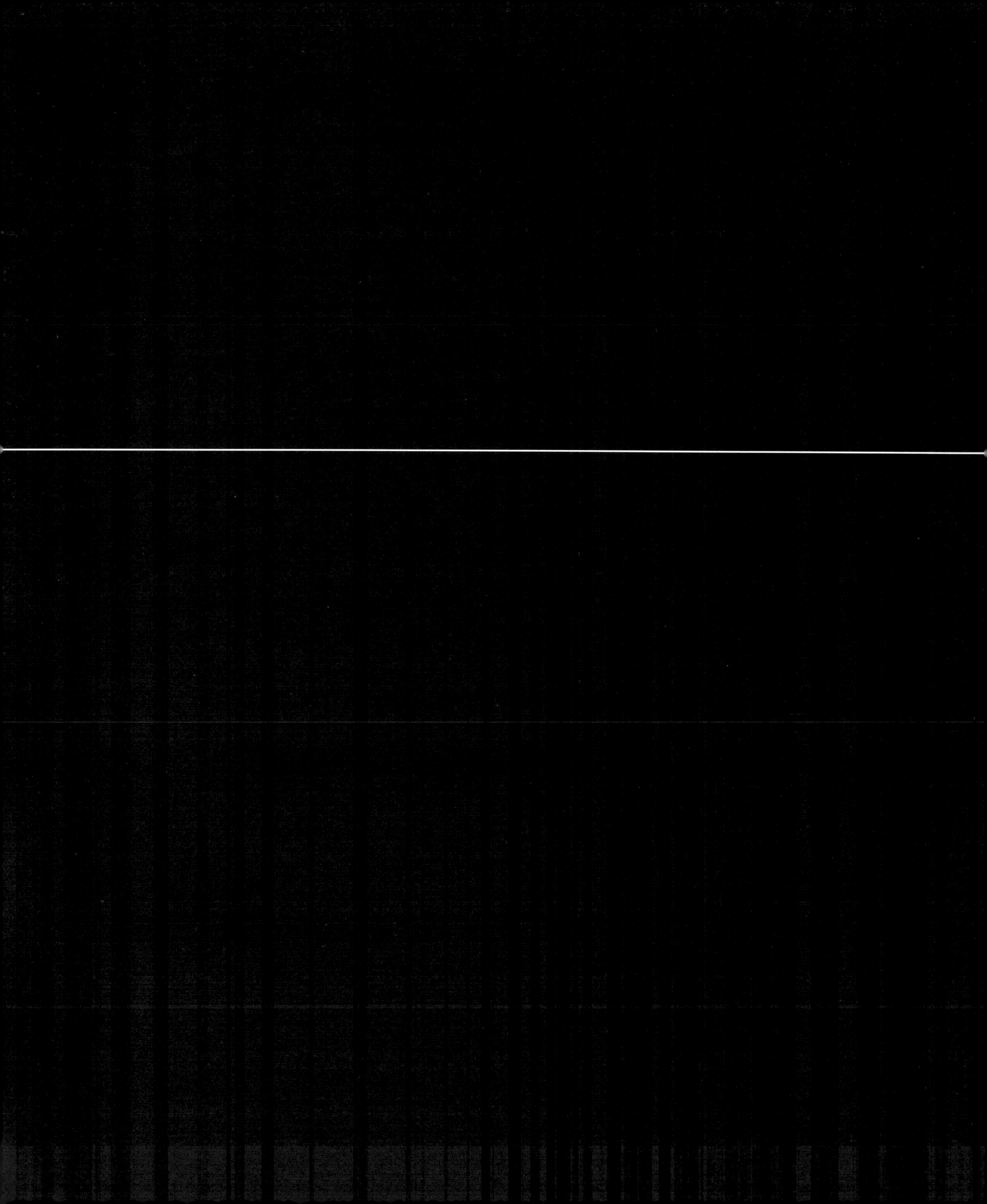

CHAPTER 3

Patient Examination and Assessment

SUBIR BANERJI AND SHAMIR MEHTA

INTRODUCTION

As indicated in Chapter 1, there is a wealth of evidence to support the popular notion that individuals with a more attractive outward physical appearance may have a distinct advantage over their peers from the point of view of improved social acceptability, occupational prospects and interpersonal relationships, and a sense of greater self-esteem and self-confidence.[1]

It has been suggested that the face is the most readily recognizable anatomical feature of the human body.[2] According to work by Goldstein,[3] the general public appear to perceive the mouth as the second most important feature after the eyes when considering facial esthetics.

The appearance of the smile is clearly an important factor in determining the attractiveness of a face.[1] An individual's smile is a key element of facial esthetics, and plays an important role in the non-verbal communication of many different sentiments, including friendliness, agreement and appreciation, and the conveying of emotions such as happiness, fear, sadness and surprise.[4]

It is hardly surprising, therefore, that the wish to improve one's smile – to enhance the appearance of the esthetic zone of the smile – may be the principal reason for an individual to seek dental care.[5] Such a wish may be reinforced by the ready access our patients have to information on contemporary esthetic treatment modalities such as tooth whitening, 'invisible' orthodontics, esthetic restorations, dental implants and other procedures, including the use of botulinum toxin and fillers to alter the appearance of the soft tissues of the face.

It is not so easy, however, to define the 'esthetic dental ideal', as the concepts of esthetics and beauty are so intimately related and vary within and between different cultures and ethnic and age groups. Beauty may be 'in the eye of the beholder' and is highly influenced by individual preferences and personal style and experiences. So-called 'subjective concepts in dental esthetics', however, cannot be relied upon to serve as effective guidelines for the planning of esthetic dental care.[6]

Practitioners must therefore have a clear understanding of what are often collectively termed the 'universal concepts of dental esthetics' when attempting to meet the demands placed on them by patients who are seeking enhanced dental esthetics.[6] Such universal concepts are based on generic perceptions of what is considered to be esthetically pleasing. They include:

- the elimination of disease and pathology
- the need to develop symmetry, proportion and harmony

- an appreciation of tooth position and dental morphology
- an appreciation of colour variations
- an appreciation of form.

Esthetic dentistry is a rapidly growing aspect of oral healthcare provision. According to survey data obtained by the American Academy of Cosmetic Dentistry (AACD), the mean revenue generated by dental practices in the USA from cosmetic procedures grew to $495,000 in 2007, representing a sizeable 15% increase over the previous year.[7] Notwithstanding subsequent growth in the esthetic dentistry market, there is a prospect of further growth well into the future. It is also important to take note of data reported by a major multinational indemnity group (Dental Protection Limited, UK), indicating that in 2011 there was a 50% increase since 2006 in the number of complaints involving smile makeover treatments, with cases reported to have been settled for five-figure sums, excluding legal costs.[8] Esthetic dentistry may be lucrative for dentists and lawyers but it is relatively high-risk in terms of patient complaints.

Medico-legal issues often arise as a consequence of incomplete or inadequate preoperative patient assessment and examination. In such circumstances, practitioners tend to have failed to appreciate, let alone fully understand, the patient's esthetic values, concerns and perceptions, and have taken it upon themselves to impose their interpretation of the smile best suited to the patient. As discussed below, the patient must always be involved in smile design decisions.

The aim of this chapter is to provide a comprehensive guide on how to assess and plan treatment for patients with concerns about their dental appearance; these concerns may range from a simple incisal edge fracture to the extreme of the patient who presents with an unsightly, dysfunctional, extensively restored and failing dentition. In all cases, a holistic approach to the care of the patient should be adopted. To achieve this, it is imperative for the practitioner to have a thorough working knowledge of the complex interplays between the dental hard tissues, the supporting alveolar and periodontal tissues, and the underlying occlusal scheme. For a satisfactory clinical outcome and a favourable prognosis to be obtained, the patient must have not just an esthetic smile, but also a stable occlusion, a good standard of oral health, and the necessary knowledge and skills to maintain his or her new dental status.

In the process of learning how to assess and plan treatment for a patient seeking esthetic dental care, it is hoped that the reader will develop an understanding of the concept of the 'esthetic ideal', founded on the evidence-based, universal principles of dental esthetics.

PATIENT HISTORY

The taking of a patient history should commence by recording essential data such as name, gender, date of birth, address and contact details, together with any information in respect of special needs when attending for dental care.

PRESENTING COMPLAINTS AND CONCERNS

The goals of esthetic dental care include the need to:

- meet the realistic expectations of the patient
- attain long-term functional and esthetic stability
- achieve the treatment goals through the application of minimal intervention approaches.

In order to begin to fulfil these goals, a comprehensive and contemporaneous patient history must be carefully obtained and appropriately documented. Above all else, it is of paramount importance that the practitioner listens attentively to the complaints and concerns of the patient, and complements the proposed history and examination procedure as necessary, so that all the issues raised by the patient are fully investigated. Treatment planning should not be commenced until such time as all investigations and related enquiries have been completed.

CLINICAL TIP

Spend sufficient time finding out why your patient is seeking esthetic change.

According to Chalifoux,[9] there are three categories of 'dental esthetic imperfections' that encourage patients to seek esthetic intervention. These relate to anomalies in tooth:

- colour
- position
- shape.

Esthetic imperfections in colour may be caused by, amongst other factors, the presence of stains, craze lines, dentine exposure, discoloration of residual tooth tissue by pre-existing and existing restorations, and alterations in the optical properties of the remaining tooth tissues associated with ageing and wear, together with tooth discoloration associated with dental caries and loss of vitality of the tooth.[10] An example of a patient who presented with discoloured maxillary central incisor teeth is illustrated in Figure 3.1. The discoloration was multifactorial, including that acquired from the presence of stained restorations with secondary caries and leakage. While many practitioners would, in all probability, consider the defective restorations, possibly together with the incisor crowding, to be the most likely causes of the patient's esthetic concerns, careful assessment revealed that it was actually the relatively trivial circular area of white opacity present in the incisal third region of the upper right central incisor (UR1) that was causing dissatisfaction, highlighting an obvious difference in perception between the patient and the dentist.

Positional concerns may be associated with the presence of dental diastema, rotations and tipping of teeth, crowding, supra-eruption or intrusion, anomalies in arch shape and size, and, of course, loss or absence of teeth from the dental arch.[9] Unilateral positional anomalies that adversely affect symmetry tend to give rise to more esthetic concerns than bilateral anomalies, particularly if the bilateral anomalies are symmetrical.

Morphological anomalies that may be associated with esthetic concerns include the presence of fractures, cracks, tooth wear – abrasion, abfraction, attrition and erosion, dental caries, surface defects such as hypoplasia, and variations in surface texture that may vary from limited to severe, as may be seen in patients with congenital conditions such as amelogenesis imperfecta.[10] Other congenital anomalies that may contribute to esthetic dissatisfaction include unusual crown dimensions – macrodontia and microdontia, and variations in root diameter dimensions. Congenital malformations of the teeth, including peg shape, dilacerations, fusions and germination, are further examples of morphological anomalies that may give rise to esthetic concerns.[10]

In addition, as our patients become more conscious of and educated about facial enhancement treatments, which dental practitioners are increasingly providing, it is not uncommon for people to present with issues relating to facial esthetics.

It is often very helpful initially to ask those who are seeking esthetic treatment to fill out an esthetic evaluation form, designed to gain information and insight into a patient's personal perceptions concerning their dental and facial esthetics. An example of such a questionnaire, as used by Jornung and Fardal,[11] is reproduced in Table 3.1. This uses a 100 mm visual analogue scale (VAS) on

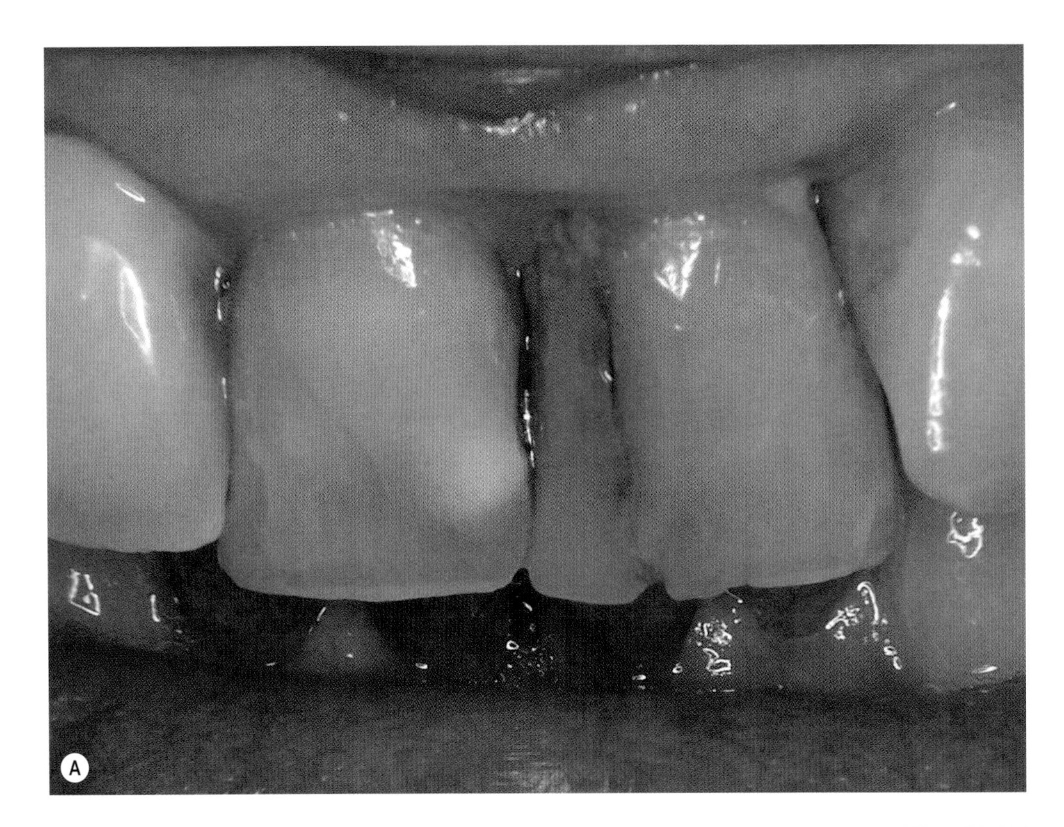

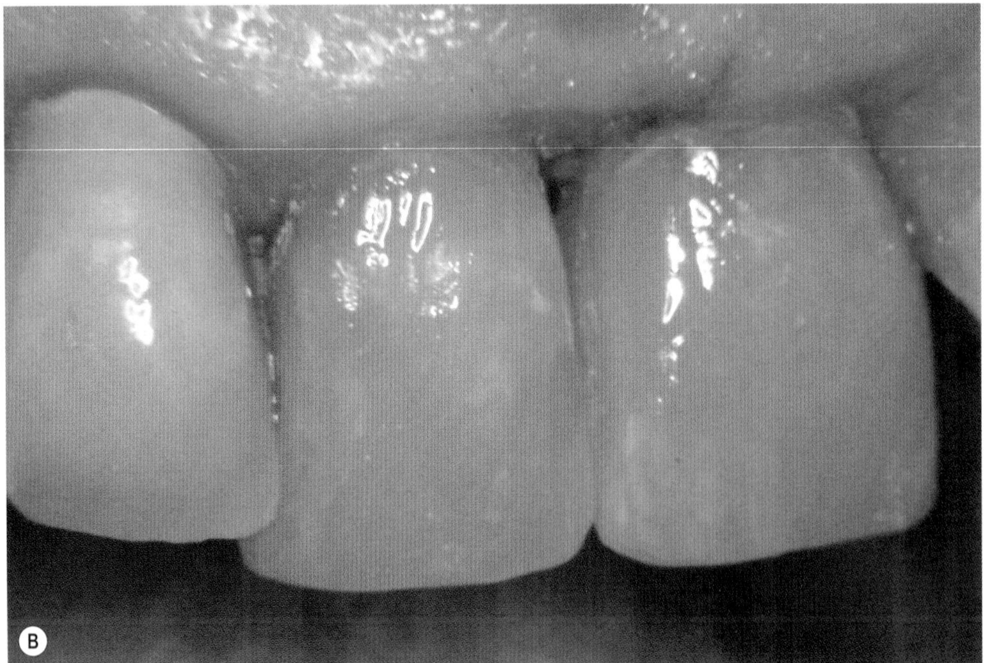

Fig. 3.1 Imperfections in colour. A. The case of a 69-year-old female patient, whose primary dental esthetic concern related to the white circular discoloration present in the incisal third of her upper right central incisor. B. Appearance following restoration with a bonded-resin composite.

TABLE 3.1 QUESTIONNAIRE USED TO RECORD PATIENT PERCEPTIONS OF AND OPINIONS ABOUT DENTAL AND FACIAL AESTHETICS*

Question	Visual analogue scale
Section 1	
How pleased/satisfied are you with your smile? Please indicate along the neighbouring line	|--| Not pleased Very pleased
How pleased/satisfied are you with the shape of your lips?	|--|
How pleased/satisfied are you with the shade (whiteness) of your teeth?	|--|
How pleased/satisfied are you with the evenness of your teeth?	|--|
How pleased/satisfied are you with the looks of your gums?	|--|
Are you aware of having receding gums? Please circle	Yes / No
If you have answered yes, how much does it affect your smile? Please indicate along the neighbouring line	|--| (Not at all) (Very much affected)
Do you have crooked teeth? Please circle	Yes / No
If you have answered yes, how interested are you in having orthodontic treatment to correct the crooked teeth?	|--| (Not interested) (Very interested)
Section 2	
How important are the following features for an attractive face? Please indicate along the neighbouring line in each case Hair	|--| (Not important) (Very important)
Hairline	|--|
Eyes	|--|
Eyebrows	|--|

TABLE 3.1 ***Continued***

Question	Visual analogue scale
Nose	|--|
Skin	|--|
Ears	|--|
Lips	|--|
Teeth	|--|
Chin	|--|
Shape of head	|--|

*Modified from Jornung and Fardal.[11]

which patients can record their perceptions according to statements relating to their dental–facial esthetics; the scale ranges from 0 to 100, indicating 'not pleased' to 'very pleased'.

The answers provided to these questions not only may help guide the clinician as to how best to satisfy the needs and expectations of the patient, but also may aid in the identification of possible underlying psychological conditions, such as body dysmorphic disorder (BDD), which may have profound medico-legal implications, as discussed below.

A detailed history of the problem should also be recorded, as it may reveal underlying conditions and pathology that may require treatment and subsequent stabilization prior to addressing the esthetic concerns. In the view of the authors, diseased tissues and structures are always considered to be unsightly. As a prerequisite to predictable esthetic treatment, any existing disease should be managed and the condition stabilized.

MEDICAL HISTORY

A detailed medical history must be obtained and recorded. The use of a template medical history form may help avoid critical omissions.

In the provision of esthetic dental care, patients' medical history and status may:

- prevent them from attending any lengthy or frequent treatment sessions that are needed

- necessitate a modification of the treatment protocol to take account of an underlying medical condition or the drugs used to treat it
- contraindicate certain types of treatment: for example, an allergy to a material or product that prevents its use
- contribute to the esthetic impairment: for example, the taking of prescription medication that may induce gingival hyperplasia, or an eating disorder, hiatus hernia or gastric reflux resulting in erosive tooth wear.

It is beyond the scope of this chapter to discuss the plethora of medical conditions that may potentially impact on the delivery of esthetic dental care. However, one condition that warrants further discussion is BDD.

BDD may be considered to be a psychiatric illness that is characterized by a preoccupation with an imagined defect in appearance; this in turn causes marked distress to the affected person. This preoccupation may cause clinically significant distress or impairment in social functioning, occupation or other important areas, with the preoccupation not being related to any other form of mental illnesses.[12] Whilst BDD has been reported to have an incidence rate of approximately 3% amongst the general population, it would appear to be more common amongst those seeking cosmetic and esthetic treatments. This is covered in detail in Volume 2 of this series as part of patient assessment.

Typical features of patients suffering from BDD include:

- onset in late adolescence
- equal prevalence amongst males and females, although unmarried individuals appear to be more susceptible[13]
- a reluctance on the part of patients to disclose their symptoms
- social phobias and obsessive–compulsive disorders (OCDs), which are common amongst sufferers
- a tendency towards alcohol dependency
- a tendency to become housebound
- suicidal tendencies.

Patients suffering from BDD appear to be most preoccupied with esthetic impairments relating to their skin, hair and nose. Indeed, a high proportion of sufferers reportedly seek cosmetic surgery involving their chins and noses. Details of such surgical intervention should be recorded as part of the medical history, which may ultimately help with diagnosis of the condition.

Clearly, patients suffering from BDD may be profoundly challenging to treat. When the dental practitioner observes behaviour that may be suggestive of BDD, referral to the patient's medical practitioner is advisable prior to considering any form of esthetic dental care, in particular any form of invasive, irreversible treatment.

DENTAL AND SOCIAL HISTORY

The patient's attitudes towards dentistry and oral health should be assessed. Oral hygiene habits, past attendance habits and previous experience of dental care should also be established. Dental phobic patients and those who lack the motivation to maintain a high standard of oral hygiene may be more suited to relatively simple, low-maintenance, minimally invasive forms of treatment that help address their concerns. Those with unrealistic expectations may require further counselling, especially prior to embarking upon complex, irreversible forms of dental treatment.

The patient's social habits, such as smoking and levels of alcohol consumption, should be ascertained. Smoking and excessive alcohol consumption not only contribute towards the initiation and progression of various forms of oral disease, but also may contraindicate certain forms of treatment, such as tooth whitening and implant therapy. The copious and frequent consumption of foods and beverages that may cause staining, including tea, coffee, red wine and turmeric, are further factors to be considered when contemplating colour-enhancing treatments such as tooth whitening.

The patient's occupation should also be noted, as it may affect their ability to attend on a frequent basis, or indeed may have an aetiological role in the causation of their esthetic concerns.

Finally, a dietary history should be obtained, taking particular note of the frequency and quantity of refined carbohydrate intakes, together with the consumption of acidic foods and drinks in the diet.

PATIENT EXAMINATION

For any given clinical condition, the reaching of a definitive diagnosis (or diagnoses) and the development of an appropriate treatment plan are primarily dependent on a meticulous patient examination. The protocols for the examination of a patient attending in the primary dental care setting are well rehearsed, and indeed form a large part of the daily routine of the practitioner.

CLINICAL TIP

Allocate a longer appointment time for your patient examination than you think you will need. This will also allow for more time to be spent on patient communication.

As many more people are seeking esthetic dental care, it should perhaps become a matter of routine to undertake a detailed dento-facial esthetic assessment of every patient, in particular those attending a practice for the very first time. This would augment the wealth of baseline information commonly acquired and provide the patient and dentist with a background understanding for any discussions pertaining to esthetic issues. A history of multiple facial esthetic procedures may alert the practitioner to the possible presence of BDD.

A patient assessment form is a particularly useful tool to help avoid any key omissions. The form advocated by the authors is reproduced in Box 3.1.

EXTRAORAL EXAMINATION

The extraoral examination should include an assessment of:

- temporomandibular joints, associated musculature and cervical lymph nodes
- facial features: facial proportions, facial symmetry, facial profile, facial shape and width
- lips: morphology and mobility
- facial skin.

The temporomandibular joints, masticatory musculature and cervical lymph nodes

The temporomandibular joints should be examined bilaterally for the presence of:

- any tenderness or pain elicited upon palpitation of the area anterior to the auricular tragi or intra-auricularly
- asynchronous movement upon mandibular opening and closure
- mandibular deviation upon opening and closure
- clicking sounds: clicks may be detected early, middle or late on opening and/or during closure
- any grating sounds, crepitation or joint locking.

BOX 3.1
TEMPLATE CHECKLIST FOR PATIENT ASSESSMENT

Personal details

- Name
- Gender
- Date of birth
- Address/contact details

Presenting complaint

- History
- Concerns

Medical history

Past dental history

- Last dental visit
- Frequency of dental attendance

Social history

- Occupation
- Habits
- Dietary preferences

Extraoral examination

- Facial asymmetry
- Facial shape
- Lymphadenopathy
- Skeletal pattern
- Temporomandibular joints
- Occlusal face height
- Resting face height
- Freeway space
- Maximal vertical opening
- Smile analysis
- Lip profile

Intraoral examination

- Soft tissues
- Muscles
- Periodontal tissues
- Existing dental charting
- Static and dynamic occlusal assessment

The use of a stethoscope may be helpful when undertaking auscultation of the joints.

The degree of maximum mandibular opening should also be determined by measuring the inter-incisal distance. Any distance of less than 35 mm is considered to be restricted. The degree of maximum lateral movement should also be determined; the normal is accepted to be about 12 mm.

Palpation of the masticatory muscles should also be undertaken. This is best accomplished by simultaneous, bilateral palpation to permit comparisons between contralateral muscles for the presence of tenderness or discomfort. Of particular importance are the anterior and posterior elements of the temporalis muscles and the superficial and deep elements of the masseter muscles. The practitioner, however, may also wish to assess the anterior digastric, sternomastoid, trapezius, and medial and lateral pterygoid muscles.

The cervical lymph nodes should be palpated, and the presence of any enlargements or tenderness documented and, where indicated clinically, investigated.

Facial features

Consensus opinion appears to suggest that there are certain proportions that are perceived to be visually pleasing.[14] Accordingly, when undertaking a smile assessment, it is important to record the extent of harmony and disharmony that exists between the facial structures and the dento-facial composition. Disharmony may require some form of intervention to create harmony; however, such interventions may change the character of the face, contrary to the wishes of the patient. Facial assessment must, therefore, be both comprehensive and careful.

The features that should be included in the facial assessment are:

- vertical facial proportions
- facial symmetry
- facial profile
- facial shape and width.

Facial proportions

In general, when viewed from a frontal direction and with the patient adopting a natural pose, the face can be divided into three distinct zones: the 'upper third', which encompasses the area between the hairline or forehead and the

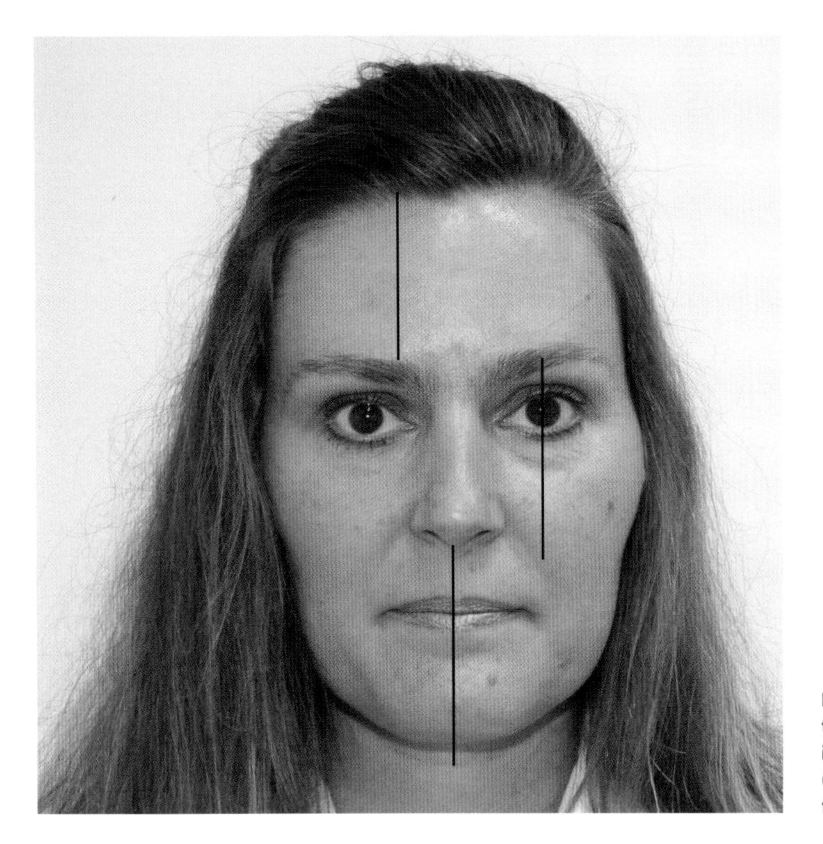

Fig. 3.2 Facial regions. The zones delineated by the vertical black lines represent the three regions into which the human face can be subdivided (upper, middle and lower thirds) when viewed from the front.

orphic line, commonly termed the brow line; the 'middle third', which spans the space between the orphic line and the inter-alar line at the base of the nose; and, the 'lower third', which includes the area between the inter-alar line and the tip of the chin. These zones are shown diagrammatically in Figure 3.2.

According to Fradeani,[15] in a well-proportioned face the three zones have similar dimensions. Dissimilarities in dimensions between the three zones, which are common, may not, however, give rise to esthetic concerns. It is generally agreed that the lower third of the face tends to determine overall facial appearance. It also happens to be the zone over which dental practitioners have most control.

When undertaking a prosthodontic rehabilitation, the practitioner should aim to subdivide the zone constituting the lower third of the face into three sections, such that the upper section is occupied by the upper lip and the lower two-thirds by the lower lip and chin.[16] This may be a useful guide when planning treatment for patients who have lost occlusal vertical height as a result of pathological tooth wear.

Facial symmetry

The facial midline and the inter-pupillary line are the vertical and horizontal reference planes employed most commonly to assess facial symmetry (Fig. 3.3). The use of a wooden spatula and a Fox's bite plane can be helpful in examining the patient for facial and dental symmetry.

It is generally accepted that esthetic harmony exists when the vertical and horizontal reference planes are perpendicular to each other, and the dental midline is co-incident with the facial midline, forming a pleasing smile.[15] Whilst it has been shown that patients can readily detect the presence of any disparity between the dental and facial midlines,[4] a more recent study by Johnston et al.[17] has demonstrated that the presence of a discrepancy of less than 2.0 mm between the facial and dental midlines may be considered to be esthetically acceptable. Accordingly, it was concluded that restorative or orthodontic intervention should, wherever possible, aim to leave the dental midline within 2.0 mm of the facial midline.

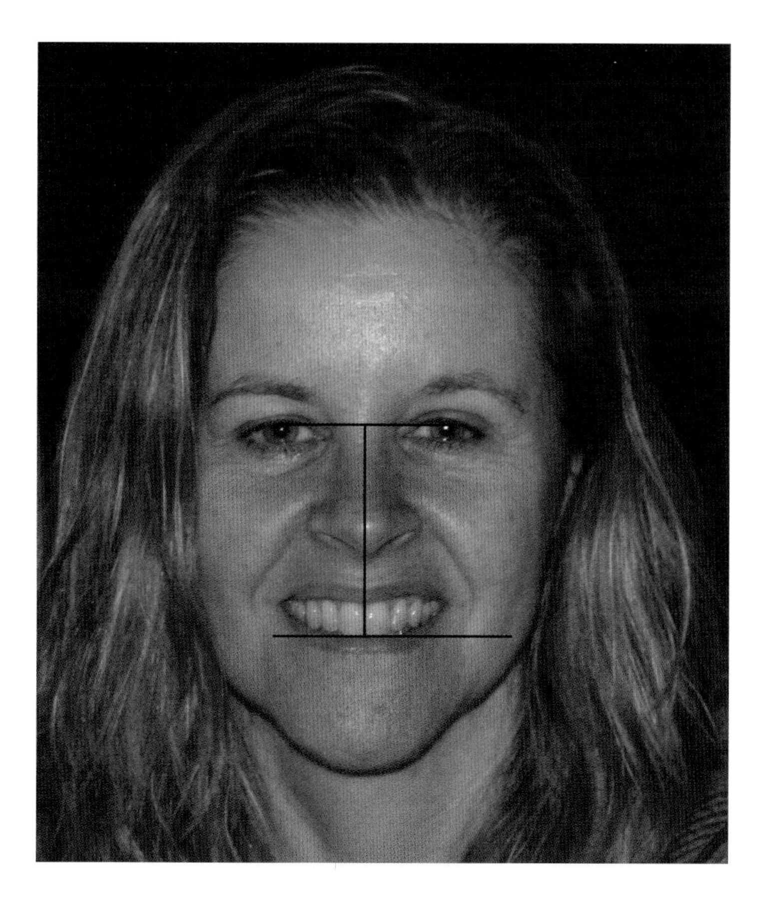

Fig. 3.3 Facial symmetry. The facial midline is determined by an imaginary line between nasion and the middle of the base of the philtrum. The inter-pupillary line is the most commonly applied horizontal reference plane when assessing facial symmetry.

The inter-pupillary line provides the operator with a key reference axis in determining the position of the incisal, gingival and occlusal planes. Traditionally, when undertaking prosthodontic rehabilitation with complete dentures, it is advocated that the incisal edges of the maxillary anterior teeth are positioned parallel to the inter-pupillary line. This concept has been extrapolated to the scenario of planning fixed prosthodontic rehabilitation for the worn anterior dentition, in particular where the tooth surface loss has resulted in a canted incisal plane, as shown in Figure 3.4. However, caution needs to be exercised where the inter-pupillary line may be canted and angled relative to the horizon, with the eyes possibly not being at the same level. In such cases, the horizon is best applied as the most appropriate horizontal reference plane.[15]

Likewise, when assessing for vertical symmetry, it is not uncommon for the tip of the nose and the tip of the chin to be divergent from the facial midline. In such circumstances the centre of the upper lip may be used as the 'ideal reference point' for determining the facial midline.[15]

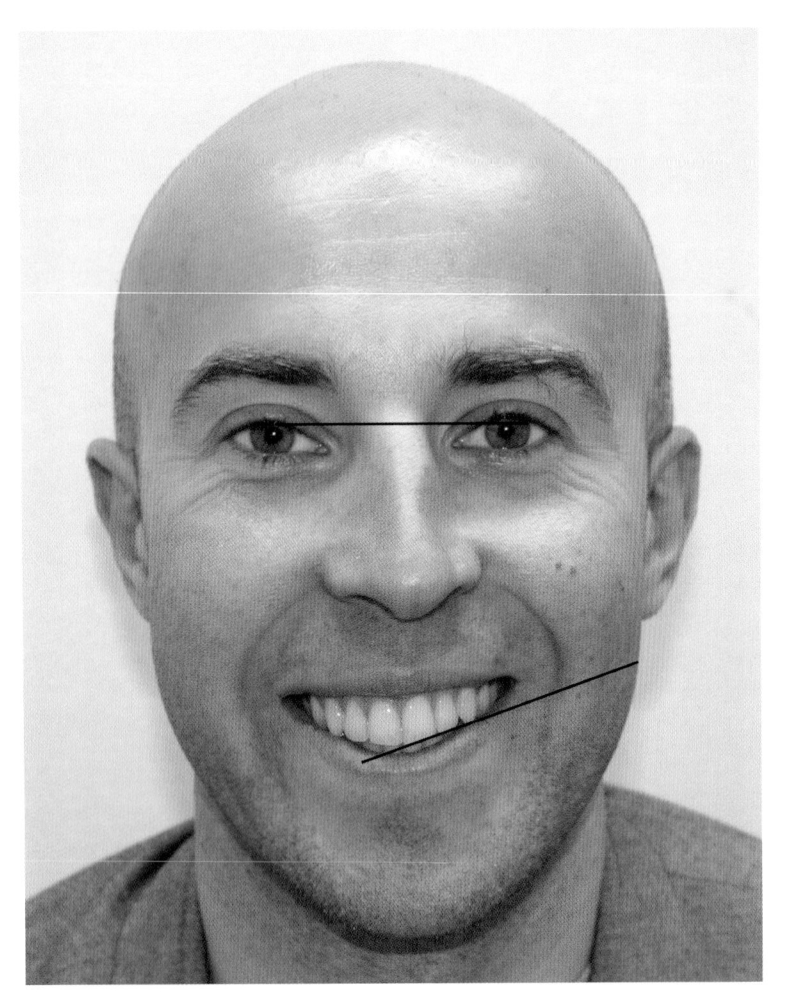

Fig. 3.4 A canted incisal plane in a patient with a worn anterior dentition.

Facial profile

The lateral facial profile is best assessed with the patient adopting a natural head posture. Some authors advocate the use of the Frankfort plane to verify the position of the head.

Three forms of facial profile are commonly described in the literature:

- normal profile
- convex profile
- concave profile.

An example of each is shown in Figure 3.5.

The 'profile angle', formed by connecting the glabella, subnasale and the soft tissue pogonion (tip of chin), may be used as a guide in determining the form of the facial profile.

It is thought that a profile angle of 165–175° corresponds to a normal (class I skeletal) profile.[18] In a convex-profile patient, the profile angle may be considerably reduced, resulting in a marked posterior divergence (often seen as a class II skeletal pattern). A profile angle in excess of 180° is most often seen in conjunction with class III skeletal patterns, with an associated marked anterior divergence. Whilst a small element of divergence may be acceptable, its absence is generally associated with esthetically pleasing facial proportions, good occlusion and superior dental esthetics.[15]

Variations in profile angles and facial profiles will not reveal which jaw is retruded or protruded; hence cephalometric analysis may be indicated.

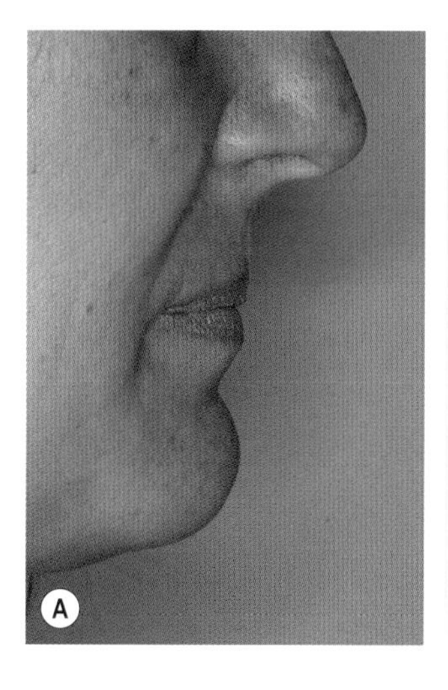

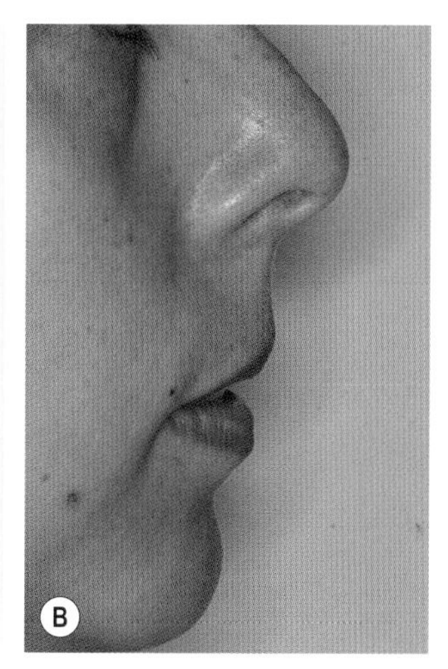

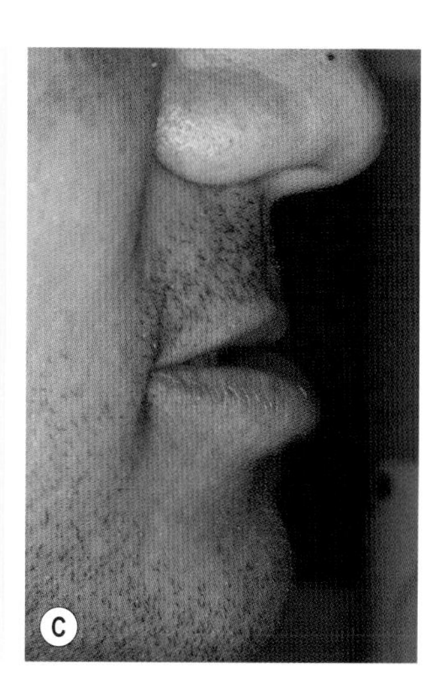

Fig. 3.5 Examples of the different facial profiles commonly observed. A. Normal profile. B. Convex profile. C. Concave profile.

The 'E-line', formed by connecting the tip of the nose to the tip of the chin, is also commonly applied in determining facial profile. A normal profile is thought to exist when the upper and lower lips are 4 mm and 2 mm posterior to the E-line, respectively.[19]

The naso-labial angle, formed by connecting the inferior nasal septum, subnasale and upper lip, can also be used to assess profile variations. Normal profiles are thought to be associated with angles in the range of 85–105°.

The application of any of the above guides in determining the lateral facial profile is subject to considerable racial variation, in particular amongst Asian–Oriental and Afro-Caribbean individuals, and between males and females. 'Normal range values' should be interpreted with caution.

It is important not to make dramatic changes to the E-line and naso-labial angles when undertaking orthodontic or prosthodontic care, as this may have a negative impact on the neutral zone formed by the equilibrium of pressures between the lips and cheeks externally and the tongue internally. Otherwise, the outcome may be an unstable arch form or prosthesis.

Facial shape and width

Traditionally, four different facial shapes have been described. Historically, these have been used with little, if any, scientific basis, to determine an appropriate tooth mould in removable denture construction. The four facial shapes are:

- ovoid
- square
- tapering
- square–tapering

In recent times, Ahmad[14] has described four typological categories to characterize a particular facial shape. These are:

- lymphatic – rounded full features with a timid personality
- sanguine – prominent thick, well-defined features associated with intransigence and spontaneity
- nervous – large forehead, thin delicate features with an anxious disposition
- bilious – rectangular and muscular features coupled with a dominant persona.

It has been suggested that the morphology of the teeth and any restorations should conform to these types.

Facial width may be crudely assessed as the width of 'five eyes'.[6]

Lips

It is important to assess lip morphology and mobility. A morphological description should take account of the width, fullness and symmetry of the lips. In general, wide lips are associated with a wide smile. A smile that is at least half the width of the face is considered to be esthetically pleasing.[6] The fullness of the lips may be described as being thin, medium or thick. Associations have been made between fullness and personality traits, which in turn may influence tooth morphology, as discussed above.

Full lips, in particular when found in a concave facial profile, are often associated with dominance of the maxillary central incisors in the esthetic zone. In contrast, a convex profile with thin lips is often associated with moderate dominance of the maxillary anterior teeth. Fullness and symmetry should be assessed across the midline. Lack of symmetry may have a significant influence on the incisal plane, which the practitioner may opt to cant slightly to mimic the asymmetrical lip profile.

Lip mobility refers to the amount of lip movement that occurs when a patient smiles. The amount of anterior tooth display should be assessed with the lips at rest and in dynamic positions. The rest position of the lips has classically been used to determine the position of the incisal edges of the anterior maxillary teeth when undertaking complete denture prosthetics. Vig and Brundo[20] determined the average ranges for tooth display at rest, according to age:

- aged 30 years: 3.0–3.5 mm
- aged 50 years: 1.0–1.5 mm
- aged 70 years: 0.0–0.5 mm.

These values may serve as a useful guide, particularly when contemplating the lengthening of the incisal edges by means of fixed prosthodontics.

As part of age-related alterations of the facial profile, changes occur to the lips, resulting in reduced tooth display in the rest position. This may be accentuated by tooth wear.

Phonetic tests, such as the enunciation of the 'F' and 'V' sounds, can help to verify the correct spatial relationship between the incisal edges of the anterior maxillary teeth and the lower lip. The length of the philtrum should be measured. In general, philtrum height should be 2–3 mm shorter than the height of the commissures. Younger patients often have a shorter philtrum height.

The mobility of the upper lip will determine the extent of the maxillary teeth and associated gingival tissue displayed on smiling, whilst the curvature of the lower lip, as discussed below, can serve as a useful guide for the arrangement of the maxillary incisal edges.

Facial skin

An assessment of the facial skin should be carried out on a routine basis, in particular when facial esthetic treatments may be indicated. Skin types may be classified according to pigmentation, tendency to burn, and likelihood of reaction to treatment, in particular heat-based treatments such as lasers. The Fitzpatrick skin phototype classification[21] provides a particularly useful way of looking at skin types to assist with treatment planning, where certain skin types, such as those of the thin, transparent variety (category 1), are less suited to dermal filler therapies. In such situations, there is a risk of developing a green/yellow discoloration if fillers are injected superficially.

The presence and distribution of skin wrinkles may also be noted, both at rest and during dynamic movements. The Glogau index[22] can provide a particularly useful tool for categorizing skin wrinkles and for quantifying improvement following treatment. This index also provides a platform for planning future re-treatments.

INTRAORAL EXAMINATION

A thorough intraoral examination should be conducted in a systematic manner. It should include an assessment of:

- soft tissues
- periodontal tissues
- dental hard tissues
- occlusion and arch form
- esthetic zone
- edentulous spaces, if any.

Soft tissues

The soft tissues of the lips, cheeks, tongue, vestibule, soft palate, hard palate and floor of the mouth should be meticulously examined for the presence of any anomalies. When present, any anomaly should be carefully described and recorded; if required, the patient should be referred for a specialist opinion. The presence of a tongue thrust or high frenal attachments should be noted.

Periodontal tissues

It is of paramount importance that signs of periodontal tissue pathology are successfully managed prior to embarking upon any form of esthetic dental treatment. It is therefore critical to assess the periodontal tissues for the presence of any disease and to determine the patient's standard of oral care. The potential impact of any restorative intervention on the periodontal tissues must also be considered. Dental restorations must be planned and designed to ensure that they are conducive to maintaining good periodontal health. This may, however, be difficult to achieve. By way of example, almost all ceramic veneers induce gingivitis to some, albeit very limited, extent; thus, a high level of oral hygiene should be a preoperative requisite.

The patient's overall standard of oral hygiene should be documented as being good, moderate or poor. The presence and extent of any plaque and calculus deposits should also be described and recorded. Any local factors that may encourage plaque and calculus accumulation and stagnation should also be determined, including overhangs and other defects in restorations. The presence and extent of extrinsic tooth stains should be noted.

The gingival tissues should be examined for the presence of any inflammatory changes, including erythema, swelling, loss of stippling, blunting of the gingival papillae, bleeding on probing and the presence of any exudates.

A basic periodontal examination (BPE) should be conducted on a routine basis.[23] Where a score of '3' is recorded for two or more sextants, a full-depth, six-point periodontal charting may be indicated. It may also be important to document the levels of attachment to determine the amount of periodontal destruction and recession that has occurred. This is achieved by measuring the distance between the most apical extent to which the periodontal probe may be placed and a fixed reference point, usually the cemento-enamel junction (CEJ).

Other periodontal features to note include:

- the presence of any tooth mobility
- furcation involvement
- bleeding on probing – immediate or late
- plaque scores.

Details of how to perform an esthetic assessment of the gingival tissues are discussed in more detail below.

Dental hard tissues

Accurate charting should aim to record the presence and absence of teeth, dental caries, sound and defective restorations, tooth fractures, cracks, wear of abrasive, erosive, abfractive and attritional varieties, and any tooth malformations.

The extent and location of any caries should be noted, as should the type and extent of all dental restorations present. Dental restorations should be further assessed for their marginal integrity and adaptation, structural integrity, form, function and esthetic appearance. The presence of any secondary caries, open contacts and other food traps and wear facets, present on either the remaining dental tissues or the functional surfaces, should be documented.

Occlusion and arch form

It is important to carry out a detailed occlusal assessment to establish the ways in which the patient's occlusal scheme differs from what may be considered to be the ideal – a mutually protected occlusal scheme[24] – and to determine the constraints the occlusal scheme may place on fulfilling the patient's esthetic expectations. One of the key aims of whatever treatment may be provided is to ensure a functionally stable dentition. The occlusion should be assessed in both static and dynamic positions.

Static occlusal examination

The static occlusal examination should seek to identify the presence of any of the following features:

- tooth rotations, tilting, drifting and supra-eruption
- crowding
- spacing, including the presence of any diastema

- abnormal overjet and overbite, including open bites and cross-bites
- atypical occlusal vertical dimension – freeway space (FWS)
- atypical arch form and relationships.

Assessment of these features will help to elicit the nature of any malocclusion.

The inter-arch occlusal relationship may be qualified by information on incisor, canine and molar segment relationships. In general, in an incisor class I case, in which the incisal edges of the mandibular incisors occlude or lie directly below the cingulum plateau of the maxillary anterior incisors, both the overjet and overbite should have a value of 2–4 mm.[25] The class I incisor relationship is considered to be the functional ideal.

An FWS assessment should be undertaken, particularly when the patient presents with a worn dentition. A plethora of different methods have been described to determine the FWS; however, a Willis gauge is widely used to measure the difference between the resting vertical dimension (RVD) and occlusal vertical dimension (OVD), as shown in Figure 3.6.

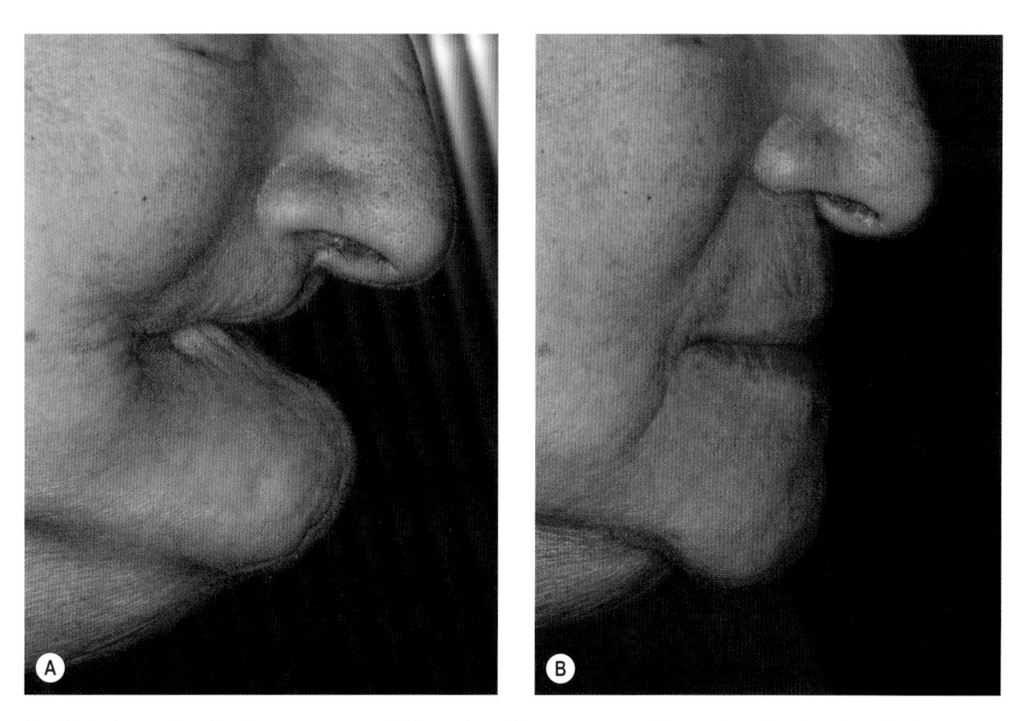

Fig. 3.6 Assessing the freeway space. A. 'Overclosed' appearance with a reduced occlusal vertical dimension. B. The resting vertical dimension.

Dynamic occlusal examination

The dynamic occlusal examination should first establish the inter-cuspal position (ICP), also commonly referred to as the maximal inter-cuspal position (MIP) or centric occlusion (CO). It is generally accepted that when a limited number of restorations are being undertaken, which may involve some minor modifications to the anatomy of the occlusal table, the occlusal endpoint should conform to the existing ICP, unless the ICP is unstable. Signs of occlusal instability include:

- mobility of teeth and fremitus
- atypical and pathological wear of teeth
- tooth fractures and chipping
- fractured restorations
- localized periodontal bone loss and recession
- occlusal discomfort
- temporomandibular joint dysfunction (TMD).

The ease with which the mandible can be manipulated into its retruded arc of closure should also be assessed. If the patient has established protective neuromuscular reflexes, this may be difficult. The use of a muscle-deprogramming device, such as a wooden tongue spatula, cotton wool rolls or a Lucia jig, may be helpful. If deprogramming devices do not help resolve the difficulty, a full-coverage, hard-acrylic stabilization splint may be required to allow the retruded arc of closure and, in turn, the retruded contact point (RCP) and centric relation (CR) to be reproducibly identified. This is important when a reorganized approach is indicated in the management of the occlusion, with the aim of ICP and RCP being co-incident.

In the majority of patients there will be a limited (1.25 mm), typically horizontal slide between RCP and ICP. The presence and extent of such a slide should be documented. In the management of tooth wear cases, the space provided by the slide between RCP and ICP may be used to accommodate restorative materials without the need to change the patient's occlusal vertical dimension, as illustrated in Figure 3.7.

It is important to document the anterior guidance and note the teeth that provide it. The steepness of the anterior guidance should also be recorded as being steep, moderate or shallow.

The effects of possible alterations to the anterior guidance on the posterior occlusion must be carefully evaluated, especially in cases where the form and function of the anterior teeth may be changed. Ideally, the anterior guidance

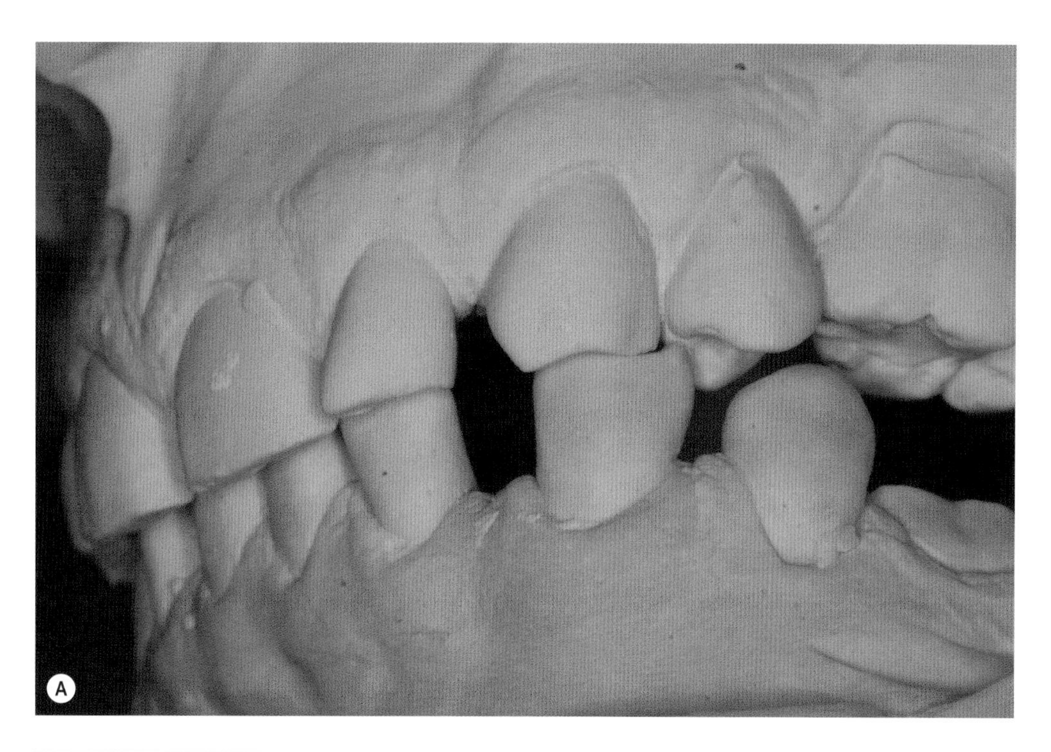

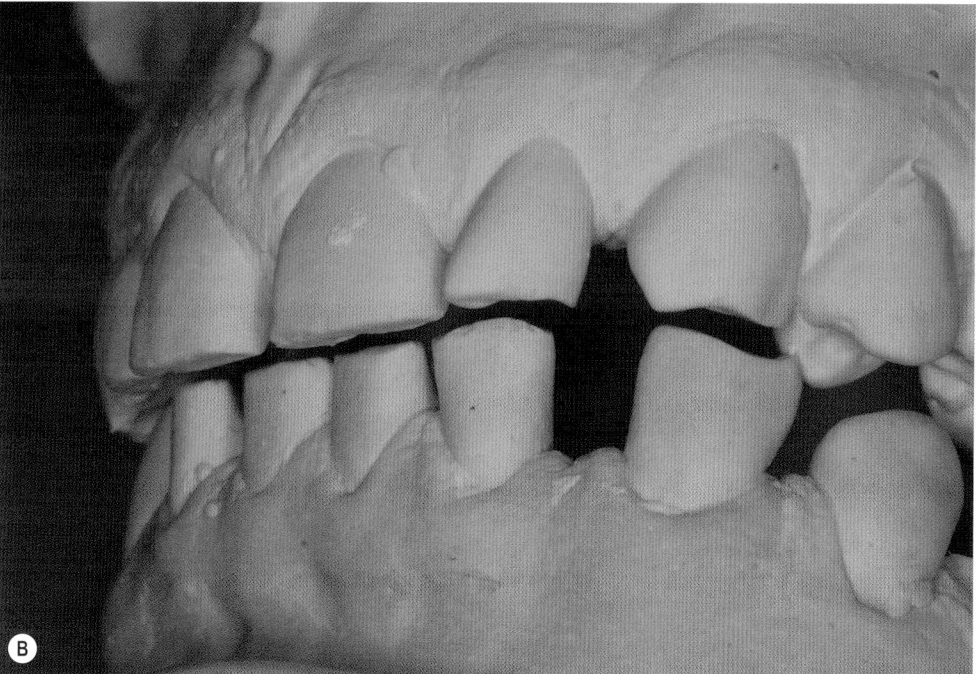

Fig. 3.7 Dynamic occlusal examination. An example of a sizeable inter-occlusal space between the upper and lower teeth when the patient is manipulated from (A) the inter-cuspal position (ICP) to (B) the retruded contact position (RCP). This space may be critical to planning restorative dental care.

should be shared between the anterior teeth to optimize the distribution of occlusal loading.

The nature of the guidance and the occlusal contacts in lateral excursion should also be assessed and noted. Lateral guidance is typically provided by the canine teeth – canine guidance – but may be premolar- or molar-guided, with teeth acting individually or in group function. The morphology of the canine tooth allows it to provide guidance during lateral excursive movements. Indeed, canine guidance is the most common form of lateral guidance in the natural dentition.[26] Canine guidance typically ensures posterior tooth disclusion during lateral excursion.

The presence of any occlusal interference on either the working or the non-working side should be noted, and investigated as indicated clinically.

The use of articulated study casts to analyse the patient's occlusion can be invaluable, if not essential, particularly when a reorganization of the occlusion may be indicated.

The esthetic zone

The esthetic zone, also known as the 'smile zone', includes all the hard and soft tissues that are visible when the patient makes a broad smile. The examination and assessment of the esthetic zone should include evaluation of:

- smile zone shape
- dento-labial relationships
- dental midlines
- tooth colour, texture and form
- tooth size, shape, proportion, symmetry and axial inclination
- contact areas and embrasures
- gingival esthetics.

Smile zone shape

Six smile zone shapes are commonly described in the literature. These are straight, curved, elliptical, bow-shaped, rectangular and inverted. Smile zone analysis should start with determining the smile zone shape.

Dento-labial relationships

There is considerable variation in tooth exposure during smiling, both by and between individuals.

The term 'lip line' or 'smile line' is used to describe the relationship that exists between the inferior border of the upper lip, the maxillary teeth and the gingival soft tissues on smiling, or when a patient is asked to make the sound 'E', commonly referred to as the 'E test'. Tjan et al.[4] have described three types of lip line (Fig. 3.8):

- low smile line – where the maxillary anterior teeth are exposed by no more than 75%, with no display of gingival tissue on smiling
- medium smile line – where 75–100% of the clinical crowns of the maxillary anterior teeth and the associated interdental gingival papillae are exposed on smiling
- high smile line – where all of the clinical crowns of the maxillary anterior teeth and the adjacent gingival tissues, beyond the gingival margins, are exposed on smiling.

Low smile lines are the most forgiving: for example, when there is an exposed cervical margin to a restoration, or an alveolar ridge defect in the anterior region, necessitating the placement of an artificial tooth with an abnormal inciso-gingival dimension and associated asymmetrical gingival profile.

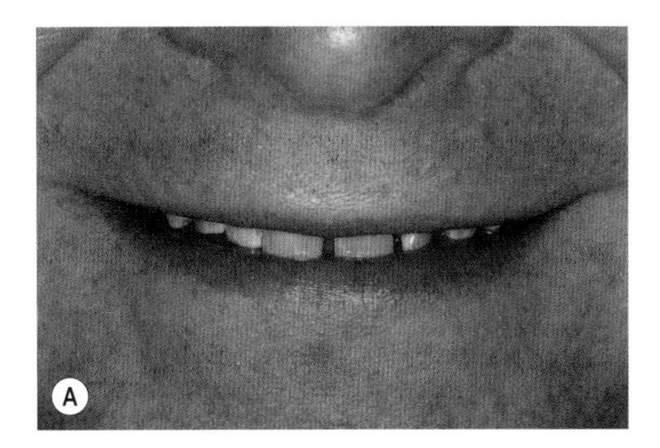

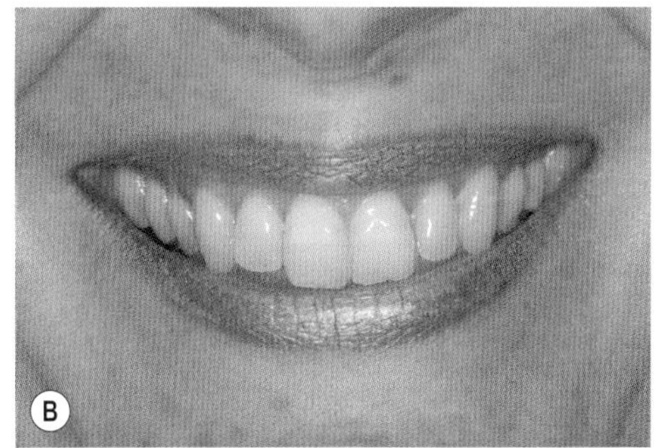

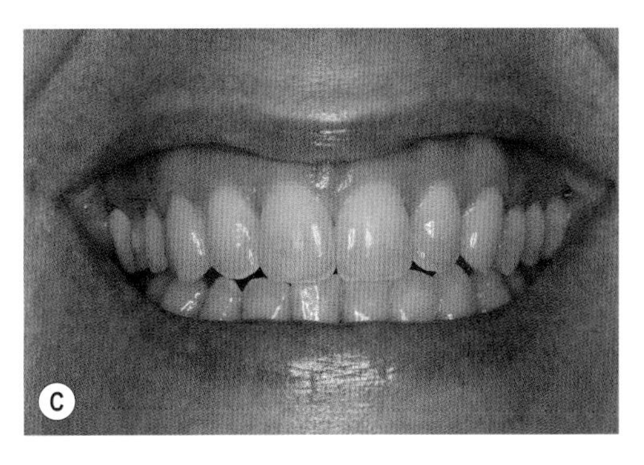

Fig. 3.8 Examples of the different 'smile line' profiles. A. A 'low smile line'. B. A 'medium smile line'. C. A 'high smile line'.

In contrast, high smile lines – the 'gummy smile' – are the least forgiving. High-smile-line smiles can give the impression of relatively small teeth set in excessively large, long gums, or of maxillary teeth positioned too low relative to the upper lip.

Tjan et al.[4] describe the 'average lip-line profile' as the most common smile-line variation. The high-smile-line appearance has been reported to be twice as common amongst females as amongst males,[4] possibly related to the slightly shorter mean length of the philtrum in females. Lip lines may be asymmetric.

Whilst the display of 2–3 mm of healthy gingival tissue, together with the maxillary anterior incisors, is considered to be esthetically acceptable when smiling, the display of 1 mm of gingival tissue has been suggested to conform to the esthetic ideal.[27] In contrast, an excessive display of gingival tissue of more than 3–4 mm is generally considered to be the least acceptable. In such cases the patient may need to be assessed for periodontal 'plastic surgery', orthodontics, the use of botulinum toxin in the levator labii and levator angularis muscles, or, in extreme cases, orthognathic surgery. The aim of any such treatment should be to provide the patient with a pleasing, symmetrical gingival profile on smiling.

The incisal display, when the lips and lower jaw are at rest, may be assessed by asking the patient to say 'M' or 'Emma'. A 'youthful smile' is associated with a greater level of incisal display. After 40 years of age, the incisal edge display at rest decreases by approximately 1 mm every 10 years.[20] The average incisal display for males is slightly less than that for females, in the order of 1.5 mm.[28] This may serve as a useful guideline when attempting to restore worn anterior maxillary segments, or when contemplating smile makeovers to attain a youthful appearance.

The width of the smile should also be assessed. A smile displaying ten maxillary teeth – the incisors, canines and premolars – is the most common smile width pattern.[29] Up to 20% of patients may display their first permanent molar teeth on smiling. Racial variations in smile width are common. The smile width may have a key bearing on the selection of restoration, restorative material and crown margin placement – sub- or supra-gingival – in cases requiring operative intervention.

For optimum esthetics, the dental hard tissues should fill the corners of the mouth to produce a 'full smile'.[30] Where a large negative (black) space exists between the buccal surfaces of the maxillary posterior teeth and the labial commissures – the buccal corridor, smile esthetics may be suboptimal (Fig. 3.9). This may occur when the cross-sectional width of the dental arches is reduced, or

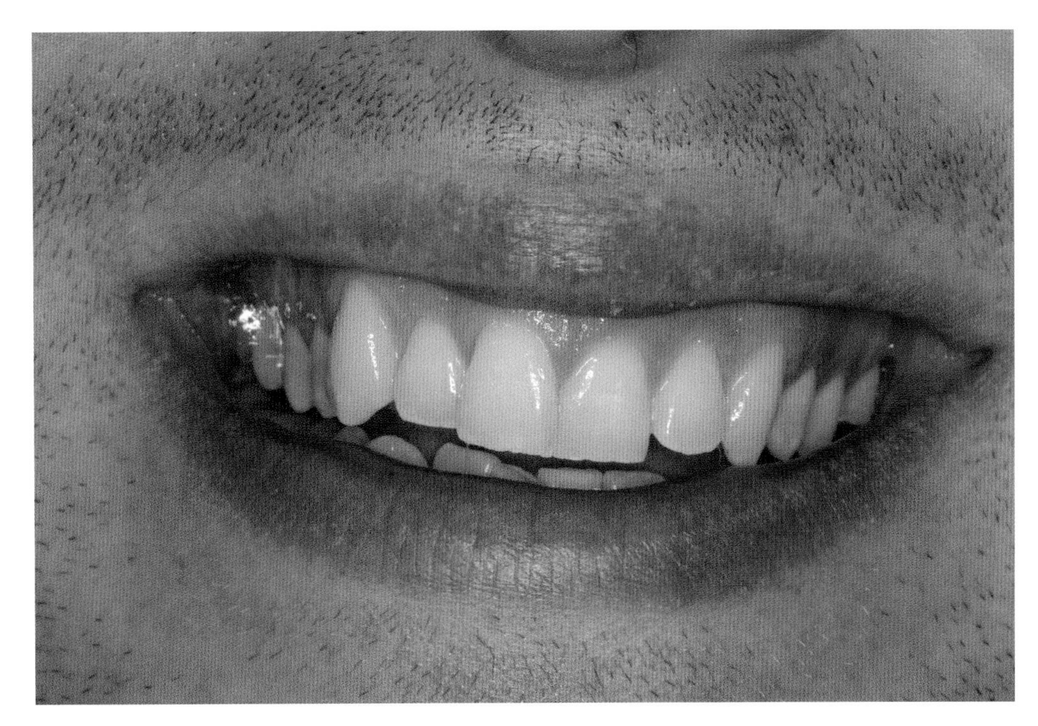

Fig. 3.9 An example of a patient with a prominent 'negative buccal corridor'.

the arches are retropositioned. Under these circumstances, such orthodontic intervention, possibly together with orthognathic surgery, may be indicated.

The smile arc must also be assessed. This term refers to the relationship between the curvature of the lower lip and the curvature of the incisal edges of the maxillary incisor teeth in a posed smile. Ideally, the curvature of the lower lip should follow the curvature of the incisor edges, with the superior border of the lower lip being slightly below the incisal edges. This is commonly termed a 'convex incisal curve'. An example of a smile displaying a convex incisal curve is shown in Figure 3.10. In contrast, a flat smile arc (Fig. 3.11) or a reverse smile arc, often observed with worn dentitions, is generally deemed to be less attractive than a convex incisal curve, and is associated with ageing. An example of a reverse smile arc associated with a worn anterior maxillary dentition is illustrated in Figure 3.12. A reverse smile can have a profound effect on the 'emotion of ageing' and, as such, is considered to be undesirable.[31]

Dental midlines

The dental midline (DM) should, ideally, coincide with the facial midline (FM). The maxillary midline is best assessed against the midpoint of the philtrum. The labial frenum and facial midline are co-incident in approximately 70% of the

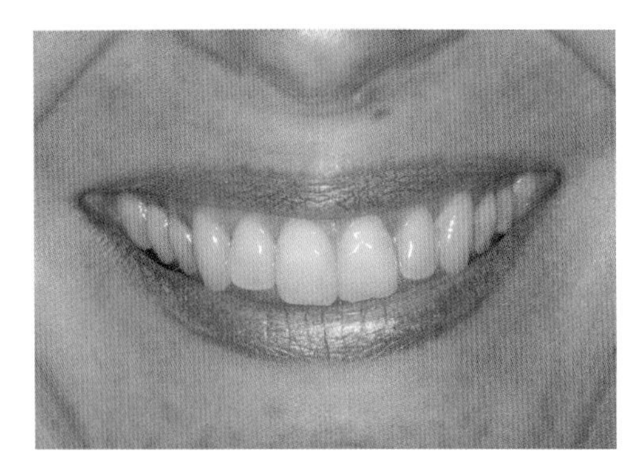

Fig. 3.10 An example of a smile displaying a convex incisal curve.

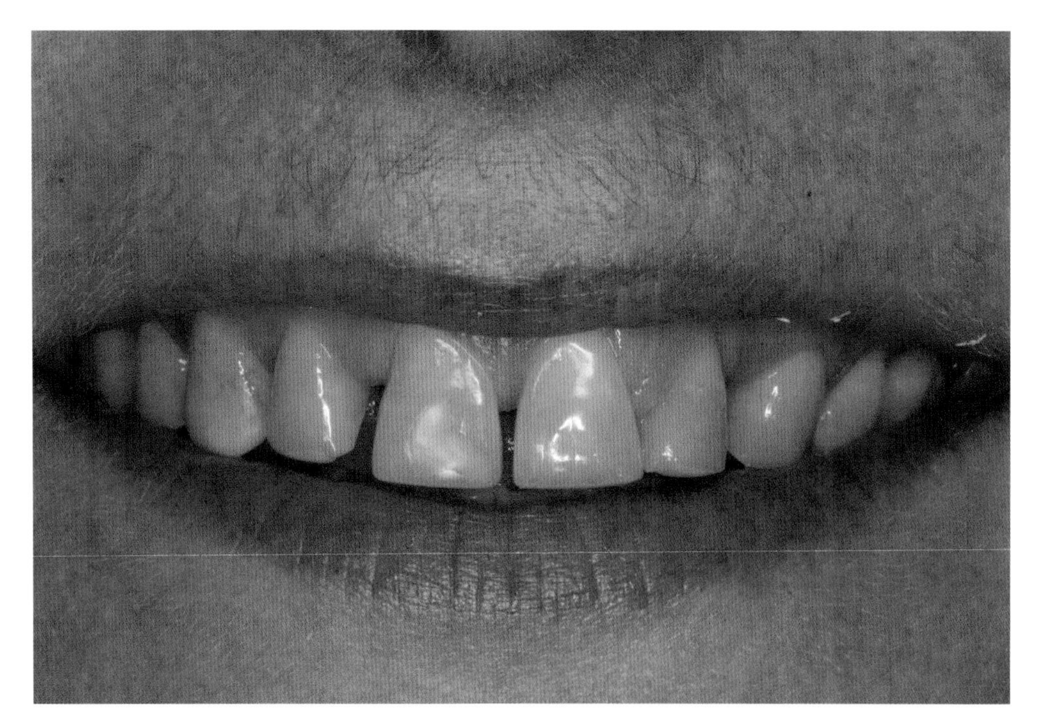

Fig. 3.11 An example of a smile displaying a flat incisal curve.

population.[14] A discrepancy of less than 2 mm between the maxillary midline and facial midline is generally considered to be esthetically acceptable. A variation of more than 4 mm is associated with a suboptimal esthetic appearance, and perfect co-incidence of the DM and FM may result in an artificial appearance. Where there is a discrepancy between the DM and FM that is of concern to the patient, orthodontic treatment may be indicated.

The mandibular midline should ideally be co-incident with the maxillary midline. This, however, occurs in only 25% of the population.[32] A small discrepancy between the two midlines may therefore not have a negative impact on the overall esthetic acceptability of a smile.

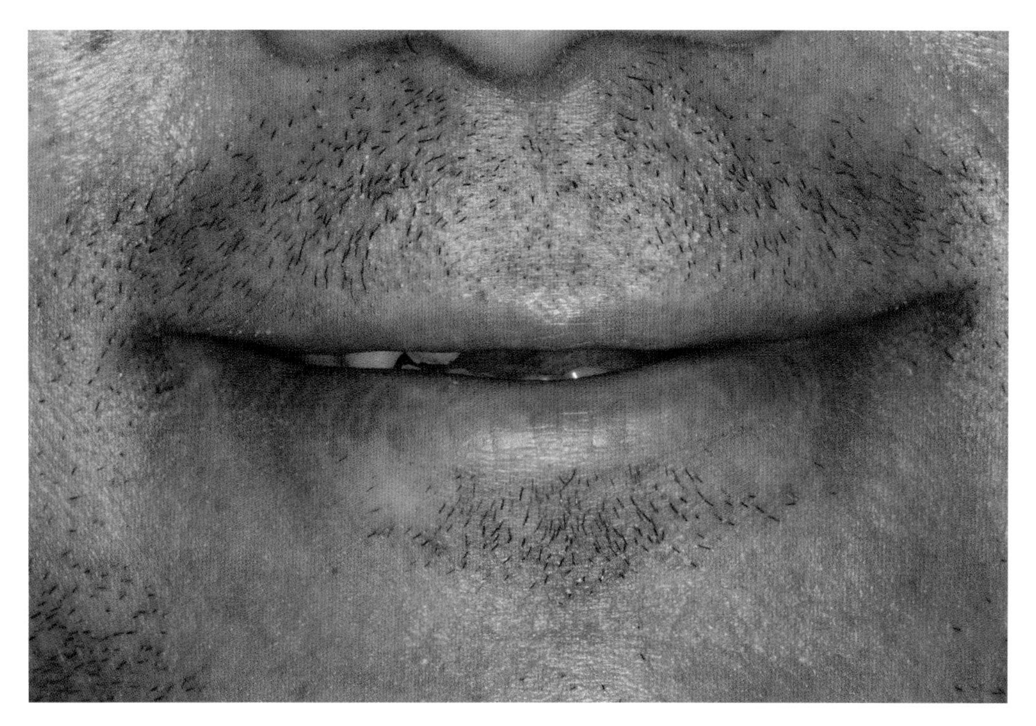

Fig. 3.12 An example of a reverse smile arc associated with tooth wear.

Tooth colour, texture and form

Tooth colour

The colour of teeth should be evaluated according to:

- hue – base colour
- chroma – saturation of the base colour
- value – brightness.

There are many shade analysis systems available in the dental marketplace. The base shade should be recorded using a preferred shade guide. Colour variations within and between different teeth in each arch, in particular the maxillary canines, should be assessed and noted. Chroma variations also occur within and between teeth; hence the concept of 'polychromacity', with the incisal third of teeth often displaying low chroma, and a tendency towards translucency, and the gingival third displaying higher chroma than the middle third.

The colour of a tooth may be influenced by many different factors. These include the presence of restorations, loss of vitality, discoloration following trauma and endodontic treatment, caries, areas of hypomineralization and hypocalcification, staining (extrinsic and intrinsic), and cracks and corrosion products from metallic restorations and steroid-based intra-canal materials.

A cross-sectional survey by Kershaw et al.[1] reported that the visible presence of dental caries may be associated with a lower overall rating of physical attractiveness. Clearly, operative interventions to eliminate factors such as caries and leaking, stained restorations will help to enhance the esthetics of a given tooth and, in turn, the dentition.

Interestingly, the above study provided evidence that a whitened tooth appearance may be associated with a higher level of attractiveness than a natural enamel appearance.[1] A youthful dental appearance is generally associated with a dentition that displays a relatively high value and low level of chroma. Ageing is usually associated with a reduction in the thickness of the enamel layer and yellowing of the dentine layer, with narrowing of the lumen of the dentinal tubules and the absorption of stains, resulting in a relatively high level of chroma and low level of value. In addition, ageing is associated with the loss of translucency of the incisal edges, and a reduction, if not loss, of the mamelons.

It is hardly surprising that vital bleaching treatments have become so popular in contemporary dental practice, with an increasing number of patients seeking a more youthful appearance, perceived to be associated with a high level of physical attractiveness.

When assessing patients for possible esthetic dental treatment, it is important to discuss their views on colour variation in the dentition, and to ascertain their perception of dental attractiveness. The patient's skin complexion may also influence colour perception, tooth shade and skin colour having an inverse relationship.

Tooth texture

Tooth surface texture and lustre should also be documented, particularly when planning indirect restorations. A good-quality study cast provides an excellent record of surface texture, amongst other features.

Tooth form

Three common tooth forms have been described in the dental literature. These relate primarily to the form of the maxillary central incisor teeth – the most dominant teeth in the smile. The three forms are:

- ovoid – egg-shaped
- square – quadrangular
- triangular – tapering.

Variations in these forms have been described: for example, square–tapering. Whilst there is little evidence to support the notion, some believe that the form of the maxillary central incisors may reflect the gender, personality and strength index of a patient. Tooth form may change with age, as a consequence of tooth wear.

Tooth size, proportion, shape, symmetry and axial inclination

Consensus opinion suggests that the size, shape and arrangement of the maxillary anterior teeth are the most influential factors in characterizing the anterior dentition.[33]

Tooth size and proportion

A plethora of studies have investigated the average dimensions of maxillary central incisor teeth. The average lengths and widths of these teeth have been reported to be between 10 mm and 11 mm, and 8 mm and 9 mm, respectively.[34] These data indicate that an average maxillary central incisor should have a height-to-width ratio of 1.2 : 1, with the width being approximately 75–80% of the height, as shown in Figure 3.13A. It is also frequently stated that the length of the maxillary central incisor should be approximately one-sixteenth of the height of the face (Fig. 3.13B).

Average values may serve as a useful guide when restoring the anterior dentitions, particularly a worn dentition. However, it is important to remember that average values are subject to certain variations among ethnic and minority groups.

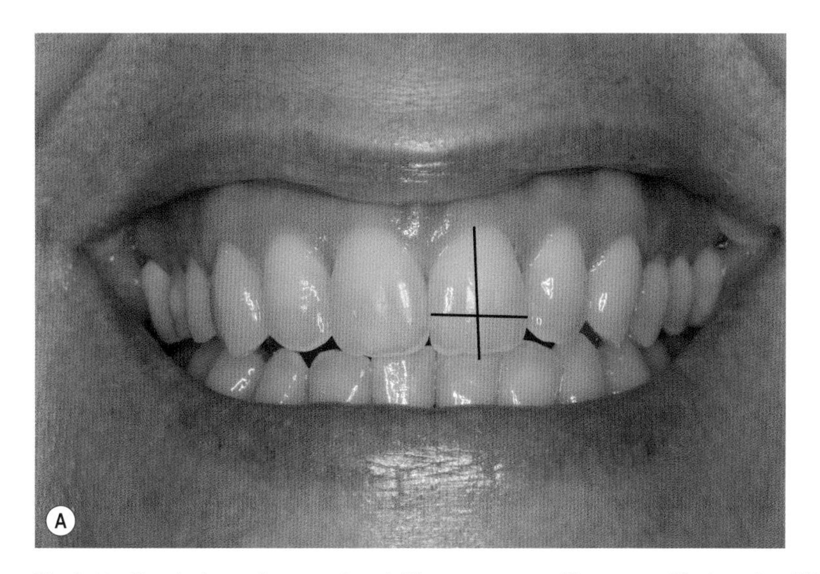

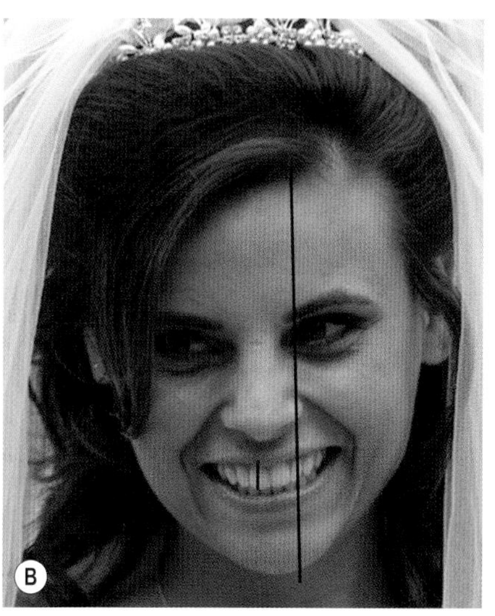

Fig. 3.13 Tooth size and proportion. A. The average maxillary central incisor should have a height-to-width ratio of 1.2 : 1. B. The average maxillary central incisor length should be approximately one-sixteenth of the facial height.

In the case of a patient presenting with an anterior edentulous space, the bizygomatic width and inter-alar width may serve as useful guidelines in determining the most esthetically pleasing width for the maxillary anterior teeth, particularly amongst female patients.[5]

As discussed in Chapter 1, the Golden Proportion is a concept that has been widely applied in esthetic dentistry (see Fig. 3.13A).[35,36] However, the Golden Proportion may only exist in just under one-fifth of all natural dentitions.[37] Accordingly, the concept must be applied with caution when examining and assessing patients for esthetic dental treatment, in particular when the individual has an atypical arch form.[34]

Accordingly, the use of resin mock-up techniques, as described below, or the use of provisional restorations may be the most effective means of determining the most esthetically pleasing tooth dimensions for a patient. Volume 2 of this series covers such mock-up techniques.

Tooth shape

In axial section, the crowns of maxillary central incisor teeth typically display two or three planes in the labial face, as shown in Figure 3.14. The gingival third or half is typically in the same plane as the gingival tissues. The middle and incisal third or, in many cases, half of the labial face has a tendency to curve palatally. This is thought to facilitate phonation and swallowing.[34]

It is important to avoid altering these profiles, as over-contouring in the labial–gingival portion, frequently seen following inappropriate tooth preparation for

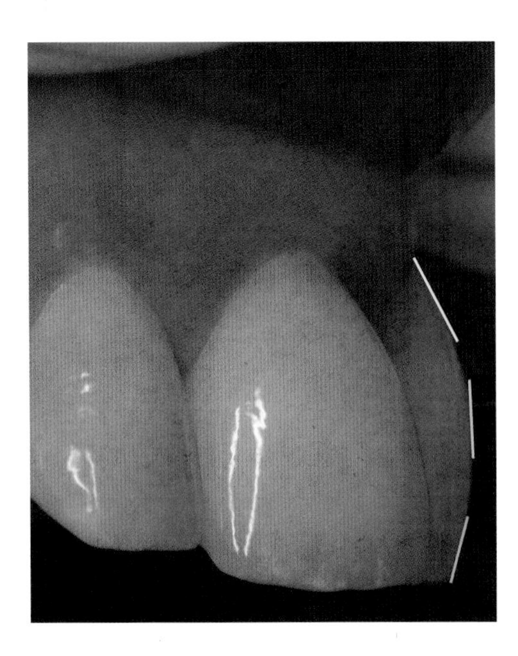

Fig. 3.14 The labial face of the maxillary central incisor. When viewed in vertical section, this face is typically formed of two or three planes.

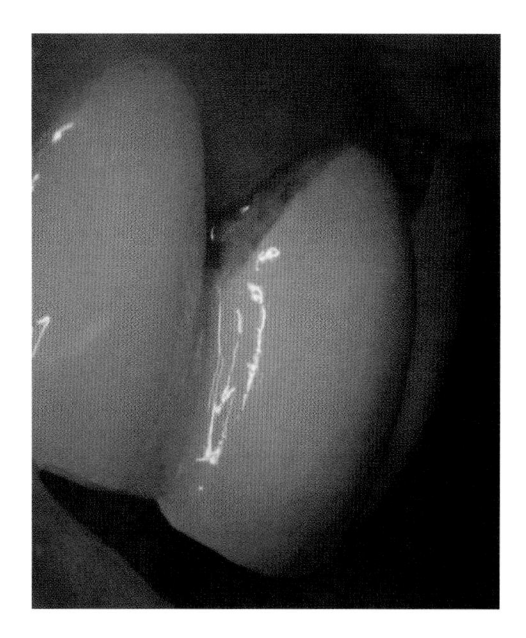

Fig. 3.15 Over-contoured restorations. Over-contoured restorations may compromise dental esthetics, gingival architecture and lip function.

indirect restorations, results in poor esthetics and may contribute to gingival recession, revealing an unsightly restoration margin (Fig. 3.15) In extreme circumstances, over-contouring of the gingival third may result in palatal tipping of teeth and interference with the function of the lip.

Attention should also be paid to the palatal profile of the maxillary incisor teeth. Alterations in this profile may result in a lisp when the patient makes the 'S' sound – a useful phonetic guide when using provisional restorations to verify esthetic and functional satisfaction with planned restorations.

The shape of the incisal edges of the anterior teeth should also be noted. The incisal edge of these teeth should have a tapered, flat form in vertical section. With ageing and physiological wear, incisal edges have a tendency to develop a sharper facio-palatal profile. The iatrogenic creation of a rounded profile often results in poor appearance.

Note should also be taken of the morphology of the central incisors in the frontal plane. Lateral incisors are seldom central and flat when viewed facially; rather, the facial profile should be convex with distinct line angles.

Maxillary lateral incisors often display considerable variations in morphology. Peg-shaped lateral incisors are commonly encountered, and may be present unilaterally or bilaterally. Alternatively, lateral incisors may appear small in comparison to adjacent central incisor and canine teeth.

The morphology and positioning of the maxillary canine tooth have an important role in determining the progression of the patient's smile from the anterior to posterior regions.

The shape of the mandibular anterior teeth should be assessed, with particular attention to the profile and appearance of the incisal edges.

Tooth symmetry

It is widely accepted that a key determinant of the esthetic consideration of a smile is symmetry of the central incisor teeth.[36] However, some asymmetry between the maxillary central incisors is common. It is suggested that differences of more than 0.3–0.4 mm in the dimensions or positioning of these teeth may be readily noticed. The esthetics of asymmetric central incisors may be enhanced if the disto-incisal line angles of the teeth appear symmetrical.

The presence of unilateral peg-shaped lateral incisors, let alone missing teeth, may have a profound effect on the symmetrical arrangement of the anterior maxillary region (Fig. 3.16).

Axial inclination

The maxillary anterior teeth have a tendency to be mesially inclined (see Fig. 3.14). The angle of inclination tends to increase in moving from the central

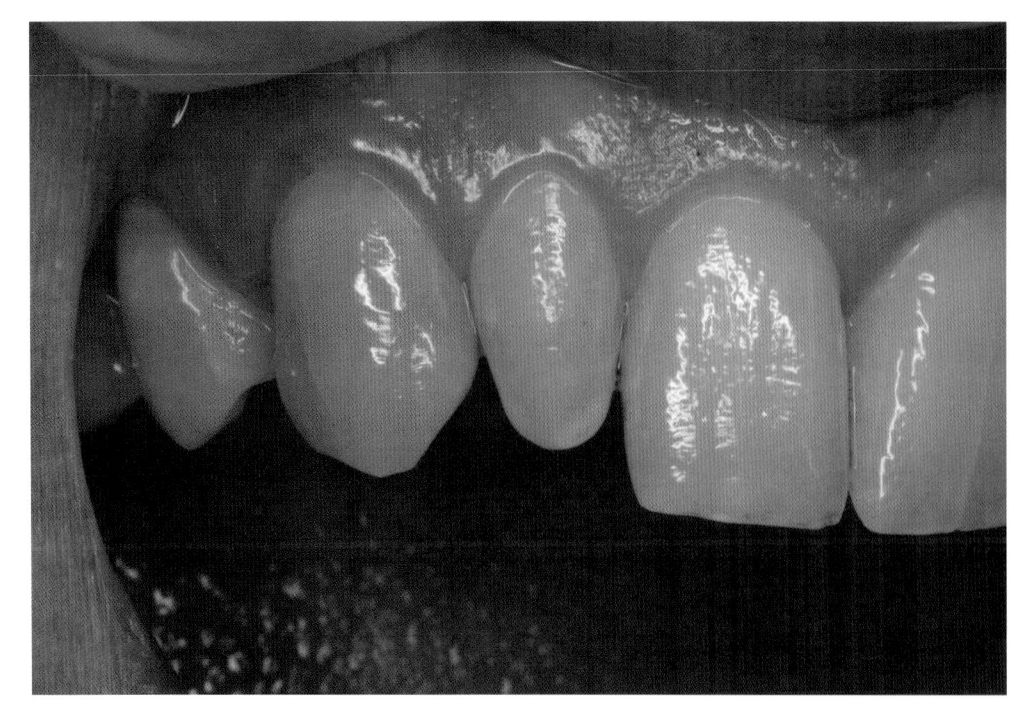

Fig. 3.16 An example of a patient presenting with a peg-shaped lateral maxillary incisor tooth. This impacts significantly on the esthetic zone.

incisors to the canines. A noticeable lack of symmetry in the axial inclination of the anterior teeth may contribute to poor esthetic appearance. Subtle anomalies in the axial inclination of the lateral incisors may not be displeasing.

Contact areas and embrasures

Embrasure spaces (as in Figure 3.17) should increase in size in moving distally from the midline.[38] When assessing the anterior maxillary dentition, it is important to record details of the embrasure spaces and to consider the ways, if any, in which these spaces may be changed during treatment.

In general, the contact areas between the maxillary central incisors should be in the incisal third. The contacts between the central and lateral incisors should be positioned at the junction of the incisal and middle thirds of the teeth (Fig. 3.18).

Dias et al.[39] have suggested the application of the '50–40–30' rule in defining the esthetic relationship between the anterior maxillary teeth, whereby the ideal contact area between the central incisors is 50% of the length of the clinical crowns; that between the central incisor and lateral incisors 40% of the length of the crown of the central incisor; and 30% of the length of the central incisor tooth between the lateral incisor and canine (Fig. 3.19).

Contacts should be symmetrical.

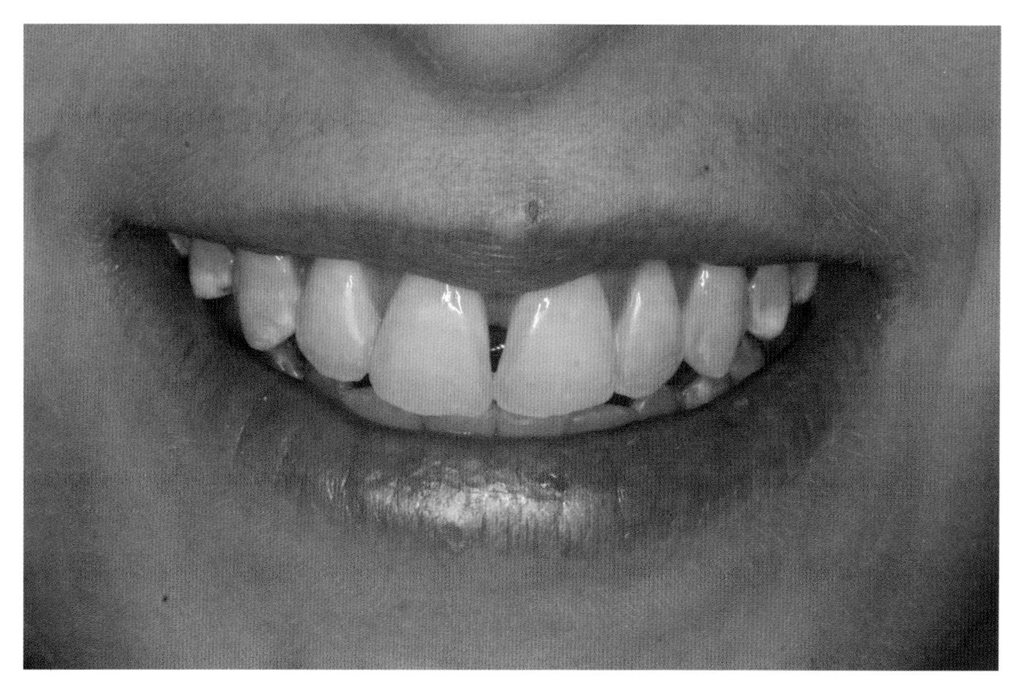

Fig. 3.17 Black triangles depict 'embrasure spaces' present in the smile zone.

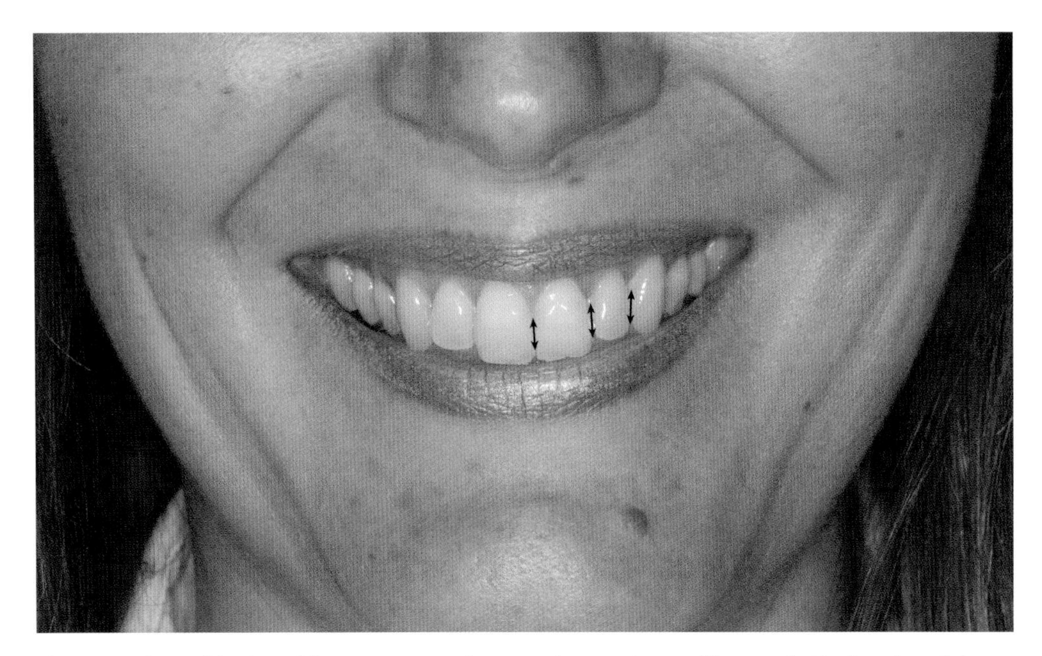

Fig. 3.18 The positioning of the contact areas between the anterior maxillary teeth. The location of the contact area moves apically when moving distally from the midline.

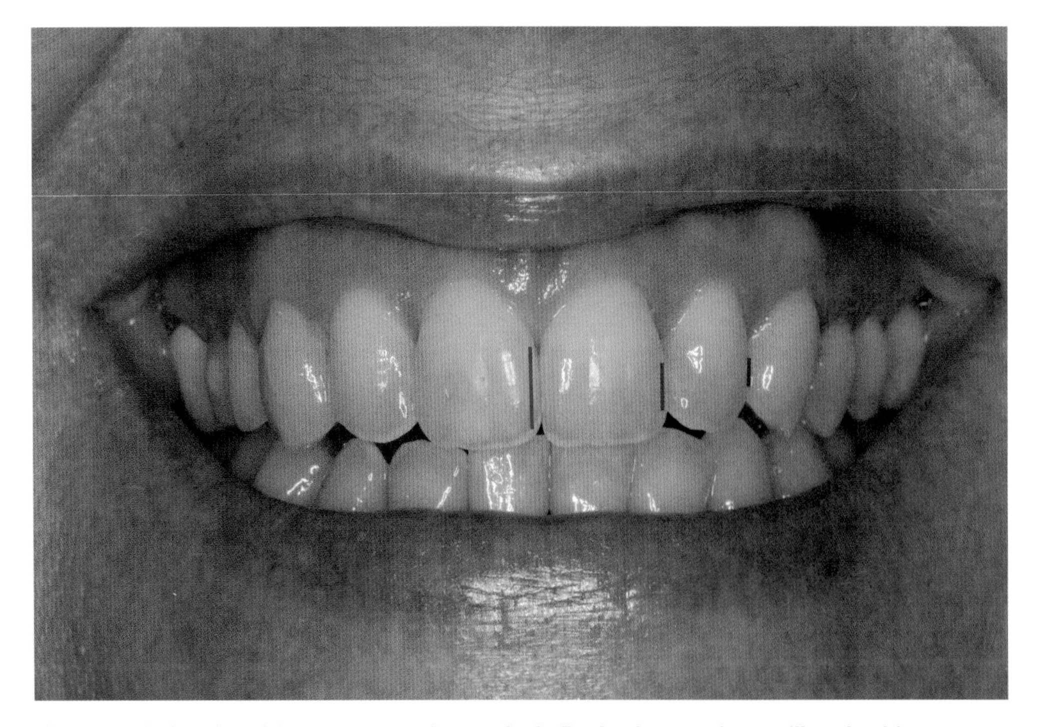

Fig. 3.19 The location of the contact areas in an esthetically pleasing anterior maxillary dentition.

Gingival esthetics

It has been suggested that, for optimum esthetics, the gingival levels of the anterior maxillary segment should be symmetrical, with the gingival margins on the central incisor and canine teeth being slightly (less than 1 mm) higher than on the lateral incisors (Fig. 3.20).[38] Disparities in gingival symmetry are frequently observed in association with localized dento-alveolar compensation, severe crowding, ankylosis, periodontal disease and the substitution of a canine for a maxillary lateral incisor.[38]

The presence of 'black triangles' between the teeth is usually considered to be highly unattractive. Ideally, the space apical to the contact area should be occupied by an interdental papilla of healthy appearance. High smile lines are particularly unforgiving to black triangles. If present in a patient being examined and assessed for esthetic dental treatment, the extent of the triangles should be carefully documented and discussed with the patient.

The morphology of the gingival tissues around each tooth may be found to be very variable. Around maxillary incisors and canines, the gingival outline

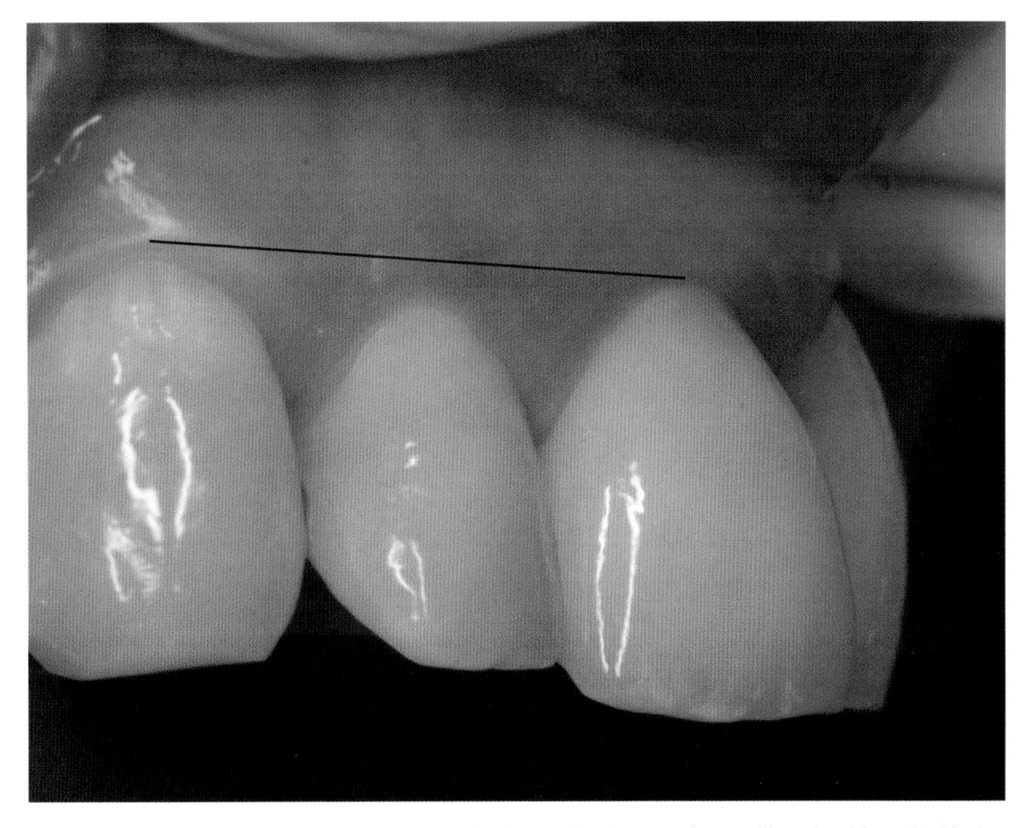

Fig. 3.20 Gingival profile associated with an esthetically pleasing anterior maxillary dentition. The black line demonstrates the relative positions of the gingival zeniths of individual teeth in the esthetic zone.

should be elliptical, with the gingival zenith being distal to the long axis of the tooth. Around maxillary lateral and mandibular incisors, the gingival contour should be rounded.[38] It is not uncommon to consider pre-restorative periodontal plastic surgery to enhance the gingival outline.

The gingival biotype – thick or thin – should be noted, as this may influence the ways in which the gingival tissues respond to the placement of dental restorations. In general, thin biotypes are associated with triangular tooth forms, and thick biotypes are commonly associated with square tooth forms.[40]

Edentulous spaces

A number of classification systems have been described for edentulous spaces. The Kennedy classification, which takes account of the location of the saddle(s) (anterior or posterior) and whether they are bounded or unbounded (unilaterally or bilaterally) is widely used.

Edentulous ridges should be assessed for form (rounded, flat, inverted or knife-edged) and for the presence of any hard or soft tissue undercuts. The overlying mucosa should also be examined for thickness and consistency (thick, thin, soft, firm or mobile).

Any existing removable prostheses should be assessed for retention, stability, support, base form, polished surface contours, occlusal function and esthetics.

SPECIAL TESTS

To complete an examination and patient assessment, it is common to have to undertake various special tests. Those typically performed in esthetic dental practice include:

- radiographs – to ascertain, amongst other features, the presence of any existing hard tissue and bony pathology, root morphology, crown : root ratios, the quality of the alveolar bone and any existing endodontic treatments
- cephalometric analysis
- vitality, sensitivity and sensibility tests
- colour photographs
- study casts, typically mounted on an appropriate form of dental articulator
- diagnostic wax and resin mock-ups
- Kesling set-ups.

RESIN MOCK-UPS

The provision of a resin (composite) mock-up is of particular value when planning esthetic and occlusal changes. A resin mock-up allows the clinician and patient to assess planned changes as part of a fully reversible process. A mock-up is also invaluable in transferring a wealth of information to the dental technologist.

The clinical protocol involves drying the anterior teeth, followed by the placement of resin composite of an appropriate shade, without any conditioning or bonding of the tooth tissues. In this way, resin composite can be added, subtracted and contoured to assess changes in the following features:

- tooth size, shape, axial inclination
- co-incidence of the dental and facial midlines
- parallelism between the anterior occlusal plane and the inter-pupillary or commissural lines
- contact areas, embrasure form and connector morphology
- dental proportions and symmetry
- buccal corridor.

Dento-labial relationships can also be assessed, together with phonetic tests, by asking the patient to enunciate the 'E', 'F', 'V' and 'S' sounds.

CLINICAL TIP

Have a laminated sheet of prose for the patient to read out loud.

The effect of any changes to the shape of the anterior teeth on the anterior guidance may also be assessed, as may any proposed change in the occlusal guidance.

The reversibility of resin mock-ups also enables the clinician to determine whether the needs and expectations of the patient, and possibly the patient's partner and family, are realistic and attainable. Treatment planning should be delayed until all parties are satisfied with the mock-up.

Once a mock-up has been accepted and is considered feasible, an over-impression should be taken and dispatched to the dental laboratory, together with

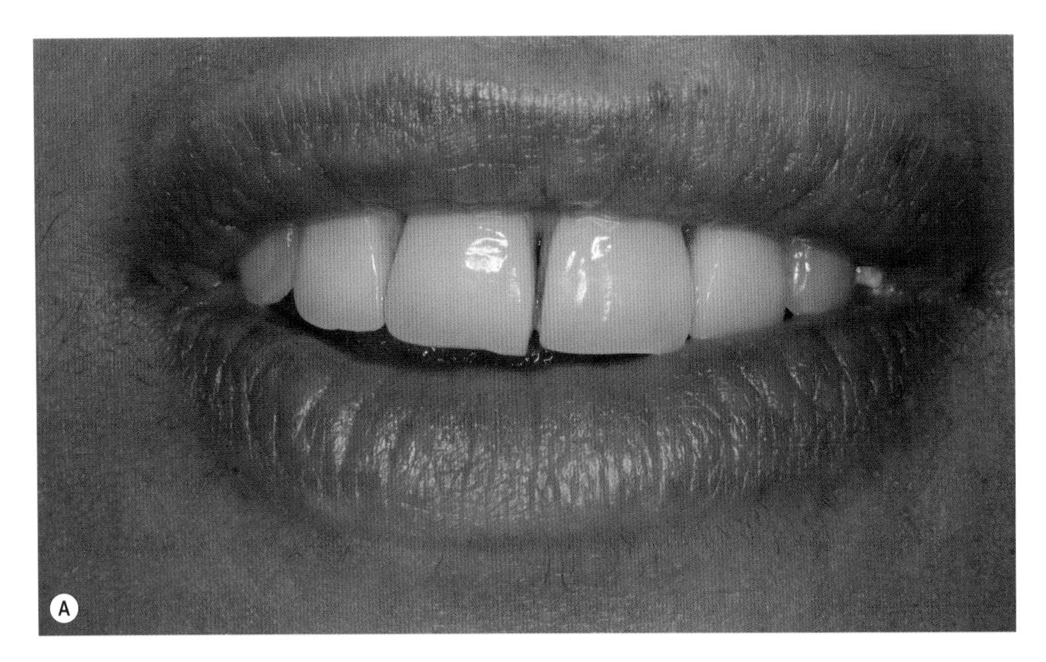

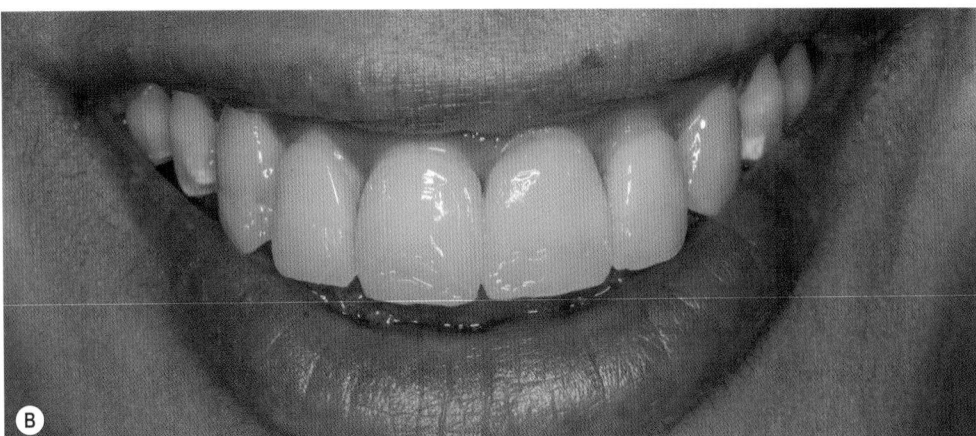

Fig. 3.21 Using mock-ups. A. Preoperative view of a patient with esthetic concerns in relation to the anterior maxillary dentition. B. Completed intraoral mock-up as part of the information provided to the dental technician.

photographs of the mock-up in situ. This information allows the dental technologist to create wax mock-ups and to refine the planned esthetic and functional changes at the appropriate stages in the treatment (Fig. 3.21).

The 'Snap-On Smile' is a recent innovation by DenMat (USA) that enables the reversible evaluation of the acceptance of esthetic alterations. It is a custom-made removable appliance similar to an orthodontic retainer, which engages undercuts present in the gingival third of the teeth. Whilst bulk, lack of stability and bad taste are commonly reported with the use of this type of appliance, it can serve as a useful diagnostic tool and an interim solution to an esthetic problem.

CONCLUDING REMARKS

Meticulous patient assessment and examination are pivotal to achieving successful outcomes in esthetic dental practice. The clinician must have a clear understanding of the concepts of symmetry, proportion, shape, function and form that underpin treatments aimed at achieving an esthetically pleasing dento-facial appearance. The clinician must, however, refrain from stereotyping and judging patients relative to 'ideals'. Each and every patient must be attentively listened to and assessed as an individual, according to their concerns, needs and expectations.

The use of reversible mock-up techniques can help to establish whether it is possible to meet the patient's needs, as well as serving as a most useful means of conveying essential information to the dental technologist.

In examining and assessing a patient for possible esthetic dental treatment, clinicians must draw on all their understanding, knowledge and clinical experience in the interests of best serving the patient. If, at the conclusion of the examination and assessment, the clinician has uncertainties, the best interests of the patient may require referral for further investigation.

CLINICAL TIP

The first treatment option should be no treatment, particularly when considering options for managing esthetics, which is not, after all, a disease!

REFERENCES

1. Kershaw S, Newton J, Williams D. The influence of tooth colour on the perceptions of personal characteristics among female dental patients: comparisons of unmodified, decayed and 'whitened' teeth. Br Dent J 2008;204:E9, 1–7.
2. Myers D. Psychology. New York: Worth; 1998.
3. Goldstein R. Study of need for esthetics in dentistry. J Prosthet Dent 1969;21:589–98.
4. Tjan A, Miller G. Some esthetic factors in a smile. J Prosthet Dent 1984;51:24–8.
5. Hasanreisoglu U, Berskum S, Aras K, et al. An analysis of maxillary anterior teeth: facial and dental proportions. J Prosthet Dent 2005;94:530–8.
6. Davis N. Smile design. Dent Clin N Am 2007;51:299–318.
7. Millar BJ. MSc Aesthetic dentistry, module 2 unit 1 (II), Smile design – clinical applications. King's College London: Learning resources; 2010.
8. Dental protection: veneers. Riskwise UK 2001;41:2–4.

9. Chalifoux P. Practice made perfect. Perception esthetics: factors that affect smile design. J Esthet Dent 1996;8:189–92.

10. Dietschi D. Optimizing smile composition and esthetics with resin composites and other conservative esthetic procedures. Eur J Esthet Dent 2008;3:14–29.

11. Jornung J, Fardal O. Perceptions of patients' smiles. A comparison of patients' and dentists' opinions. J Am Dent Assoc 2007;138:1544–53.

12. American Psychiatric Association. Diagnosis and statistical manual of diseases (DSM-IV). Washington, DC: American Psychiatric Press; 1994. p. 466–9.

13. Phillips K, Dias S. Gender differences in body dysmorphic disorder. J Nerv Ment Dis 1997;185:570–7.

14. Ahmad I. Anterior dental aesthetics: facial perspective. Br Dent J 2005;199:15–21.

15. Fradeani M. Esthetic rehabilitation in fixed prosthodontics, vol. 1. Esthetic analysis. Chicago: Quintessence; 2004. p. 35–62.

16. Proffit W. Diagnosis and treatment planning. In: Proffit W, editor. Contemporary orthodontics. St Louis: Mosby; 1986. p. 128.

17. Johnston C, Burden D, Stevenson M. The influence of facial midline discrepancies on dental attractiveness. Eur J Orthodont 1999;21:517–22.

18. Arnett G, Bergmann R. Facial keys to orthodontic diagnosis and treatment planning: part III. Am J Orthod Dentofac 1993;103:395–411.

19. Ricketts R. Planning treatment on the basis of the facial pattern and an estimate of its growth. Angle Orthod 1957;27:14–37.

20. Vig R, Brundo G. The kinetics of anterior tooth display. J Prosthet Dent 1978;39:502–4.

21. Fitzpatrick T. The validity and practicality of sun reactive types I–VI. Arch Dermatol 1988;124:869–71.

22. Glogau R. Aesthetic and anatomic analysis of the aging skin. Semin Cutan Med Surg 1996;15:134–8.

23. Aiamon J. Assessment of periodontal treatment needs. Adaptation of the WHO Community Periodontal Index of Treatment Needs (CPITN) to European conditions. Public health aspects of periodontal disease in Europe. Berlin: Quintessence; 1983.

24. Staurt C, Sallard H. Concepts of occlusion. Dent Clin N Am 1963;7:591.

25. Fradeani M. Esthetic rehabilitation in fixed prosthodontics, vol. 1. Esthetic analysis. Chicago: Quintessence; 2004. p. 63–116.

26. D'Amico A. The canine teeth – normal functional relation of the natural teeth of man. J South Calif Dent Assoc 1958;26:6–23.

27. Blitz N, Steel C, Willhite C. Diagnosis and treatment evaluation in cosmetic dentistry – a guide to accreditation criteria. Madison: American Academy of Cosmetic Dentistry; 2008. p. 8–10.

28. Rufenacht C. Principles of esthetic integration. Chicago: Quintessence; 2000. p. 109–11.

29. Dong J, Jin T, Cho H, et al. The esthetics of the smile: a review of some recent studies. Int J Prosthodont 1999;12:9–19.

30. Moore T, Southard K, Casko J, et al. Buccal corridors and smile esthetics. Am J Orthod Dentofac 2005;127:208–13.

31. Ahmad I. Anterior dental aesthetics: dentofacial perspective. Br Dent J 2005;199:81–8.

32. Miller E, Bodden W, Jamison H. A study of the relationship of the dental midline to the facial median line. J Prosthet Dent 1979;41:657–60.

33. Al-Johany S, Alqahtani S, Alqahtani F, et al. Evaluation of different esthetic smile criteria. Int J Prosthodont 2011;24:64–70.

34. Summit J, Robbins J, Hilton T, et al. Fundamentals of operative dentistry, a contemporary approach. 3rd ed. Chicago: Quintessence; 2006. p. 68–80.

35. Lombardi R. The principles of visual perception and their clinical application to denture esthetics. J Prosthet Dent 1973;29:358–82.

36. Levin E. Dental esthetics and the golden proportion. J Prosthet Dent 1978;40:244–52.

37. Preston J. The golden proportion revisited. J Esthet Dent 1993;5:247–51.

38. Gill S, Naini F, Tredwin C. Smile aesthetics. Dent Update 2007;34:152–8.

39. Dias N, Tsingene F. SAEF – smile's aesthetic evaluation form: a useful tool to improve communication between clinicians and patients during multidisciplinary treatment. Eur J Esthet Dent 2011;6:160–75.

40. Fradeani M. Esthetic rehabilitation in fixed prosthodontics, vol. 1. Esthetic analysis. Chicago: Quintessence; 2004. p. 243–6.

CHAPTER 4

Psychology of Dental Esthetics

J. TIMOTHY NEWTON

INTRODUCTION

Why is facial attractiveness so important and what are the psychological determinants of 'attractiveness'? Why are some faces perceived as attractive whereas others are not? In this chapter the advantages of facial and, more specifically, dental attractiveness will be explored, and the possible mechanisms by which beauty exerts its widespread effects will be outlined.

THEORIES OF FACIAL ATTRACTIVENESS

There are three broad categories of theories to explain the attractiveness of facial traits:

- those emanating from evolutionary psychology, which suggest that in some way facial attractiveness is an indicator of genetic fitness – the so-called 'good genes hypothesis'
- the 'cognitive hypothesis', which suggests that the human brain is equipped with specific mechanisms for identifying prototypes such as 'male' and 'female' faces, and that facial beauty is related to the degree of match between the face observed and the prototype
- social explanations, which place an emphasis on the acquisition of perceptions of facial attractiveness through social and cultural norms that will vary across time and society.[1]

While all three theories are plausible explanations of the importance of attractiveness, they are primarily *post hoc* explanations of the phenomenon and do not necessarily provide testable predictions. Furthermore, evidence cited in support of one theory can often be interpreted to support the alternative hypotheses.

KEY POINT SUMMARY

Is the increased concern about facial esthetics in part due to the increased availability of camera phones and their use on social networking sites?

GOOD GENES HYPOTHESIS

Central to the good genes hypothesis are two assumptions: that facial attractiveness judgements are related to the individual's phenotype, and that attractive people have a phenotype more strongly related to survival than less attractive individuals. Supporters of this theory cite evidence suggesting that faces that appear to be 'average' are more attractive, and symmetrical faces are also rated as more attractive than asymmetrical faces, proposing that both averageness and symmetry suggest a genome free from mutations.[2] Further, Symons[3] suggests that the 'average' face is most likely to be associated with above-average performance in tasks such as chewing and breathing, and hence would be favoured during evolution.

KEY POINT SUMMARY

An attractive appearance is associated with averageness, symmetry and characteristics related to youth.

COGNITIVE HYPOTHESIS

According to the cognitive hypothesis and following the work of Jean Piaget, human thought develops by first defining a prototype of each construct. For example, a child may start by drawing a 'prototype' of a house that contains those elements that the child conceives to be necessary for a house; only later, as the child's knowledge and conception of 'houses' are modified through experience, can they develop the conception to include other kinds of houses. In the same way, the cognitive hypothesis proposes that the child defines the concept of 'face' according to a simple prototype. The prototype or 'average' face is perceived as attractive since it will elicit strong responses from perceptual systems, as it is most strongly related to the 'core' concept of a face. Further evidence in support of this hypothesis is the finding that young infants look longer at attractive faces that are prototypical and hence easier to classify.[4]

FACIAL ATTRACTIVENESS AND 'AVERAGENESS'

Both the good genes hypothesis and the cognitive theory of facial attractiveness draw on evidence to suggest that 'averageness' should be found attractive. Langlois and Roggman[5] digitized male and female undergraduate student faces of Hispanic and Asian origin and asked adults to judge the attractiveness of both the individual faces and the computer-generated composite images. Both male and female composite faces were judged more attractive than almost all the individual faces comprising the composites. In addition, the composite faces became more attractive as more faces were entered. Alley and Cunningham[6] argue, however, that although 'average' is attractive, it is not the most attractive and, furthermore, composite images are characterized by a 'soft focus' effect as well as smooth uniform skin tones, free of blemishes, with a high degree of facial symmetry. Perrett et al.[7] also argued against the overwhelming importance of 'averageness', by demonstrating that a face derived from the composite of 60 females was rated as less attractive than a face representing the average of the 15 most attractive female faces from the same group. In addition, attractive composites can be made more attractive by exaggerating the shape differences from the sample mean. They concluded that highly attractive facial configurations are not wholly 'average' and that small deviations from average enhance attractiveness.

In conclusion, it is clear that while 'averageness' plays a large role in ratings of attractiveness, other traits can enhance the effect of 'averageness', in particular those that are related to the appearance of youthfulness.[1] For a further discussion of the importance of 'youthful' features in attractiveness, see below.

FACIAL ATTRACTIVENESS AND SYMMETRY

Measures of human body symmetry correlate with attractiveness. Perrett et al.[8] showed that increasing the degree of symmetry within a face (while holding skin textures constant) increases ratings of attractiveness for both male and female faces. Evolutionary psychologists have suggested that symmetry may be an indicator of ability to tolerate environmental stress, the argument being that asymmetry would arise from disease or injury.[9]

FACIAL ATTRACTIVENESS AND FEATURES SUGGESTING YOUTHFULNESS

Facial features associated with youthfulness – in particular, those most often seen in infants, including large eyes, smooth skin and a small nose – have been associated with increased ratings of attractiveness,[10] possibly because they promote nurturance. Similarly, white teeth are rated as more attractive than darker teeth, in particular teeth that have become more yellow in appearance with age.[11]

In conclusion, it would appear that facial attractiveness is related to a degree of 'averageness' in the face and to symmetry, though distinctive features can make a face appear more attractive, particularly if they are associated with a youthful appearance. The reasons for these preferences amongst observers are unclear, though they have been the source of some theoretical discussion.

IMPACT OF DENTO-FACIAL APPEARANCE

Facial appearance plays a key role in human interaction. In the absence of other information, facial attractiveness is used as a guide to infer a variety of characteristics about a person, including personality, integrity, social and intellectual competence, and mental health.[12] The impact of appearance on perceptions of personal characteristics is not limited to initial meetings – such perceptions may have a lasting effect.[13] Moreover, individuals rated as attractive tend to earn more, have more successful life outcomes and have greater self-worth than less attractive individuals.[14-16] Good dental appearance is thought to be a requirement of prestigious occupations among some professional groups.[17]

IMPACT OF DENTO-FACIAL ANOMALIES ON PERCEIVED PERSONAL CHARACTERISTICS

An important component of facial appearance is the appearance of the mouth and teeth. In face-to-face situations, studies of eye movement show that the eyes primarily scan the other person's eyes and areas of the mouth, with little time spent in observation of other features.[18] It is not surprising, therefore, that poor dento-facial appearance produces negative perceptions of personal characteristics.[19,20] Individuals with less dental disease are judged to be more socially competent, to show greater intellectual achievement and to have better psychological adjustment.[21] The impact of dento-facial esthetics upon perceptions of personal characteristics may vary according to cultural traditions and social background.[20]

KEY POINT SUMMARY

Facial appearance is important in social interactions. The presence of facial and dental anomalies can result in negative social judgements.

Shaw et al.[19] found that the presence of orthodontic (dental) abnormalities was associated with lower expectations by a teacher and lower ratings of attractiveness, as well as bullying. Given the extent to which these impacts may have a major influence upon an individual's life, it would suggest that orthodontic anomalies may give rise to quite severe consequences.[21,22] Lovegrove and Rumsey[23] found that 75% of 11–13-year-olds had been teased or bullied about their appearance. Furthermore, there is some evidence that social skills training for individuals with facial abnormalities is effective in reducing the stress they experience.

Physical attractiveness is important in teachers' expectations. Children rated as less attractive are judged by teachers to be poorer performers academically. This is in spite of the fact that there is little relationship between physical attractiveness and absolute levels of intelligence. Furthermore, children tend to judge their peers as less popular if they are less attractive. Juries are more likely to find an attractive defendant to be innocent than an unattractive defendant, and finally, of course, physical attractiveness plays a major role in interpersonal attractiveness.[12]

There is experimental evidence to suggest that visible dento-facial anomalies may have an impairing effect on facial attractiveness. Such anomalies may influence interpersonal relationships in both children[19] and young adults.[20,24] In these studies, facial photographs have been used, giving the benefit of standardization and artificial modification of different facial cues whilst controlling for non-manipulated variables.[21,24] In these studies, visible anterior malocclusion, such as severe crowding and broad midline diastema, was seen to have a detrimental influence on a person's perceived social success, characterized by intelligence, beauty, social class and sexual attractiveness.[21] Similarly, neutral and protrusive teeth were significantly preferred in comparison to retrusively positioned teeth, even at the level of millimetres.[24]

In experimental research using digitally modified photographs, it has been shown that dentally influenced social judgements are affected by factors such as the presence of visible dental decay,[21] the whiteness of teeth[11] and also the position of the dental caries.[25] Participants judged those with less dental disease to be significantly more socially competent, to show greater intellectual achievement, and to have better psychological adjustment than those with a higher degree of dental disease.[23] Similarly, another study[11] found that tooth colour exerted an influence on social perceptions, where more negative judgements were made about people's social competence, intellectual ability, psychological adjustment and relationship satisfaction for a decayed dental appearance in comparison to unaltered images. The authors suggested the results might be explained by negative beliefs about dental decay, such as its link with poor oral hygiene. More recently, the position of visible dental decay and/or the extent of the lesion were found to be determining factors in social judgements of digitally modified photos of targets (Fig. 4.1), where a more central position of dental caries was predictive of poor social judgements in the constructs of intellectual ability, extroversion and care for one's personal appearance than just the presence of decay or even twice the amount of decay.[25]

CLINICAL TIP

Understand the patient's reason for seeking change in their attractiveness. Are they hoping for *more* than a beautiful smile?

As a consequence of the pervasive finding that attractiveness is related to the judgements other people make about us, it has been suggested that individuals with facial abnormalities must experience an impaired quality of life and psychological distress; however, this does not appear to be the case, certainly for major facial abnormalities. Hunt et al.[26] concluded that the majority of children with cleft lip and palate do not appear to experience major psychosocial

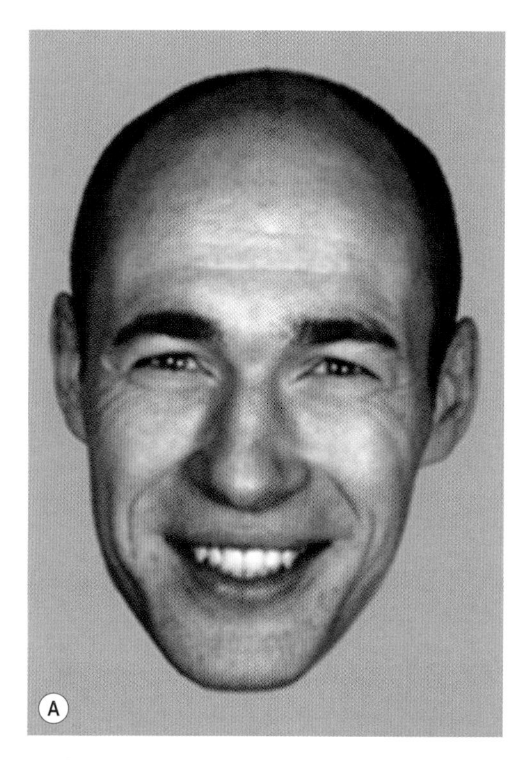

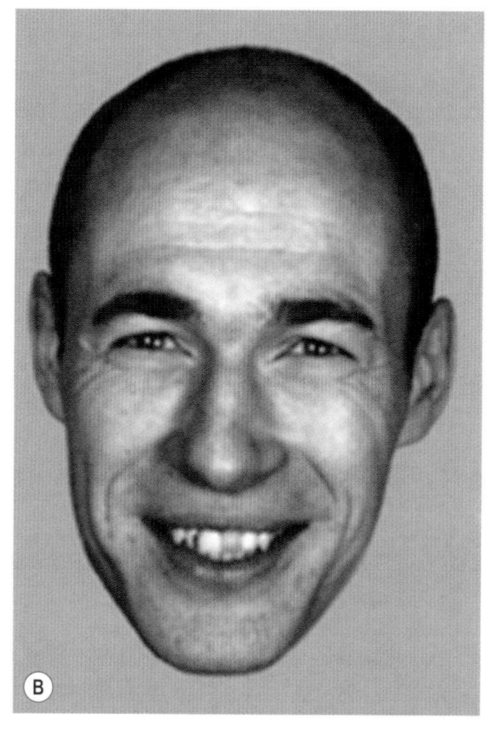

Fig. 4.1 Images used to assess the viewer's judgement of the person's social status and intelligence. Picture A shows the unmodified image, while Image 2 has been digitally modified to suggest the presence of decay and discolouration. Ratings of social status and intelligence are on average lower for image B.

problems. Liu et al.[27] found no difference in global quality of life between individuals with cranio-facial abnormalities and control groups, although there was some difference in terms of functional oral health measures. Furthermore, there is some evidence that in families where a member has a cleft lip and palate there are positive consequences. Locker et al.[28] found that self-rated oral health was higher amongst individuals with an oral facial abnormality. Topolski et al.[29] found that the relationships amongst family members were better in the group where the child had a cleft lip and palate. Similarly, Marcusson et al.[30] found that there were increased quality of life ratings in individuals with cleft lip and palate for their use of leisure time and their social life.

A number of studies have looked at the relationship between the presence of orthodontic anomalies and oral health-related quality of life. By and large, these studies have been cross-sectional investigations and have found some relationship. For example, De Oliveira and Sheiham[31] found in a cross-sectional survey that adolescents that had completed orthodontic treatment had better oral health-related quality of life than those who had not. O'Brien et al.[32] found differences in quality of life across groups divided by the index of orthodontic treatment need, and Johal et al.[33] found that individuals with either increased overjet or increased spacing had poorer oral health-related quality of life in comparison to controls. Using a stronger longitudinal design, however, Shaw et al.[34] found that lack of orthodontic treatment when there was need did not lead to psychological difficulties in later life. This study has been criticized for using measures that were unlikely to show any difference, given the nature of orthodontic need. It does seem to suggest, however, that orthodontic treatment has no major impact upon psychological characteristics.

In conclusion, it would appear that, in cross-sectional studies, differences in orthodontic conditions do relate to oral health quality of life, but not to levels of general quality of life. This suggests that there may be some differences between individuals with different oral conditions. Many studies, however, have found, both for orthodontic anomalies and for more major anomalies, such as cleft lip and palate, that individuals with these conditions do not show a major psychological impact. This would seem to suggest that individuals with these anomalies are learning to cope, and therefore do not experience psychological impact. Indeed, there may even be a positive impact, bringing the family together and enhancing communication between family members. While this seemingly positive image of the impact of orthodontic anomalies may give hope to individuals with such conditions, what does seem to be particularly important is not the reaction of the individual themselves, but the reaction of other people who are looking at that individual. There is a pervasive process of perceiving other people with such anomalies to have a range of negative characteristics. This is something beyond the control of the individual with a cranio-facial anomaly and does suggest that managing the esthetic condition of these individuals is important, not for the people themselves but for the reaction of other people interacting with them.

KEY POINT SUMMARY

An improvement in dental attractiveness often leads to an increase in self-confidence, which in itself may then bring about other benefits.

CONCLUDING REMARKS

Physical attractiveness, especially facial attractiveness, is an important component of human interaction. The social benefits of an attractive appearance are widespread and marked. The underlying mechanisms for this are unclear, though it would appear that facial characteristics associated with genetic fitness are rated as more attractive – for example, averageness and symmetry. Furthermore, characteristics associated with youth are also rated as attractive. While there is little evidence to suggest that facial attractiveness influences individuals' appraisal of themselves, it is clear that the judgements made by other people of facial and oral appearance, in particular the presence of facial and dental anomalies, may give rise to perceptions of negative characteristics.

KEY POINT SUMMARY

The clinician should be cautious: while improved dental attractiveness may lead to a changed lifestyle, this should not be implied by the clinician as an outcome of altering the smile.

REFERENCES

1. Rhodes G, Zebrowitz LA. Facial attractiveness. Evolutionary, cognitive and social perspectives. Westport: Ablex; 2002.
2. Thornhill R, Gangstead SW. Facial attractiveness. Trends Cogn Sci 1999;3:452.
3. Symons D. The evolution of human sexuality. Oxford: Oxford University Press; 1979.
4. Langlois JH, Roggman LA, Casey RJ, et al. Infant preferences for attractive faces: rudiments of a stereotype? Dev Psychol 1987;23:363.
5. Langlois JH, Roggman LA. Attractive faces are only average. Psychol Sci 1990;1:115.
6. Alley TR, Cunningham MR. Averaged faces are attractive, but very attractive faces are not average. Psychol Sci 1991;124:124.
7. Perrett DI, May KA, Yoshikawa S. Facial shape and judgements of female attractiveness. Nature 1994;368:239–42.
8. Perrett DI, Burt DM, Penton-Voak I, et al. Symmetry and human facial attractiveness. Evol Hum Behav 1999;20:295–307.
9. Moller AP. Sexual ornament size and the cost of fluctuating asymmetry. P Roy Soc Lond 1991;243:59–62.
10. Grammer K, Fink B, Juette A, et al. Female faces and bodies: N-dimensional feature space and attractiveness. In: Rhodes G, Zebrowitz LA, editors. Facial attractiveness. Evolutionary, cognitive and social perspectives. Westport: Ablex; 2002.
11. Kershaw S, Newton JT, Williams DM. The influence of tooth colour on the perceptions of personal characteristics: comparisons of unmodified, decayed and 'whitened' teeth. Br Dent J 2008;204:E9.
12. Eagly AH. 'What is beautiful is good, but ...': a meta-analytic review of research on the physical attractiveness stereotype. Psychol Bull 1991;110:109–28.
13. Berscheid E. An overview of the psychological effects of physical attractiveness and some comments upon the psychological effects of knowledge of the effects of physical attractiveness. In: Lucker W, Ribbens K, McNamera JA, editors. Logical aspects of facial form. Ann Arbor: University of Michigan Press; 1981.
14. Dion K, Berscheid E, Walster E. What is beautiful is good. J Pers Soc Psychol 1972;24:285–90.
15. Loh ES. The economic effects of physical appearance. Soc Sci Quart 1993;74:420–38.

16. Hamermesh DS. Beauty pays: why attractive people are more successful. Princeton: Princeton University Press; 2011.

17. Jenny J, Proshek J. Visibility and prestige of occupations and the importance of dental appearance. J Can Dent Assoc 1986;52:987–9.

18. Miller AC. Role of physical attractiveness in impression formation. Psychol Sci 1970;19:231–4.

19. Shaw WC, Rees G, Dawe M, et al. The influence of dentofacial appearance on the social attractiveness of young adults. Am J Orthodont 1985;87:21–6.

20. Kerosuo H, Hausen H, Laine T. Influence of incisal malocclusion on the social attractiveness of young adults in Finland. Eur J Orthodont 1995;17:505–12.

21. Newton JT, Prabhu N, Robinson PG. The impact of dental appearance on the appraisal of personal characteristics. Int J Prosthodont 2003;16:429–34.

22. Seehra J, Newton JT, Dibiase AT. Bullying in school children: an update for general dental practitioners. Br Dent J 2011;210:411–15.

23. Lovegrove E, Rumsey N. Ignoring it doesn't make it stop: adolescents, appearance, and bullying. Cleft Palate-Cran J 2005;42:33–44.

24. Schlosser JB, Preston CB, Lampasso J. The effects of computer-aided anteroposterior maxillary incisor movement on ratings of facial attractiveness. Am J Orthodont Dentofac 2005;127:17–24.

25. Somani A, Newton JT, Dunne S, et al. The impact of visible dental decay on social judgements: comparison of the effects of location and extent of lesion. Int Dent J 2010;60:169–74.

26. Hunt O, Burden D, Hepper P, et al. The psychosocial effects of cleft lip and palate: a systematic review. Eur J Orthodont 2005;27:274–85.

27. Liu Z, McGrath C, Hagg U. The impact of malocclusion/orthodontic treatment need on the quality of life. A systematic review. Angle Orthodont 2009;79:585–91.

28. Locker D, Jokovic A, Tompson B. Health-related quality of life of children aged 11 to 14 years with orofacial conditions. Cleft Palate-Cran J 2005;42:260–6.

29. Topolski TD, Edwards TC, Patrick DL. Quality of life: how do adolescents with facial differences compare with other adolescents? Cleft Palate-Cran J 2005;42:25–32.

30. Marcusson A, Akerlind I, Paulin G. Quality of life in adults with repaired complete cleft lip and palate. Cleft Palate-Cran J 2001;38:379–85.

31. de Oliveira CM, Sheiham A. Orthodontic treatment and its impact on oral health-related quality of life in Brazilian adolescents. J Orthodont 2004;31:20–7.

32. O'Brien K, Wright JL, Conboy F, et al. The child perception questionnaire is valid for malocclusions in the United Kingdom. Am J Orthodont Dentofac 2006;129:536–40.

33. Johal A, Cheung MY, Marcene W. The impact of two different malocclusion traits on quality of life. Br Dent J 2007;202:E2.

34. Shaw WC, Richmond S, Kenealy PM, et al. A 20 year cohort study of health gain from orthodontic treatment: psychological outcome. Am J Orthodont Dentofac 2007;132:146–57.

CHAPTER 5

Treatment Planning and the Delivery of Care in Esthetic Dentistry

BRIAN MILLAR

INTRODUCTION

By now you will be aware of the importance of esthetics to your patients. It may be sufficient motivation for them to seek advice and esthetics, rather than more important oral health factors, may be the reason for them coming to your practice. Whatever the motivation, it gives the practitioner an opportunity to provide comprehensive oral healthcare, while still meeting the patient's esthetic aspirations.

Treatment planning should both satisfy the professional responsibilities of the practitioner – achieving oral health – and meet the needs of the patient – obtaining an esthetic smile. This may need to be explained, as patients typically prefer to go direct to the esthetic stage and use their funds for anterior esthetics, rather than for posterior restorative care. Your patient may have to be made aware of the fact that oral health is linked to general health, that oral disease is unesthetic, and that loss of posterior teeth and support may compromise anterior teeth and any esthetic work that has been carried out.

There may need to be explanation, discussion and compromise to meet both the practitioner's requirements and the patient's expectations. Patients often do not appreciate the risks and irreversible damage associated with most dental treatments. A clear explanation of the long-term risk of tooth damage, or even tooth loss, following invasive procedures is essential. Discussion must include the need for long-term maintenance and its associated costs, including repair and salvage.

Treatment planning can only begin once a full and detailed history has been recorded and a clinical examination has taken place. The techniques involved and the importance of the patient assessment have been covered in Chapter 3.

As well as providing an opportunity to establish the patient's needs and esthetic aspirations, the initial examination appointment is a chance to obtain good records, comprising:

- written documentation
- medical history proforma
- photographs
- radiographs
- study casts.

KEY POINT SUMMARY

The clinical examination should cover the following points:

- Reason for attendance
- History of past care
- Medical history
- Examination
- Extraoral assessment
- Intraoral assessment
- Special tests
  - Radiographs
  - Vitality tests
  - Transillumination
  - Mobility
- Occlusal analysis
  - Study casts
  - Load tests
  - Fremitus
  - Manipulation into centric relation

You may also wish to use an esthetic self-assessment proforma to save chairside time while giving your patients more time to reflect on their concerns, esthetic desires and treatment aims.

Volume 2 in this series is dedicated to the esthetic assessment. Some aspects of the assessment will need to be rechecked periodically: given any change in symptoms, the medical history or medication in particular.[1] Revisiting the patient's esthetic desires is important, as some individuals will start to be more forthcoming once they relax and begin to know and trust the clinician. Their aspirations may change during the course of a treatment plan, and this is particularly relevant to esthetic procedures that tend to be carried out during the latter stages of the treatment. Inhibitions may be reduced and less information may be held back as people relax.[2] Furthermore, a patient's socioeconomic position or priorities may change over time, and this may have an influence on their dental aspirations.[3]

KEY POINT SUMMARY

- *Symptoms* are what the patient describes
- *Signs* are what a suitably trained clinician can observe and detect
- *Diagnosis* is the recognition of pathology or a specific disease

The examination may lead to a straightforward and obvious *diagnosis* – for example, a fractured upper lateral incisor – or a more complex group of conditions, creating a *differential diagnosis*. Special tests are often used to narrow down this list of possible conditions, leaving a single diagnosis. Of course, many patients will present with multiple conditions and so have multiple *diagnoses*.

The history-taking and clinical examination, including any special investigations, are two of the most important aspects of the patient assessment process, and must come together if they are to lead to a diagnosis and provide the foundations on which to build a satisfactory treatment plan.[4]

The skilled clinician will avoid jumping to any conclusions. The fractured mesial corner and displacement of the UL2 (22) shown in Figure 5.1 happened for a reason. Was it direct trauma? What about that over-erupted third molar and mandibular displacement?

The aim of the assessment should be information gathering, leading to a diagnosis. From the diagnosis stems consideration of the treatment options as part of treatment planning, which must be followed through prior to commencing treatment (Fig. 5.2). Do not feel pressured to provide treatment immediately. Take a measured approach and collect the necessary records. Think the findings and assessments over and reflect; create a written treatment plan in your own time and present this to the patient. Any immediate dental problems can be dealt with while treatment planning takes place. Take time to assess the records in detail. One advantage in taking impressions to analyse study casts is that it gives you time to establish a treatment plan. This may provide a much-needed opportunity to study the options or speak to colleagues. However, bear in mind the need to maintain confidentiality when discussing cases.

Chapter 3 has covered the upper part of the flow chart shown in Figure 5.2. This chapter will deal with the process summarized in the lower half of the chart:

- diagnosis
- treatment options and planning
- prognosis
- overview of techniques.

The very important topic of maintenance is covered in the following chapter. It is essential for the patient to be made aware of the risks of treatment, including the inevitable failure of restorations, salvage potential and what comes next. The practitioner's focus should be on survival of the remaining dental tissues, not of the restorations.

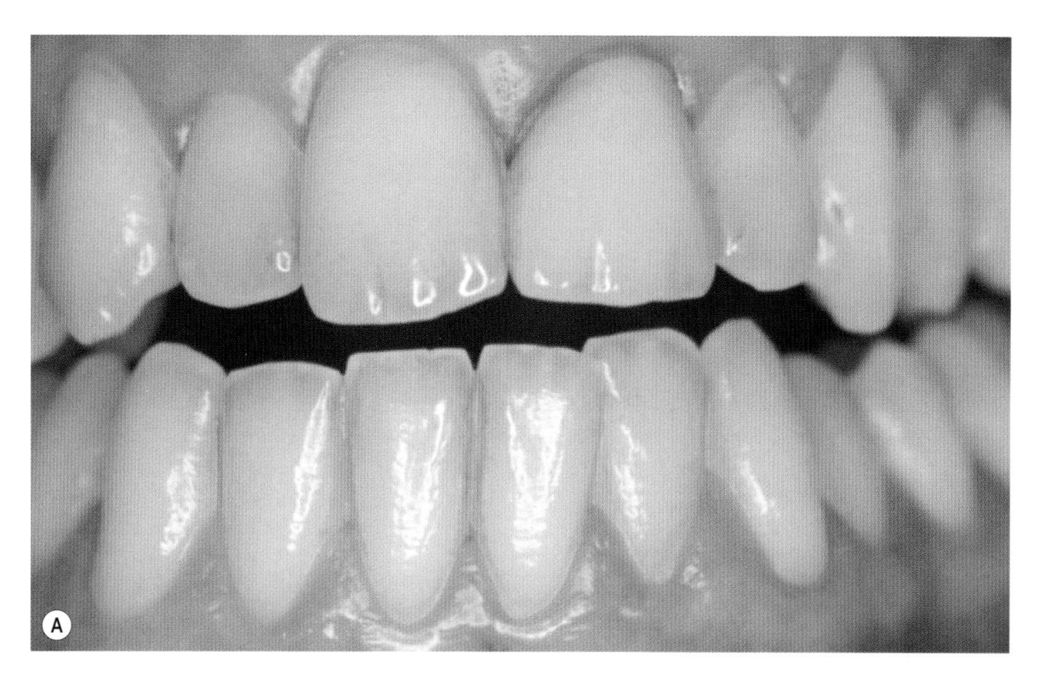

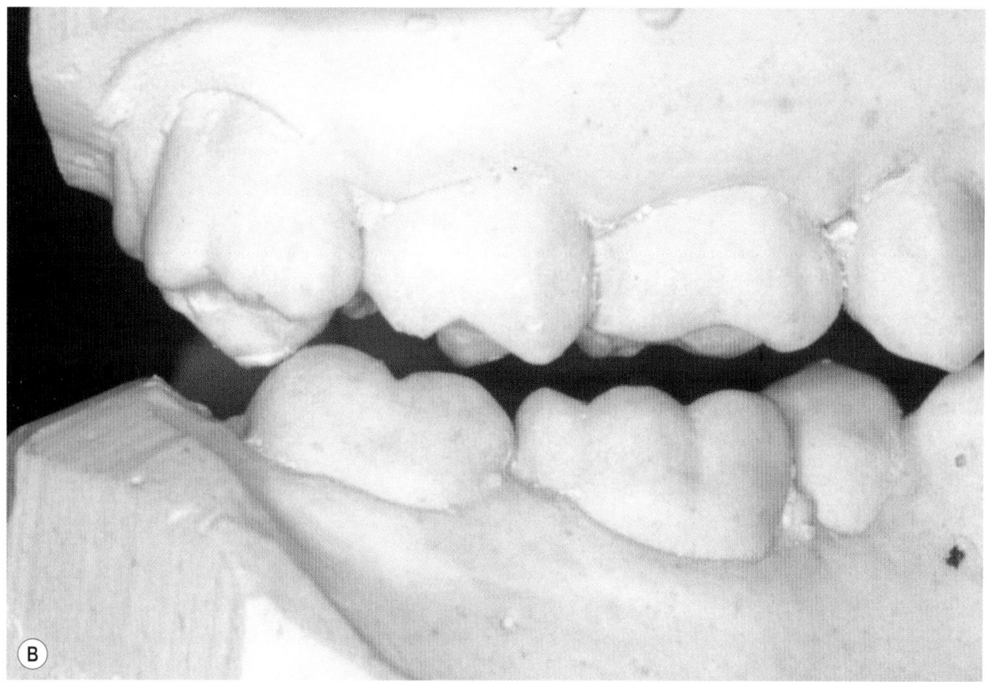

Fig. 5.1 Importance of occlusal analysis. A. Labial drifting of UL2 (22). B. This is due to the over-erupted UR8 (18) visible on articulated models mounted in centric relation.

KEY POINT SUMMARY

Survival is important, of course, but is your focus on survival of your restoration or the patient's tooth?

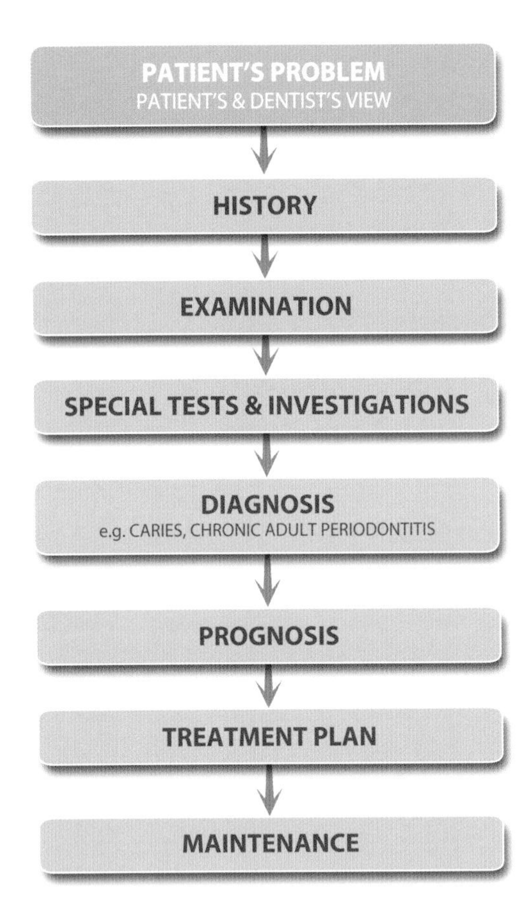

Fig. 5.2 Pathway from initial visit to completion.

Patients easily understand that, when more tooth material is cut away, less tooth is left behind. Tooth failure is related to the amount of remaining dentine. As dentists, we can call it residual dentine thickness (RDT). As RDT is reduced, the risks increase – 'risk' meaning failure of the remaining tooth tissue, pulp death, root or coronal fracture, apical pathology and tooth loss. We must add to that the fact that most restorations cause iatrogenic damage to surrounding tissues, both gingival tissues and adjacent teeth, and sometimes opposing teeth. However, it is known that improved esthetics in a demanding patient may encourage invasive techniques and so patients must be made aware and records kept.

Fortunately, it has been found that, when given a choice, twice as many patients choose non-invasive composite veneers to more invasive ceramic veneers, yet record equal levels of esthetic satisfaction with the outcome.[5] Given that some dentists, while preparing teeth for ceramic veneer preparations, used in pursuit of a uniform bright white smile, remove 30% of coronal tooth tissue,[6] due consideration has to be given to the no-preparation composite veneer options, which have the advantage of ease of repair and adjustment while providing a natural smile look.

We now practise the art of esthetic dentistry in an era in which skilled clinicians have access to a broad range of materials and techniques, offering a variety of non-invasive and invasive esthetic procedures.

THE IMPORTANCE OF DIAGNOSIS

Diagnosis should take into consideration the aetiology, distribution and extent of any existing disease: for example, erosive tooth wear affecting palatal surfaces of all upper anterior teeth into dentine. Recognition of the aetiology is the key to prevention. The extent and severity of the problem are the keys to establishing treatment options and estimating the likely prognosis.

Diagnosis is important to enable the patient to:

- understand the cause of the condition
- appreciate the severity of the condition
- take ownership of the disease
- take responsibility for preventative measures
- give informed consent to treatment.

Diagnosis is important to enable the practitioner to:

- design a suitable prevention strategy
- understand the complexity of the treatment and offer solutions
- provide a treatment plan
- estimate the prognosis
- cost the treatment accurately
- answer the patient's questions.

THE PATIENT'S CONCERNS

How important is it to inform the patient of the diagnosis? Whether the patient is more interested in the *diagnosis* or the *solution* is debatable.

THE TREATMENT PLAN

While treatment plans will clearly vary according to clinical situations, health-care systems and socioeconomic factors, there is a generic structure that many find useful to apply and then adjust to suit a particular case.

KEY POINT SUMMARY

The generic treatment plan comprises:

1. Disease control and pain relief
2. Stabilization phase
   a. Prevention
3. Basic restorative care
4. Advanced oral care
   a. Periodontal factors
   b. Endodontics
   c. Prosthodontics: prostheses, implants, esthetics
5. Maintenance

The initial stage of the treatment plan is to render the patient symptom-free, or at least pain-free. This is followed by eradication of any existing disease processes and stabilization where possible, achieved by managing the primary disease factors by adopting a preventative approach. Usually, this will focus on plaque control and dietary and lifestyle factors. Next comes a restorative phase, during which missing and damaged tissue is repaired or replaced. In common with all other aspects of dental care, this should be delivered with esthetics in mind. Why would we carry out dentistry that is unsightly – 'unesthetic'? The guiding principles in esthetic dentistry, as covered in the present series of books, help us to focus on esthetics as an integral element of routine restorative care.

INITIAL TREATMENT

Pain relief may require the practitioner to deal urgently with:

- pulpal inflammation
- periapical pathology
- caries removal
- sensitivity
- gingival inflammation
- trauma, fractures
- other conditions, such as pericoronitis.

This aspect of dental care is covered in many textbooks. From an esthetic perspective, bear the long-term possibilities in mind, even at this early stage of treatment. Save strategic tooth tissue and teeth where possible. There may be a good reason to remove irreversibly damaged, diseased tissue immediately: for example, pulp by extraction or pulpotomy. Wherever possible, tooth tissue should be preserved, as no synthetic material matches the esthetics or performance of the original dental tissues.

PREVENTION

Following pain relief, the focus should be on the prevention of further damage and loss of tooth tissue. A prevention strategy should comprise three levels:

- Primary prevention: preventing the occurrence of primary disease through, for example, oral hygiene instruction, health education and dietary advice.
- Secondary prevention: ensuring early detection and intervention as appropriate to prevent the progression of disease by means of regular oral health assessments (dental recalls), including radiographs and measures to arrest or eliminate early lesions, as indicated clinically.
- Tertiary prevention: limiting the effects of the disease on function and preventing its recurrence. This includes rehabilitation measures to replace missing tissues.

This may take some time to carry out. It is essential for patients to buy into the strategy, taking responsibility and ownership of the aetiological factors. It is their oral health, their disease, their preventative programme and their responsibility.

Patients must be clear that planned restorative treatment is doomed to fail without their co-operation. Monitoring, reassessment and reinforcement of the strategy must be carried out prior to embarking on complex treatment. It must be unethical to provide complex and expensive restorative care, knowing that the patient is unlikely to be able to maintain it in the long term, or to afford to have it repaired when it fails, as this may create an even more complex problem in the future when the individual is even less able to manage it (Fig. 5.3).

Prevention includes avoiding cutting teeth now for esthetic gain, knowing that pathology will follow that is difficult to manage, and will often be forced on to another clinician to explain and manage (Fig. 5.4).

KEY POINT SUMMARY

Prevention includes refraining from cutting away tooth tissue when alternatives exist, and not providing restorative work that is likely to fail, creating more complex problems in the future.

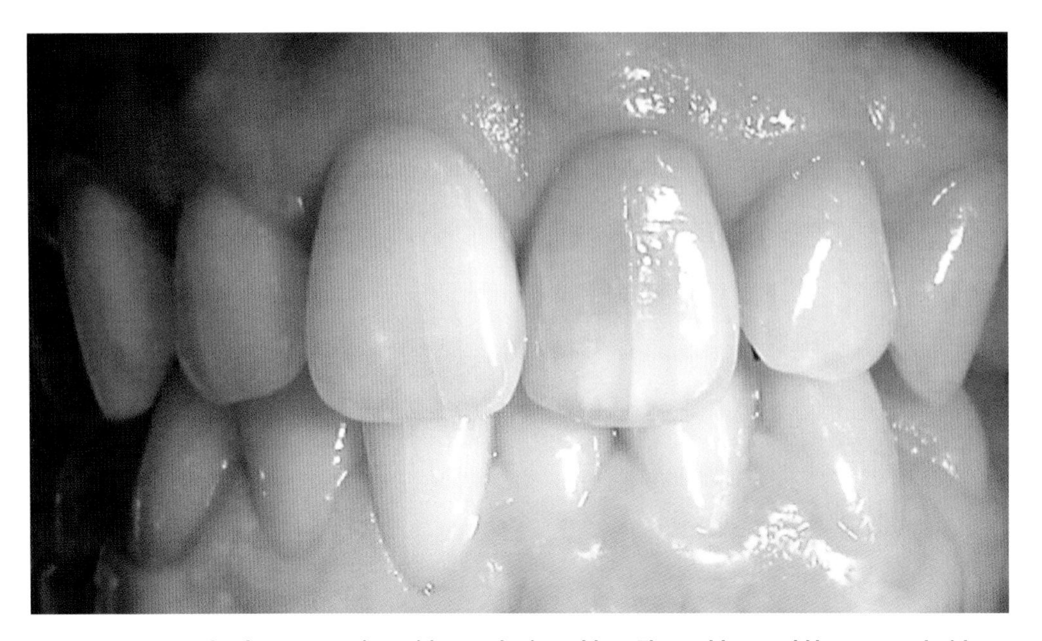

Fig. 5.3 An example of a young patient with an esthetic problem. The problem could be managed with: (a) a post, core and crown, or (b) internal bleaching and possibly a composite veneer. Which is likely to result in earlier tooth loss?

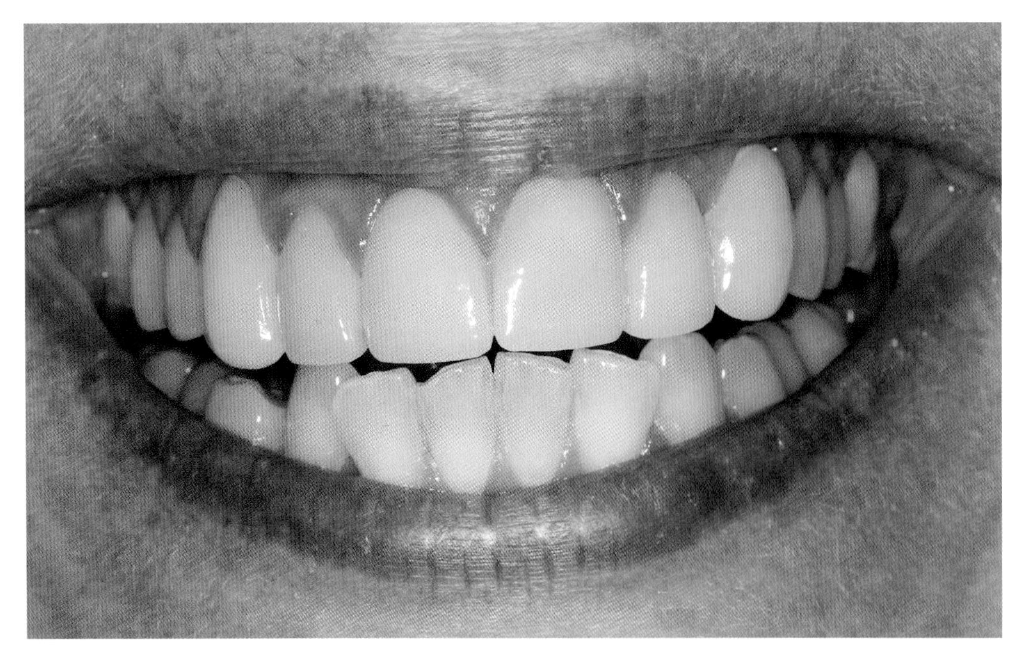

Fig. 5.4 An example of ceramic veneers associated with gingivitis.

NATURE OF TREATMENT

There are three factors that determine the direction that the treatment plan takes:

1. *patient factors*, including expectations and attitudes, socioeconomic factors, ability to control disease risk factors, medical history and ability to attend and pay for treatment
2. *dentist factors*, related to experience, training, type of practice and ethical philosophy, together with ability to understand the needs of the patient
3. *dental factors*, including periodontal status, endodontic status, quantity and quality of remaining tooth structure, length of span of any edentulous spaces, and angulation and position of any abutment teeth.

If patients cannot or will not comply with a prevention programme, then they may be unable or unwilling to maintain complex esthetic dentistry. Your work may fail and you may be responsible, not having informed or educated the patient suitably prior to providing the treatment.

Periodontal factors

Periodontal assessment is mandatory, even in what might seem to be a straightforward case involving simple changes to one or more teeth. Bleeding on probing and deep probing depths are indicative of the presence of periodontal disease. Approximately 20% of the population are susceptible to attachment loss of the supporting tissues, with half of these people able to reduce the damage through meticulous oral hygiene. The risk factors for periodontal disease are:

- plaque
- smoking
- medical conditions affecting the immune system, such as diabetes.

The ability to control these risk factors will affect the progression of the periodontal disease. Control of plaque will have the most important effect on the prognosis of periodontal breakdown.

Anatomical difficulties, such as furcation involvement and deep probing depths, can make access difficult for the patient and it will be hard to maintain good levels of plaque control. Esthetic restorations, such as labial veneers (see Fig. 5.4), often demonstrate a combination of poor marginal fit with small overhangs, bulbous contours and emergence angles, exposed composite lute and rough edges. All of these features provide a safe haven for bacteria, which oral hygiene measures cannot reach. Many photographs in dental magazines illustrate this: showing images of patients with good preoperative gingival health and a mild esthetic problem are shown side by side with postoperative images showing multiple bright uniform veneers, potential over-treatment and a loss of gingival health.

Recession also affects the appearance of the teeth and is more likely with thin gingival biotypes. Crown preparation on such elongated teeth is difficult and more destructive. Minimal intervention (MI) techniques are more appropriate. Margins should always be carefully chosen and patient consent must be given prior to tooth preparation.[7]

All oral tissues should be free from disease prior to complex restorative work. Overhangs and poorly fitting crowns should be removed, or trimmed as a short-term measure, to aid the patient to clean more effectively supra- and subgingivally.

Endodontic status

Esthetics can be dramatically affected by non-vital teeth, both restored and unrestored (see Fig. 5.3). Determining the apical and pulpal status of teeth is therefore an important part of the oral assessment.

Non-vital teeth restored with posts make unpredictable abutments and often compromise esthetics. Colour change is usually present, including darkening visible through the gingival tissues. Moreover, there is evidence to suggest that approximately 13% of teeth prepared for full-coverage crowns became non-vital postoperatively, compared to approximately 5% for partial-coverage restorations.[8] Cheung et al.[9] reported that over 50% of anterior bridge abutments had loss of pulp vitality – another good reason to adopt MI techniques. However, endodontically treated teeth often require occlusal protection. This is the focus of Volume 3 in this series.

The marginal ridges of posterior teeth are important in maintaining the strength of teeth undergoing endodontic procedures. The loss of one marginal ridge reduces tooth rigidity by approximately 5%, whereas the loss of both marginal ridges reduces rigidity by approximately 60%.[10]

Where post and cores cannot be avoided, it is best not to use such teeth as abutments in bridge design. In single, post-crowned tooth units, as much sound tooth as possible should be retained as a ferrule. Parallel-sided serrated cemented posts allow for maximal retention with the least stress induced to the remaining root. Approximately 3–5 mm of gutta percha should be left in the root canal to prevent leakage into the peri-radicular tissues.

Where the pulp status is questionable and extensive restorative work is planned, it may be prudent to carry out root canal treatment beforehand – elective endodontics – to prevent opening up of the tooth afterwards. It is known that coronal seal is more important than the technical quality of the endodontic obturation.[11] A difficult decision revolves around compromised broken-down teeth: is it best to provide endodontic treatment and restore, or extract and replace with an implant-retained restoration?

Tooth structure factors

Residual dentine thickness (RDT) is a key factor. The quality and quantity of remaining tooth structure have a significant effect on the ability to restore. Sound tooth structure should be preserved wherever possible. Where tooth structure is limited, the prognosis is reduced, although techniques utilizing adhesives and crown-lengthening can improve the situation. Tooth wear can substantially reduce RDT and conventional restorative techniques often remove even more dentine. Modern restorative procedures tend to work more with existing tooth tissue, preserving what remains and using adhesive material to restore lost volume. These adhesive materials have the additional benefit of being adjustable and repairable.

KEY POINT SUMMARY

Bond to enamel before it is lost through tooth wear and do not cut more of it off.

Figure 5.5 illustrates a case of advanced tooth wear in a 23-year-old man with correction of the esthetics and occlusion, and prevention of further damage through the use of bonded composite restorations to cover exposed dentine surfaces. At no stage was any enamel or dentine cut away from the already damaged teeth. The application of composite anteriorly to replace missing tissue was used to create space and restore vertical height, allowing the posterior teeth to over-erupt. This occlusal adaptation is sometimes referred to as the Dahl technique. The building-up of anterior teeth with an initial set of palatal veneers discludes the posterior teeth. This enables the patient to distalize the mandible and adopt a more comfortable and anatomically correct temporomandibular relationship, closer to centric relation (CR), within a few weeks. Intrusion of the restored teeth and extrusion of the other teeth typically take place over 4 months as part of occlusal adaptation to the new occlusal position. Research going back to the early 1960s[12] shows that high metal crowns do not cause pain, and intentionally high restorations have become a recognized method of treating tooth wear by replacing lost tissue.[13–15]

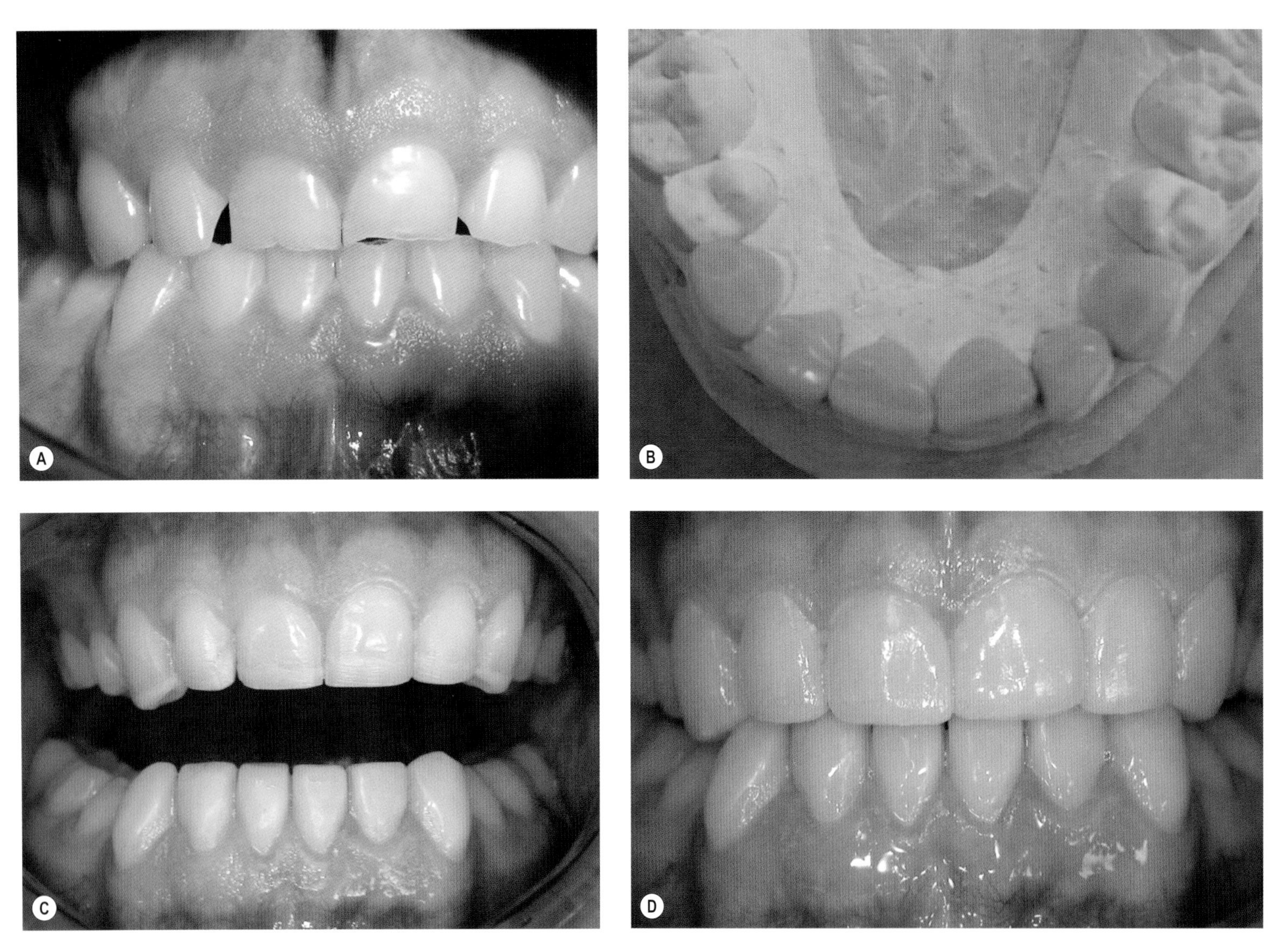

Fig. 5.5 Advanced tooth wear. A. Preoperative view of tooth surface loss. B. Casts with indirect composite veneers. C. Eight months later, following occlusal adaptation and restoration of the lower anterior teeth with non-invasive composite veneers. D. Restoration with non-invasive labial veneers.

Occlusal factors

Dental occlusion involves significant forces, complex movements and a range of vulnerable hard and soft tissues. These forces can be written off as destructive or made to work for us.

CLINICAL TIP

Look for signs of occlusal problems:

- wear
- fractured teeth
- fractured restorations
- unexplained tooth movement or mobility
- temporomandibular joint (TMJ) symptoms

Occlusal assessment

Assess the occlusion for two important features:

1. All teeth should meet when the patient closes into the inter-cuspal position (ICP), which should be at or close to CR.
2. Posterior disclusion is provided by anterior guidance.

Looking at this further: all teeth should come into occlusion simultaneously, but with provision for the posterior teeth to contact initially, and for the anterior teeth to come into contact close to, if not in, the ICP. A common error in esthetic dentistry is to adjust anterior restorations to contact at the same time as the posterior teeth. This results in displacement during clenching, giving rise to fracture, mobility and drifting.

The position into which the patient naturally closes should be close to CR. The ICP, or centric occlusion (CO), should be stable and not too far from CR, therefore maintaining the condyle in the correct position within the TMJ. Determining CR is difficult to achieve with precision and reproducibility. It has been beautifully described as the 'bite *du jour*',[16] indicating its daily variability and therefore the difficulty of recording it accurately.

Posterior disclusion is possibly the most important occlusal feature to maintain or create in restorative dentistry. It protects the posterior teeth (and TMJs) from adverse, damaging forces. This important feature is obtained through anterior guidance: simply, the way that the size, shape, contour and position of the anterior teeth bring about a separation of the posterior teeth. In other words, the posterior teeth must only contact in ICP, or ideally CR. Hence the use of bonded anterior restorations, such as the palatal composite restorations illustrated in Figure 5.4, which provide a fixed anterior repositioning splint with posterior disclusion to create a 'Lucia jig effect', allowing the patient to close in a position near to CR as part of their occlusal adaptation.

KEY POINT SUMMARY

The most important feature is disclusion. It has two key components:

- closure into CR or close to it with all teeth touching
- anterior guidance providing posterior disclusion

Adverse occlusal contacts – that is, any contact that prevents the above features being present – should be identified. Occlusal management is beyond the scope of this chapter but should be additive where possible, accentuating anterior guidance rather than reducing posterior cusps. After all, it is often the wear of canines that reduces anterior guidance, resulting in reduced disclusion and the formation of destructive non-working side contacts. In some cases (see Fig. 5.1), an interference preventing closure into CR, or close to it, should be removed with the patient's full understanding and consent. Unopposed, over-erupted teeth can cause significant occlusal interferences, mandibular repositioning with an adverse ICP, and varying degrees of occlusal damage.

Canine guidance has no advantage over group function, other than for restorative convenience. The occlusion should be carefully evaluated using articulated study casts, and any working and non-working interferences must be carefully assessed. If occlusal interferences exist and require removal, the proposed reduction should be carried out on duplicate articulated study casts prior to making any adjustments in the mouth.

Parafunctional patients should have splint therapy to reduce attritional tooth wear and the risk of failure of any restorative work. Often splints need to be provided postoperatively. Deep overbites often allow early posterior disclusion, facilitating posterior reconstructions, whereas shallow overbites require more prosthetic care to maintain posterior disclusion and avoid excursive interferences.

Restorative care can be either *conformative*, working within existing occlusal relationships – for example, the placement of a simple composite occlusal restoration; or *reorganized*, where the occlusal relationship is to be changed intentionally – for example, building up canines to create canine guidance in a group function case, or the use of Dahl restorations to enable occlusal adaptation to take place (see Fig. 5.5).

Accept or change the existing occlusion?

The need to choose between a conformative or reorganized approach arises in many aspects of dentistry. In esthetic dentistry, when it is considered appropriate to restore an anterior tooth, the practitioner must decide whether the new restoration should be made to match the existing teeth (conformative), which may involve compromising esthetics, or whether to go for the reorganized approach of smile design, changing the overall esthetics of the smile zone.

Similarly, in restorative dentistry, there are many times when the existing occlusion is accepted and a new restoration designed to fit in. However, there

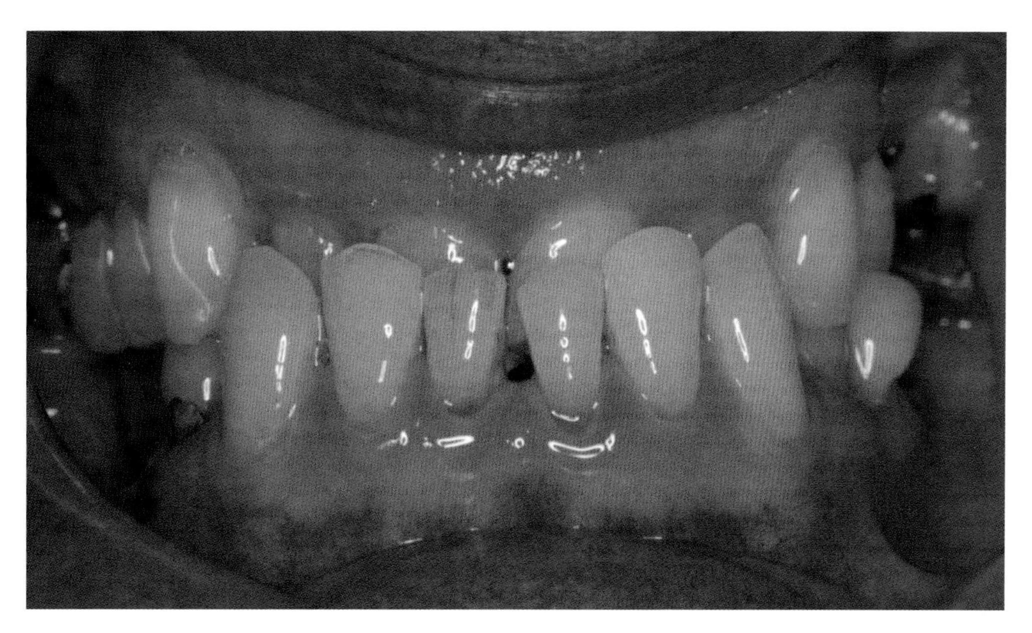

Fig. 5.6 An example of a patient who cannot be restored in centric relation.

are situations where it is preferable to take the opportunity to reorganize the occlusion: that is, when ICP is flawed, missing, compromised, unstable, too far from CR or unreproducible. If the clinician has checked both ICP and CR and is uncomfortable about restoring to the current ICP, then RCP/CR should be considered. It may not always be possible or desirable to convert the patient back into CR (Fig. 5.6).

The traditional Lucia jig is a useful concept but suffers from being removable. Nowadays, the bonded equivalent has the benefit of providing prevention, esthetic improvement and occlusal correction through rapid repositioning of the mandible by the patient into CR, as shown in Figure 5.5.

CLINICAL TIP

To obtain centric relation:

- the clinician can carry out manipulation
- the patient can insert and wear a Lucia jig or Michigan splint
- the occlusion can adapt by itself where anterior Dahl restorations are placed

The use of splints

In the management of acute episodes of pain, a full-coverage soft splint may have a place but otherwise does little more than provide a placebo effect. This,

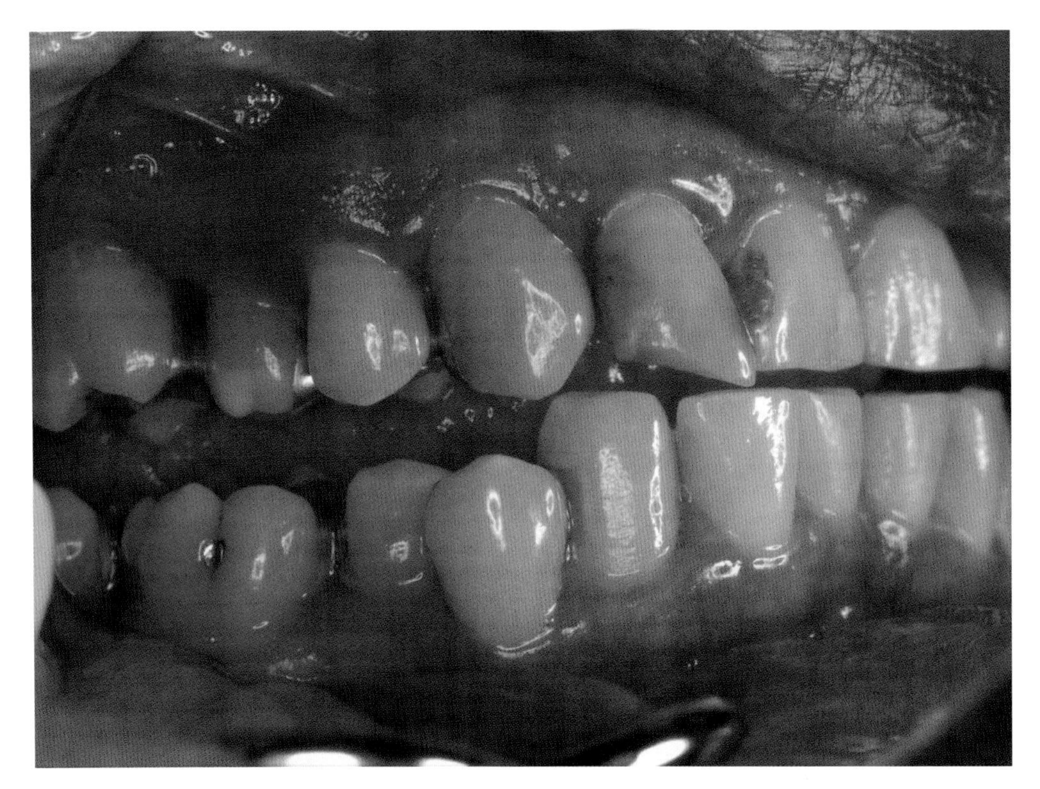

Fig. 5.7 Posterior intrusion caused by prolonged wearing of a posterior splint.

however, is not to be undervalued. Full-coverage acrylic stabilization splints to correct the occlusion, according to the features listed above, are of great value. They can be used to provide relief from temporomandibular dysfunction (TMD), headaches and muscle pain, as well as to protect restorations. They can be easily converted into repositioning splints for more advanced therapies such as disk recapture. Partial-coverage splints have some indications but must be closely monitored as tooth intrusion can occur (Fig. 5.7).

PROGNOSIS AND OUTCOMES

The decision-making process relating to whether a tooth can be restored or not, and to its potential replacement if extracted, can be summarized as shown in Figure 5.8. Assessing the tooth using these factors gives an indication of its long-term prognosis. A tooth with a poor prognosis may, however, still have some value. For example, a periodontally compromised, endodontically treated tooth reduced to gingival level may continue to have some value in maintaining what little gingival attachment remains, and provide support as an overdenture abutment. It is best to plan the loss of a tooth if it compromises the overall treatment plan; however, if is to be retained for the short to medium term, definitive plans should be laid down to deal with its eventual loss.

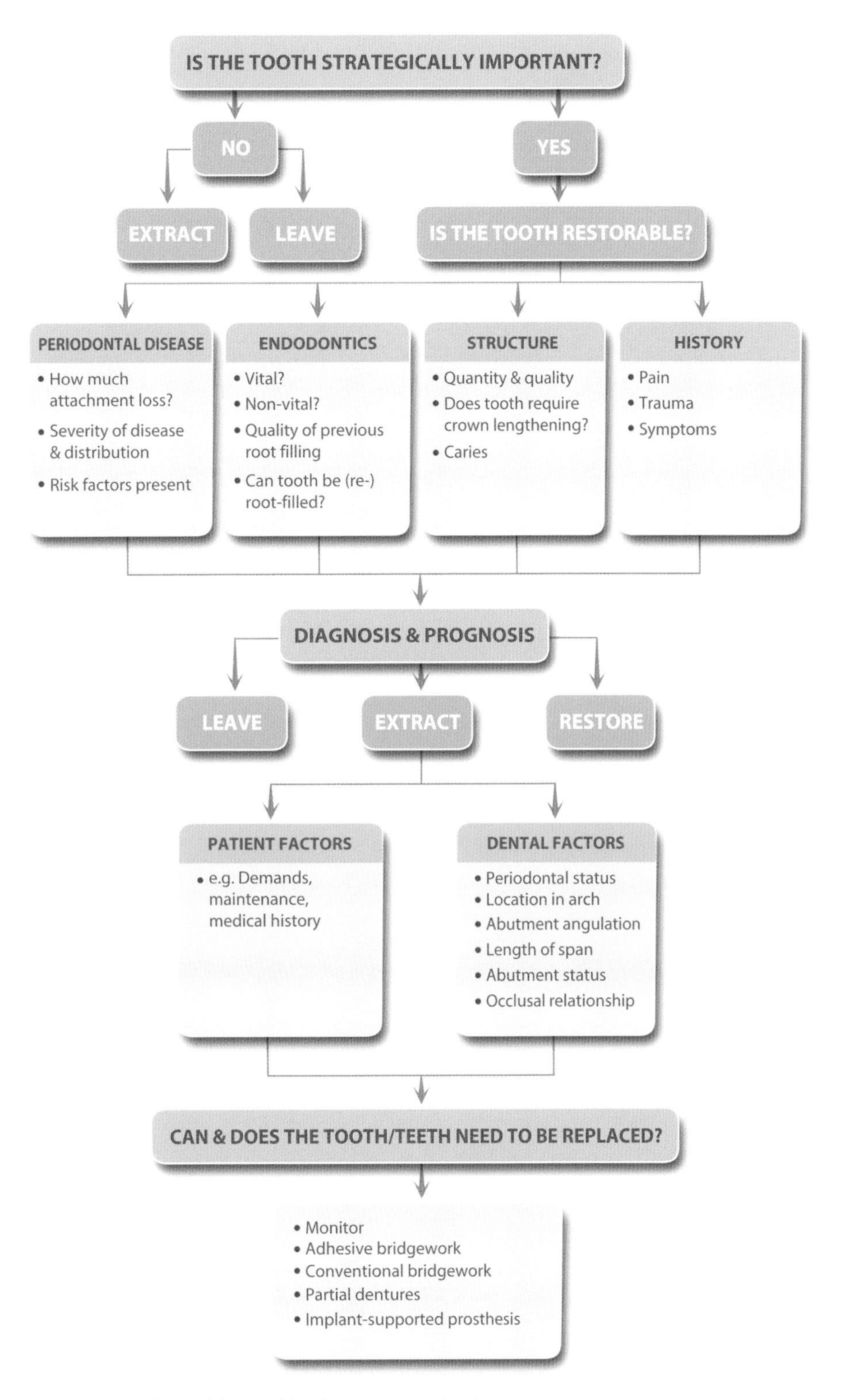

Fig. 5.8 Flow chart for decision-making in restorative dentistry.

DELIVERY OF ESTHETIC RESTORATIONS

This is the focus of the other volumes in the *Essentials of Esthetic Dentistry* series, but the main points are summarized here.

TREATMENT PRINCIPLES

KEY POINT SUMMARY

Replace what is missing without damaging what is remaining.

A patient should be offered all reasonable treatment options even if you, the practitioner, cannot carry them all out and referral to another practitioner is required. Lack of training, lack of ability, lack of enthusiasm for a particular approach or lack of equipment is no excuse for limiting a patient's treatment options.

Dental schools around the world tend not to teach advanced esthetic dentistry techniques at graduate level, despite methods in this field having been developed and validated over a number of years. Hence, practitioners interested in providing such care need to undergo suitable postgraduate training to become competent in the relevant techniques and processes. Several leading dental institutes now run Masters programmes in esthetic dentistry both as part of internal programmes and online via blended delivery.

Ethical and professional principles are often challenged in the field of esthetic dentistry, as the treatment needs of the patient tend not to be health-related. The surgical removal of diseased tissue is what surgeons, including dental surgeons, do. However, cutting irreplaceable dental tissue in the pursuit of an esthetic outcome puts practitioners in a difficult decision-making position, covered in detail in Chapter 2.

OVERVIEW OF TECHNIQUES FOR ESTHETIC TOOTH CORRECTION

Non-invasive options

Esthetic dentistry can sometimes be non-invasive, although there are only a few examples of this:

- *Tooth-whitening* – the provision of 6% hydrogen peroxide and 10% carbamide peroxide gels in close-fitting trays for home use is a proven and popular technique.
- *Orthodontics* – the use of aligners is popular, although fixed appliance therapy remains the gold standard.

- *Adhesive restorations* – this includes resin-bonded bridges without tooth preparation.
- *Direct bonding of composite resin* to reshape teeth, close spaces and cover defects – this is increasing in popularity as adhesives, composites and techniques improve.
- *Clip-on acrylic resin overdenture-type devices*, such as the Snap-On Smile (Denmat) – these can be effective where existing teeth are small or spaced, as discussed in Chapter 3.
- *Removable prostheses* without tooth preparation.

Minimal intervention options

In many cases, some irreversible tooth reduction is required but is considered to constitute minimal damage:

- correctly designed veneers, using a variety of techniques – direct composite, laboratory composite, ceramic or semi-direct systems
- adhesive bridges on minimal preparations
- removable prostheses with tooth preparation.

Significant tooth reduction

Conventional esthetic dentistry requires significant tooth reduction.

Prepared ceramic veneers

The tooth will require some reduction to accommodate the cervical 0.3 mm ceramic edge; otherwise, a ledge will be created. On many teeth, this cervical reduction will breach the enamel–dentine junction (EDJ). Full labial coverage is required, as matching ceramic to enamel on a visible surface is close to impossible. Veneers are less destructive than crowns and offer esthetic control of labial and incisal surfaces. Where a slice preparation is carried out, the clinician can also control the proximal surfaces and alter tooth width, as well as contour to eliminate gingival black triangles, as discussed in more detail in Volume 2.

Crowns

These are much more destructive of tooth tissue and should rarely be placed on teeth not already crowned. Pascal Magne has, for the past decade, stated in lectures that there are no indications for the initial placement of crowns on teeth, and the author tends to agree with this view. There is almost always a better, more conservative restoration (for example, a veneer) or treatment (for example, orthodontics). Massive tooth reduction of the type necessary for a crown will increase the likelihood of devitalization and the need for endodontics and a post, greatly reducing the tooth's chances of survival. A clinician may be tempted to crown an anterior tooth if every surface requires contour change; however, this can be achieved by the MI approach (see Fig. 5.5).

Conventional bridges (fixed prostheses)

These are less often indicated nowadays, given the risk of failure and poor salvage potential. Design should be minimal wherever possible, observing the published data, which indicate that two-unit bridges – one pontic and one retainer – offer the best survival in most cases.

Implant-retained restorations

These are often seen as the treatment of choice for a missing tooth in an intact healthy arch, provided local and systemic factors permit. However, implant failure and its devastating implications and high cost of salvage must be taken into account at the initial treatment planning stage.

ESTHETIC COMPONENTS OF TEETH

Esthetic dentistry requires control of three components of the teeth in the smile zone: colour, shape and position.

Colour

Ideally, any discoloured teeth should be whitened to match the arch. Then, perhaps, the whole arch should be whitened. The use of 10% carbamide peroxide in trays is well tested and evidence-based. Be aware, however, of the risk of over-whitening imperfect teeth. Excessive whitening draws attention to the smile. This may not be a problem, if it is a perfect smile. Otherwise, it will draw the viewer's eye to black triangles and other shape and position defects.

Shape

Today's adhesives enable practitioners to bond composite to enamel, dentine, ceramic, metal and existing composite. Composite can be used in any thickness, and can be thinned to a knife-edge when used in anterior teeth, and colour-blended to match existing tooth tissue. Generally, two layers are required; rarely, three or more. New materials have improved polish retention and better colour match. Layered shade guides are now available.

Ceramic restorations provide a long-lasting surface finish but require extensive preparation, including full labial surface coverage. This forces the practitioner to carry out enamel reduction on labial and often proximal surfaces, which may expose and remove dentine. Pulp exposure has been reported following porcelain veneer preparation.

Position

Orthodontics is the means to realign teeth, unless additive techniques will suffice. Subtractive methods should rarely be used.

TREATMENT OPTIONS FOR TOOTH REPLACEMENT

When assessing the smile, you will be aware of the three key components of colour. Missing tooth tissue appears as the colour black in the smile zone, causing patients more concern than white or pink colour problems. A missing tooth is therefore a major concern.

Monitoring

When the disease process has been stabilized and there are limited functional or esthetic effects from missing teeth, it is prudent to monitor the patient and their dentition. Poorly motivated patients may not be suitable for invasive therapy such as implants. Monitoring can take place through the use of study casts and photographs with periodic examination and assessment. Numerical indices have little value in monitoring tooth wear in individuals, as they are subjective and difficult to standardize. It is important for the patient to understand that recall is essential and that, if deterioration is recognized, further treatment may be necessary. This aspect of the treatment plan should not take the form of 'supervised neglect', allowing deterioration of the patient's condition without the dentist or the patient being aware of change. It is wise to set end points, such as establishing that when the tooth wear involves dentine, intervention is indicated.

It may be tempting to replace missing teeth with implant-retained crowns and bridges, conventional or adhesive bridges, or dentures. Patients can often function and manage with missing teeth, however, and no action may be the healthier option for them and their remaining teeth, particularly in the longer term when oral hygiene may be more difficult to maintain around complex restorations. The shortened dental arch (SDA) concept, stating that older patients can function with 10 upper and 10 lower anterior teeth, may find applications in esthetic dentistry. This requires discussion with the patient and may need to be the preferred option while disease is managed and prevention is applied and monitored. Detailed treatment planning can be undertaken while a case is being monitored.

From an esthetic viewpoint, missing teeth that create visible spaces when a person is smiling will need to be replaced. However, the patient must be made aware of the risks involved and must realize that there is unlikely to be any functional gain, despite the esthetic benefit.

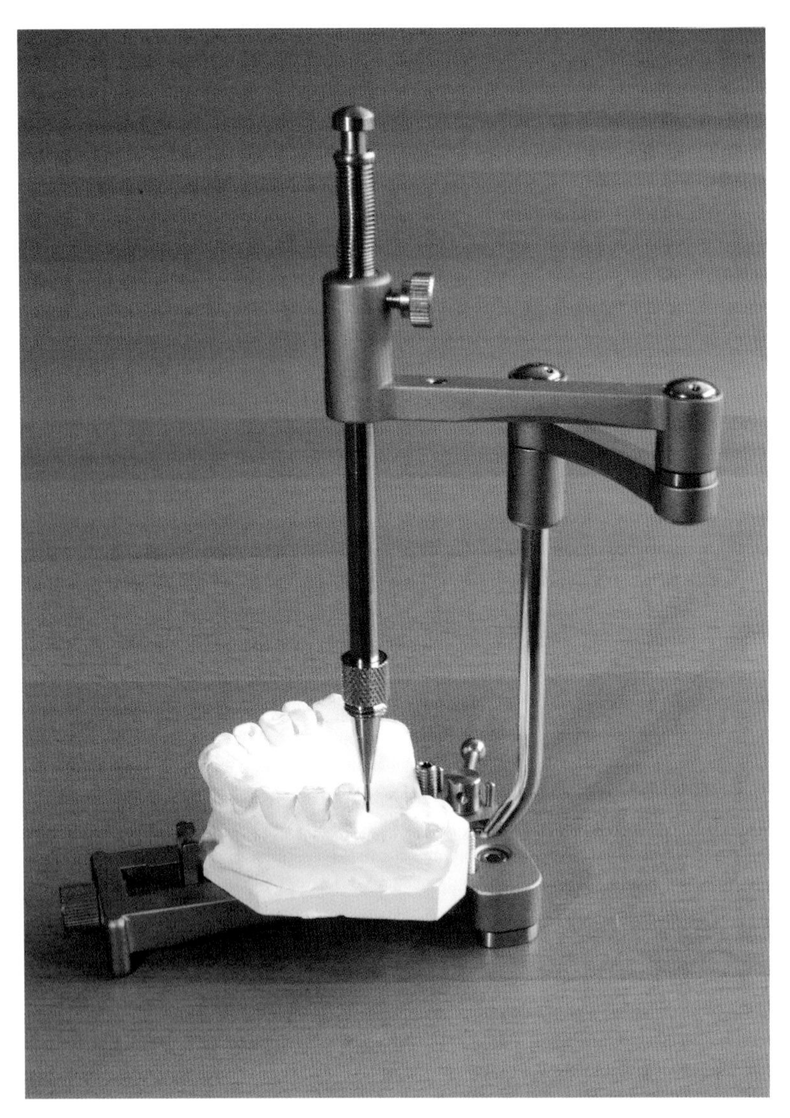

Fig. 5.9 Surveying a study cast on a portable surveyor (Micro Surveyor, Compass, Japan).

Removable prostheses

Where edentulous spaces are numerous, abutment teeth poorly angulated or teeth shortened through wear, when oral hygiene is less than ideal, or for reasons of cost, then partial dentures should be considered. These are also suitable when ridge form has been lost and requires restoration. Pre-restorative preparation of the mouth is required, with appropriately planned design of clasps and rest seats. Ideally, support should be gained from the teeth, but this is not always possible. Guide planes allow one path of insertion and should be carefully considered during the planning stages using study casts on a surveyor. The use of esthetic removable prostheses will be the subject of a later volume.

Adhesive bridgework

Bonding to the remaining tooth structure of the abutment teeth has the advantage of being the least destructive option. Ideally, little ridge form should be lost and the abutment teeth should be sound. Studies suggest single-tooth cantilever designs in comparison to fixed-fixed designs. Good-quality enamel is essential for adherence and ideally the pontic should be of similar size or smaller than the retainer. Good moisture control is also essential to avoid contamination of the adhesive surfaces. Surveying the study casts, as shown in Figure 5.9, can help select a suitable path of insertion to minimize the need for tooth reduction. In the posterior region of the lower arch, modifying the path of insertion by tilting lingually can lower the lingual survey line and avoid the need for enamel reduction.

A recent analysis of published studies[17] indicates annual failure rates to be 4.6% (±1.3%) for metal-framed adhesive bridges, 4.1% (±2.1%) for fibre-reinforced adhesive bridges and 11.7% (±1.8%) for all-ceramic adhesive bridges. The most frequent complications were: debonding for metal-framed resin-bonded bridges (93% of all failures); delamination of the composite veneering material for the fibre-reinforced bridges (41%); and fracture of the framework for the all-ceramic bridges (57%). All types of resin-bonded bridges provide an effective short- to medium-term option, with all-ceramic types performing least well and having the least favourable mode of failure.

Conventional bridgework

Where adhesive bridgework is not suitable due to large spans, compromised abutment teeth, or enamel lacking in quality and quantity, then conventional bridgework may be more appropriate. However, conventional bridgework is associated with greater tooth reduction, leaving less tooth structure for treatment in the future.

The abutments should ideally not have post cores, as these have a poor prognosis in comparison to vital abutments. Little ridge form should be lost with angulation of the abutment teeth close to parallel, unless fixed-movable connectors are to be used; this requires meticulous planning beforehand.

Salvage when a conventional bridge fails is a major concern. There is usually marginal failure, pulp death or failure of root fillings due to leakage, periapical infection and sometimes root fracture. Frequently, caries is seen to have separated the retainer from the underlying abutment tooth. The majority of failed conventional bridges are replaced with removable prostheses, as further fixed options are no longer available. Many lessons learnt from adhesive bridges can be applied to conventional bridges: single abutments and cantilever designs should be employed where possible.

Implant-supported prostheses

Implants provide options where tooth support cannot be gained without significant tooth destruction, or where other fixed options are contraindicated. All the alternatives discussed above should be considered beforehand due to the expense of implants. Sufficient bone should be present for accurate implant placement and requires meticulous planning beforehand. If experience is lacking in such an area, referral to a specialist should be considered.

Treatment planning with implant-supported restorations must be realistic. Implants can fail, sometimes catastrophically. A high standard of oral hygiene is essential. As a patient ages, the demand on that person to maintain a high level of hygiene around complex restorations must be considered.

DEVISING A TREATMENT PLAN

Clinicians will usually have an approach to formulating a treatment plan that is customized for the individual case. It should be written down for the patient, using accessible language, and integrated with the patient's photographs where possible. It will summarize the diagnosis, risks and prognosis. The treatment options should be listed and all realistic options provided. In terms of sequence, the gold standard option should be given first. Pros and cons should be given for each option in a neutral way to avoid pushing the patient in a preferred direction. Known costs and any unknown additional expense must be clearly stated.

The patient should be given adequate opportunity to discuss the options at the time and at later visits. Consent should be built into the treatment-planning documentation and signed to show agreement and that the risks have been understood; an opportunity to ask questions must be provided.

When the treatment plan has been devised, the final stage prior to treatment is to plan, step by step, all the procedures that will be carried out in the clinic and the laboratory. An estimate of the amount of time allocated to each procedure will help timing and accurate costing. Costs can be determined according to items of work required, or based on the time allocated to the case multiplied by the hourly rate plus laboratory bills.

SELECTING A TREATMENT OPTION

Posting a typed treatment plan to the patient soon after the assessment appointment and then inviting the person back to the practice to discuss the options and to ask questions seems to be the most logical approach. It has been said that the options should be financially neutral to the clinician in order to avoid bias towards the promotion of one treatment option over another. However, the clinician can state a preference: for example, towards an MI approach.

There may be an instance where an option is technically available but the clinician would be uncomfortable in going ahead with it: for example, providing extractions and dentures for an esthetic case that could be corrected by orthodontics. It is better not to treat a case and to suggest a referral rather than starting or continuing with a treatment that the clinician feels to be inappropriate.

The practitioner must avoid an uncomfortable compromise; doing it 'because the patient wants it' is not the basis for ethical and appropriate treatment. If a patient, or anyone else for that matter, requests that you do something unethical, you would have no hesitation in refusing on professional, personal or moral grounds. Yet, so often at professional meetings, we see examples of over-treatment, with the clinician attempting to justify it because 'the patient wanted it'. Figure 5.10 shows such a case.

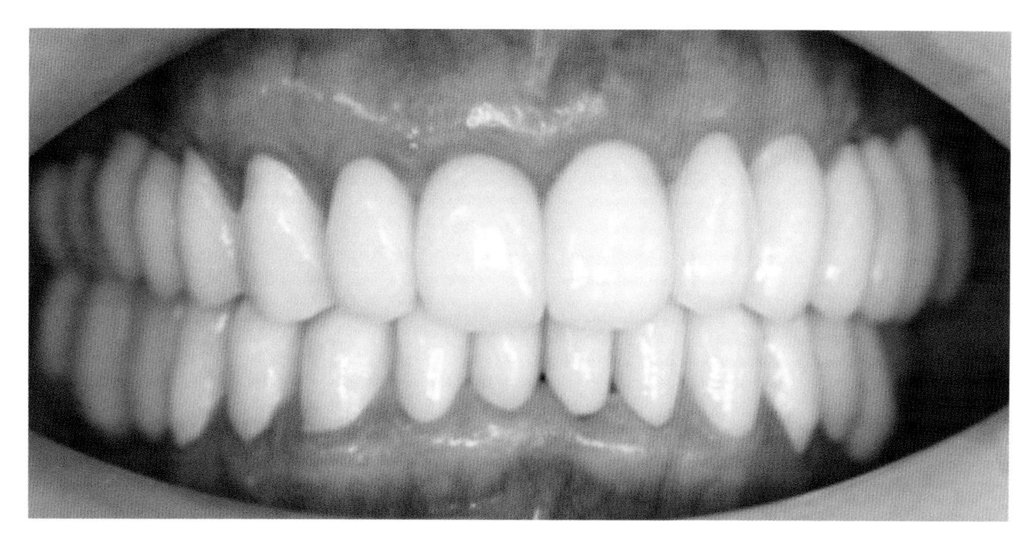

Fig. 5.10 Shade selection. This 85-year-old female patient apparently selected the shade and wanted crowns but was she poorly advised? Is it always correct to give patients what they want? Answer – NO.

A treatment plan should therefore contain only those options that are morally and ethically appropriate and can be openly defended. It must be based on what is judged to be best for the patient without consideration of the clinician's financial interest. Ideally, treatments should be cost-neutral to avoid a selling bias. Apply the daughter test.

CLINICAL TIP

Remember the 'daughter test': do not carry out treatment on one of your patients that you would not be prepared to do in an identical way on your daughter, given the same clinical scenario (Martin Kelleher).

You may, of course, include appropriate treatment options that you cannot carry out yourself and which require referral. You should not avoid presenting an option just because you or your practice cannot provide the treatment.

HELPING THE PATIENT SELECT THE OPTIONS

Who decides? Ultimately, the treatment plan to be adopted should be the decision of the patient, possibly guided by the dental team and by the information you have provided. The patient needs the clinician's expertise and guidance but, in the process, the practitioner must not overrule the patient. The patient is aware of numerous personal and financial factors that will need to be weighed up. Clear advice, the use of photographs and radiographs, and an unhurried approach invariably help the process.

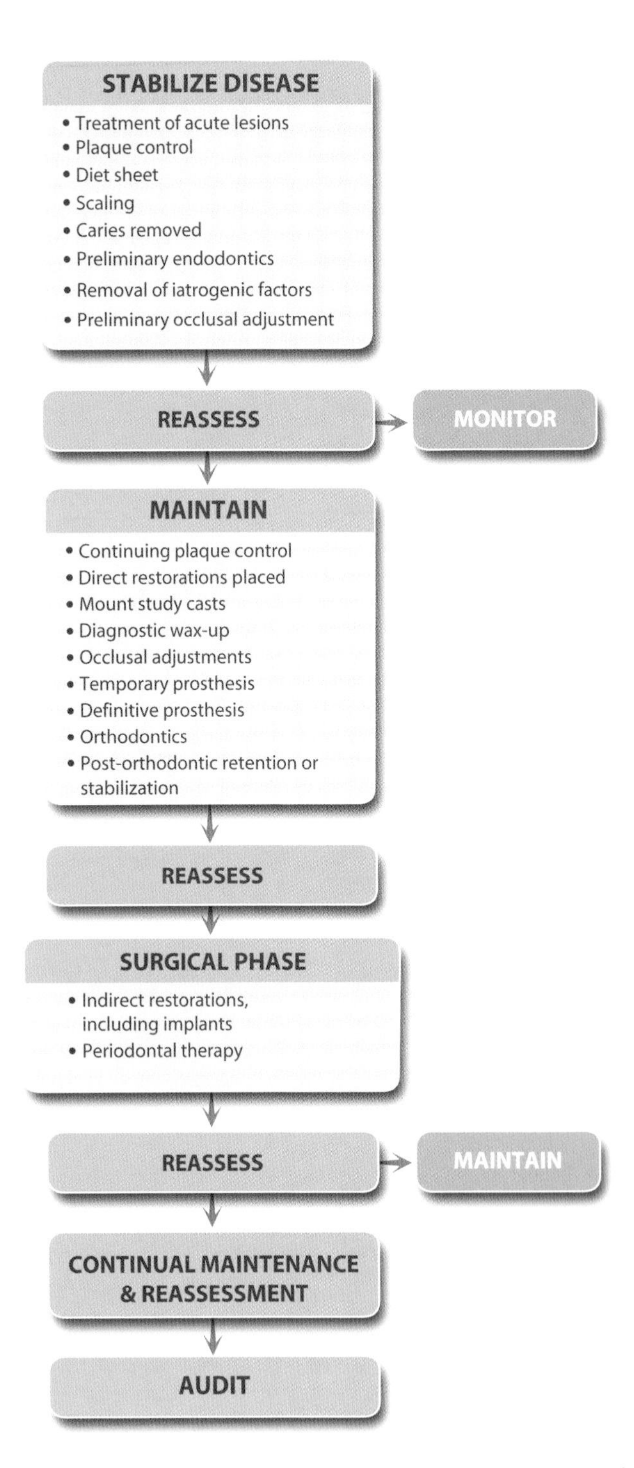

Fig. 5.11 A summary flowchart for the planning of esthetic and restorative care. Actual sequencing and detail will depend on individual cases.

COMMUNICATION OF INFORMATION TO THE PATIENT

It will often be difficult for the patient to visualize an esthetic outcome. Fortunately, there are now many techniques from digital designs on the patient's dental and facial photographs to actual physical mock-ups, many based on a diagnostic wax-up to provide squash-on and clip-on trials to visualize, assess and even test-drive the potential outcome. These are covered in detail in Volume 2.

CONCLUDING REMARKS

A suggested flowchart for the planning of esthetic and restorative dental care is reproduced in Figure 5.11.

KEY POINT SUMMARY

- Accurate diagnosis of a patient's problem is essential for effective treatment planning
- An accurate diagnosis is only possible following a detailed dental and medical history, both of which may affect the outcome of proposed treatment
- Risk factors for dental disease, such as smoking, must be recognized by the clinician early and highlighted to the patient
- Examination of a patient should always follow a systematic order to ensure that no areas are overlooked
- Clinicians should readily seek a second opinion from colleagues if a diagnosis or treatment plan is in doubt
- Whenever possible, treatment plans should be non-invasive and reversible
- A treatment plan is incomplete unless the patient has given informed consent regarding all options

REFERENCES

1. Chavez EM. Systematic review of the medication list: a resource for risk assessment and dental management. J Calif Dent Assoc 2008;36:739–45.
2. Derlega VJ. Reasons for HIV disclosure/nondisclosure in close relationships: testing a model of HIV disclosure decision making. J Soc Clin Psychol 2004;23:747–67.
3. Cohen LA, Bonito AL, Eicheldinger C, et al. Correlation of dental problem and socioeconomic situation. J Am Dent Assoc 2011;142:137–49.
4. Newsome P, Smales F, Yin XX. Oral diagnosis and treatment planning: part 1. Introduction. Br Dent J 2012;213:15–19.
5. Nalbandian S, Millar BJ. The effect of veneers on cosmetic improvement. Br Dent J 2009;207: 72–3.
6. Edelhoff D, Sorensen JA. Tooth structure removal associated with various preparation designs for anterior teeth. J Prosthet Dent 2002;87:503–9.

7. Bishop K, Briggs P, Kelleher M. Margin design for porcelain fused to metal restorations which extend onto the root. Br Dent J 1996;180:177–84.

8. Felton D, Madison S, Kanoy E, et al. Long term effects of crown preparation on pulp vitality. J Dent Res 1989;68:1009. (Abstract).

9. Cheung GSP, Dimmer A, Mellor P, et al. A clinical evaluation of conventional bridgework. J Oral Rehabil 1990;7:131–6.

10. Reeh ES, Messer HH, Douglas WH. Reduction in tooth stiffness as a result of endodontic and restorative procedures. J Endod 1989;15:512–16.

11. Ray HA, Trope M. Periapical status of endodontically treated teeth in relation to the technical quality of the root filling and the coronal restoration. Int Endod J 1995;28:12–18.

12. Anderson DJ. Tooth movement in experimental malocclusion. Arch Oral Biol 1962;7:7–15.

13. Dahl BL, Krogstad O, Karlsen K. An alternative treatment in cases with advanced localized attrition. J Oral Rehabil 1975;2:209–14.

14. Poyser NJ, Porter RW, Briggs PF, et al. The Dahl Concept: past, present and future. Br Dent J 2005;198:669–76.

15. Magne P, Magne M, Belser UC. Adhesive restorations, centric relation, and the Dahl principle: minimally invasive approaches to localized anterior tooth erosion. Eur J Esthet Dent 2007;2:260–73.

16. Becker IM. Comprehensive occlusal concepts in clinical practice. Oxford: Wiley–Blackwell; 2011.

17. Miettinen M, Millar BJ. A literature review on the success and failure characteristics of resin-bonded bridges. Br Dent J 2013;215:E3.

CHAPTER 6

Periodontal Aspects of Esthetic Dentistry: Managing Recession Defects

AMIT PATEL AND IAIN CHAPPLE

INTRODUCTION

For thousands of years men and women have been obsessed with beauty and attractiveness. An important element of dental and, in turn, facial attractiveness is the appearance of the periodontal tissues, in particular the gingivae.

Whilst advances in surgical techniques have focused on the successful management of disease, a major secondary consideration has been an acceptable post-operative appearance, particularly in the development of surgical procedures involving the face. Advances in dental procedures have been no exception, with one of the desired outcomes of oral and dental operative interventions being good facial and dental esthetics. Patients who wish to have a perfect smile are seen on a daily basis in periodontal practice. Many of these patients undergo orthodontic therapy, smile redesign or restorative reconstruction, as dealt with in detail elsewhere in this book. Success in such cases often depends on the extent to which a symmetrical gingival contour is maintained, or, more commonly, recreated and then maintained to frame the teeth. When patients seeking enhancement of their orofacial attractiveness present requesting correction of gingival recession (the most common cause of gingival tissue loss), it is essential that clinical decisions are based on careful periodontal assessment and diagnosis, and the most appropriate surgical technique is employed if complete, esthetically pleasing root coverage is to be achieved (Fig. 6.1). This requires patient engagement and cooperation, together with an informed, evidence-based, biological approach to the management of the gingival defects.

THE PATIENT'S CONCERNS

The majority of patients with recession will be unaware of it and those seeking treatment will do so because of dentine sensitivity. Patients are often concerned that the condition may get worse.

This chapter will focus on the management of gingival recession, but this is not to ignore the wider range of soft-tissue esthetic challenges that may present, and require referral to a periodontal specialist. Other challenges include excess gingival display and gingival overgrowth. These conditions may require correction by crown-lengthening surgery to augment crowns, bridges or veneers, or resective procedures, but in ways that do not compromise the biological width. This chapter, with its emphasis on the management of gingival recession within the esthetic zone, is intended to complement the other aspects of the book dealing with periodontal health and attractiveness.

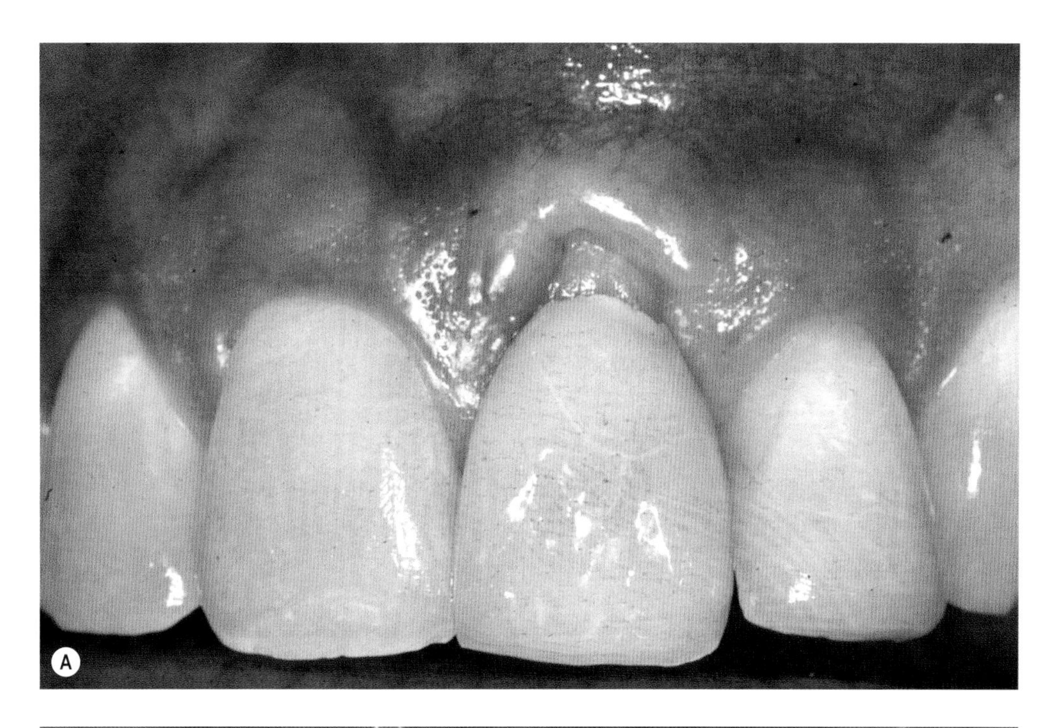

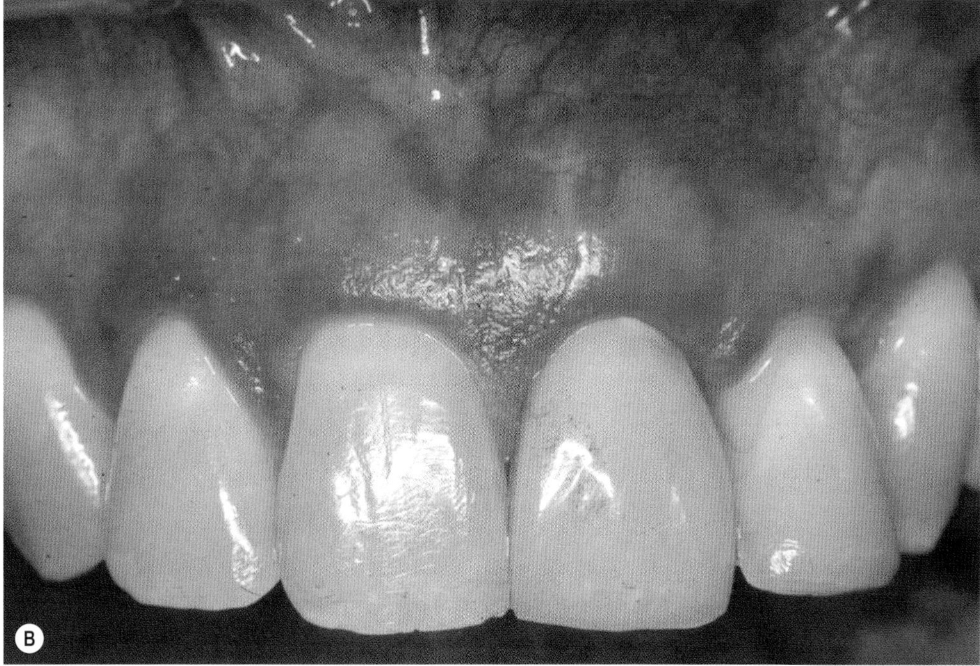

Fig. 6.1 Colour matching. A. A patient with gingival pigmentation. B. Colour matching achieved with a laterally repositioned flap.

KEY POINT SUMMARY

Biological width is the combined dimension of the junctional epithelium and connective tissue attachment: that is, the height between the deepest point of the gingival sulcus and the crest of the alveolar bone.

DEFINITION

Gingival recession is defined as the displacement of the gingival margin apical to the cemento-enamel junction (CEJ). It is characterized by the loss of the periodontal connective tissue fibres along the root cementum and by concomitant loss of alveolar bone. The causes of gingival recession include:

- inflammatory periodontal diseases
- trauma from over-zealous oral hygiene
- periods of recurrent gingival inflammation over underlying bone dehiscence or fenestration
- recurrent inflammation associated with overhanging restorations
- orthodontic tooth movement through the labial bone plate
- viral-induced ulceration of the gingival margin
- cytotoxic drug-induced ulceration of the gingival margin
- neutropenia (benign familial)
- traumatic injuries to the gingival margin
- gingival ischaemia.[1–4]

Gingival recession defects are typically treated by mucogingival surgery, aimed at the esthetic, biologically sustainable correction of defects of the morphology, position and/or dimensions of the gingiva.

Although gingival recession in itself does not appear to be associated with adverse effects on the health of the periodontal tissues, it may lead to root hypersensitivity, compromised gingival esthetics and cervical root caries. In some situations, changing the anatomy of the marginal gingival tissues – for example, repositioning the tissues coronally – may improve the effectiveness of oral hygiene aids, simplify plaque control and thereby limit the risk of adverse effects. Other approaches, when minimal, non-surgical intervention may be indicated, include orthodontic interventions.

There is some controversy regarding the prognosis of repairs of mucogingival defects. One study concluded that a minimum width of attached and keratinized gingiva of 2 mm is required to maintain gingival health and resist the trauma of tooth-brushing (Fig. 6.2).[5] Others have concluded, however, that there is no minimum width of attached and keratinized gingiva necessary to maintain gingival health.[6] These differences may be explained by the findings of a study in

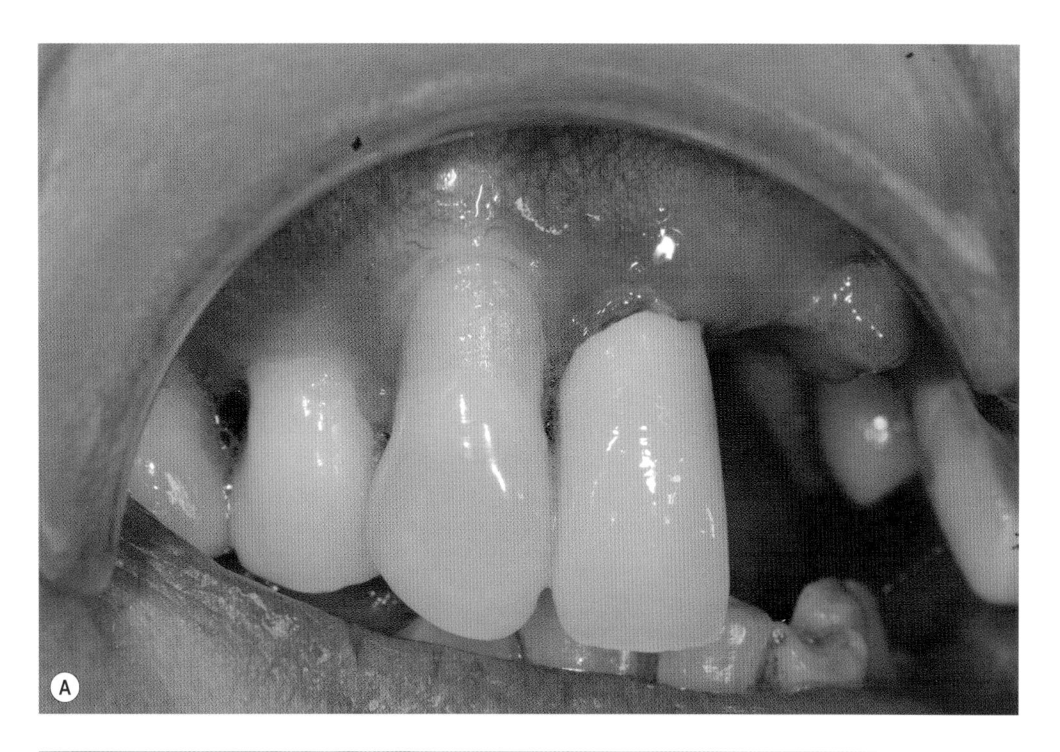

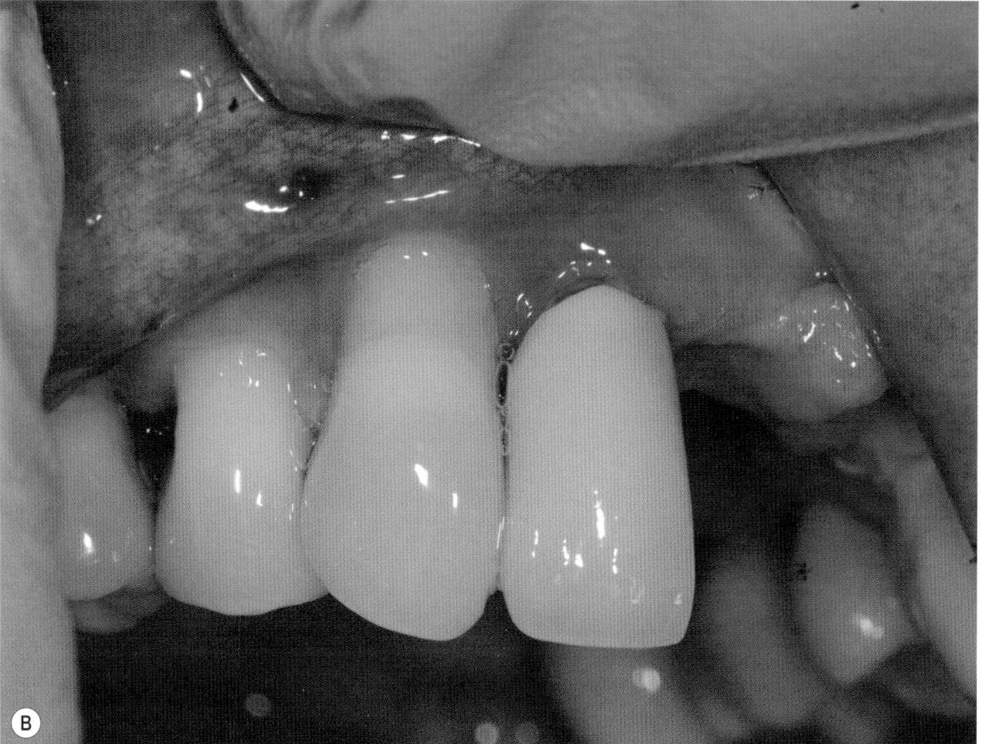

Fig. 6.2 Assessment of mucogingival defects. A. Upper right canine with no minimum width of keratinized tissue. B. By rolling the mucosal tissue one can assess the amount of keratinized tissue present.

which it was observed that mucogingival defects in the presence of plaque showed signs of inflammation clinically, but not at a histological level.[7] This implied that such areas are no more likely to develop further lesions than sites with an 'adequate' zone of attached gingiva. A further study, conducted by Dorfman, involved a split mouth design in 22 patients with bilateral recession defects. One side was treated by gingival graft surgery and the other by scaling and root planing, with prophylaxis being performed at 3 and 6 months. After a 4-year postoperative follow-up, the non-grafted sites suffered no further recession. In some cases there was tissue 'regain', so-called 'gingival creep-back'.[8] This, however, does not address the impact of the presence of recession defects in the esthetic zone.

CLASSIFICATION

Gingival recession can be categorized using Miller's classification (Fig. 6.3).[9] This classification remains the most widely employed system for local recession defects. It is based on the morphological evaluation of the defect and the likelihood of achieving full or at least partial root coverage following surgery.

Class I and class II recession defects of less than 5 mm have been shown to be favourable for complete root coverage. Class III recession defects have a poor prognosis for complete root coverage. When dealing with class IV defects, root coverage is unlikely to be achieved (Fig. 6.4).

When assessing gingival recession, it is important to view the mouth as a whole, as illustrated in Figure 6.5. In this figure, the upper left central incisor appears to be associated with a Miller class I recession defect. On close examination, however, the CEJ is at the correct level and the gingival levels are coronal to the CEJ. In such circumstances, the correct treatment option may be to crown-lengthen the upper right central incisor to achieve a more harmonious gingival contour.

FLAP THICKNESS, VASCULARITY AND POSITIONING

The gingival biotype is a good predictor of the likelihood of complete root coverage. A thick biotype, displaying a deep and wide zone of keratinized tissue, and therefore providing a thicker flap, is more likely to achieve complete root coverage. A thin biotype, where a shallow and narrow zone of keratinized tissue is present, makes the surgical procedure more difficult as the tissues are delicate and postoperative complications, such as flap necrosis, are relatively common. Studies have suggested that flap thickness is associated with complete root coverage. Whilst a thin flap is likely to break down, a thicker flap possesses greater

Class I
Recession defect not extending beyond mucogingival junction and no loss of interdental soft tissue and bone

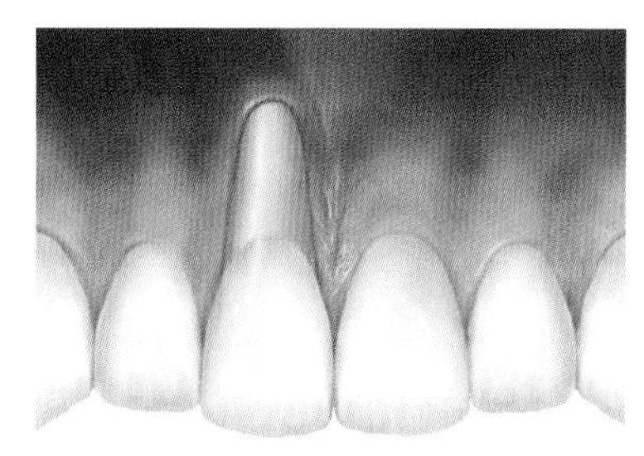

Class II
Recession defect extending beyond mucogingival junction and no loss of interdental soft tissue and bone

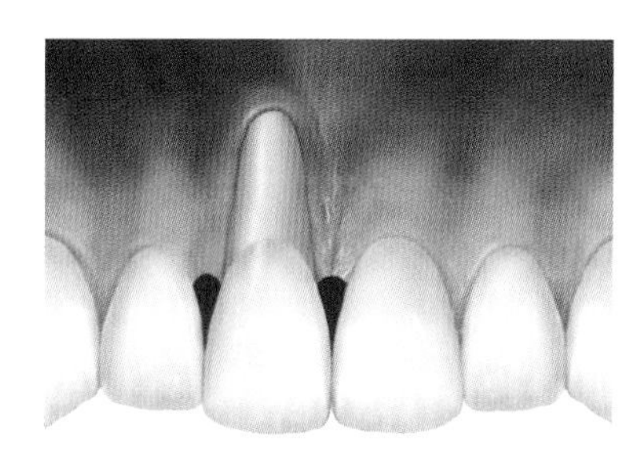

Class III
Recession defect extending beyond mucogingival junction with loss of interdental soft tissue and bone apical to the cemento-enamel junction but coronal to the recession

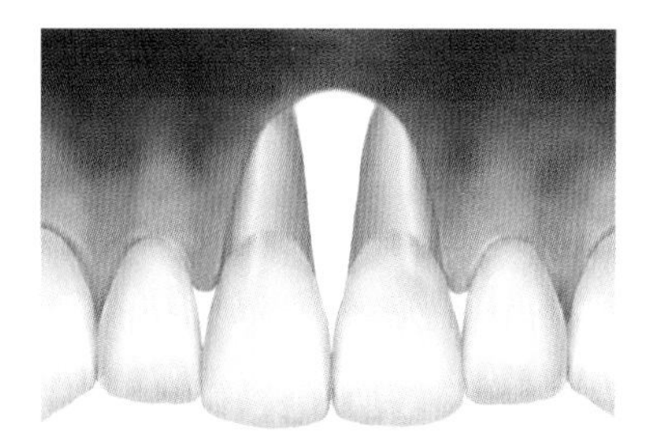

Class IV
Recession defect extending beyond mucogingival junction with loss of interdental soft tissue and bone apical to the recession

Fig. 6.3 Miller's classification of recession defects.

vascularity and is more likely to lead to a successful clinical outcome. A flap thickness of at least 0.8 mm has been suggested as the minimum required when attempting complete root coverage.[10]

Flap survival is dependent upon vascularity postoperatively and the collateral circulation from the periosteal connective tissue bed. In most root coverage

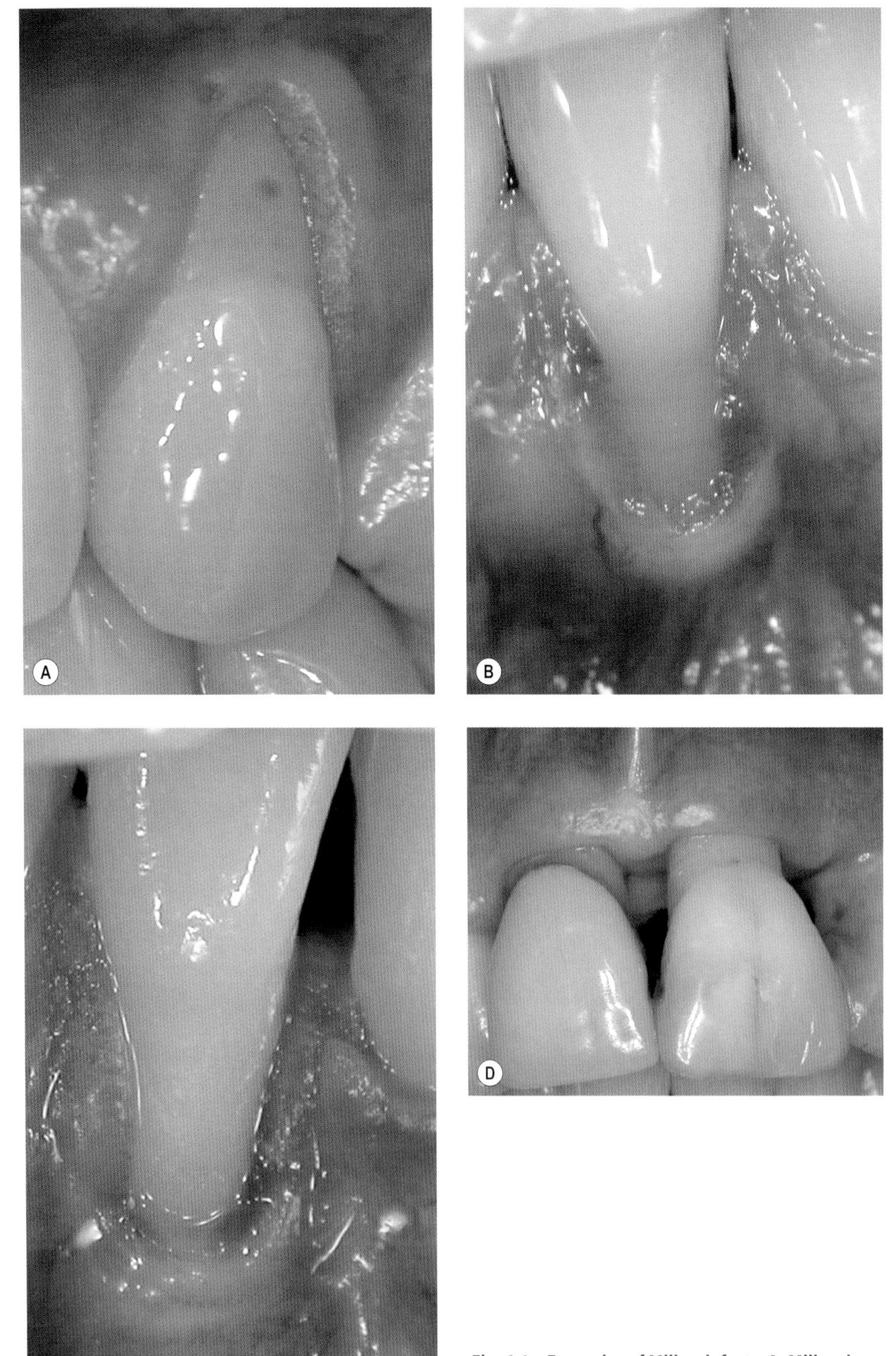

Fig. 6.4 Examples of Miller defects. A. Miller class I defect. B. Miller class II defect. C. Miller class III defect. D. Miller class IV defect.

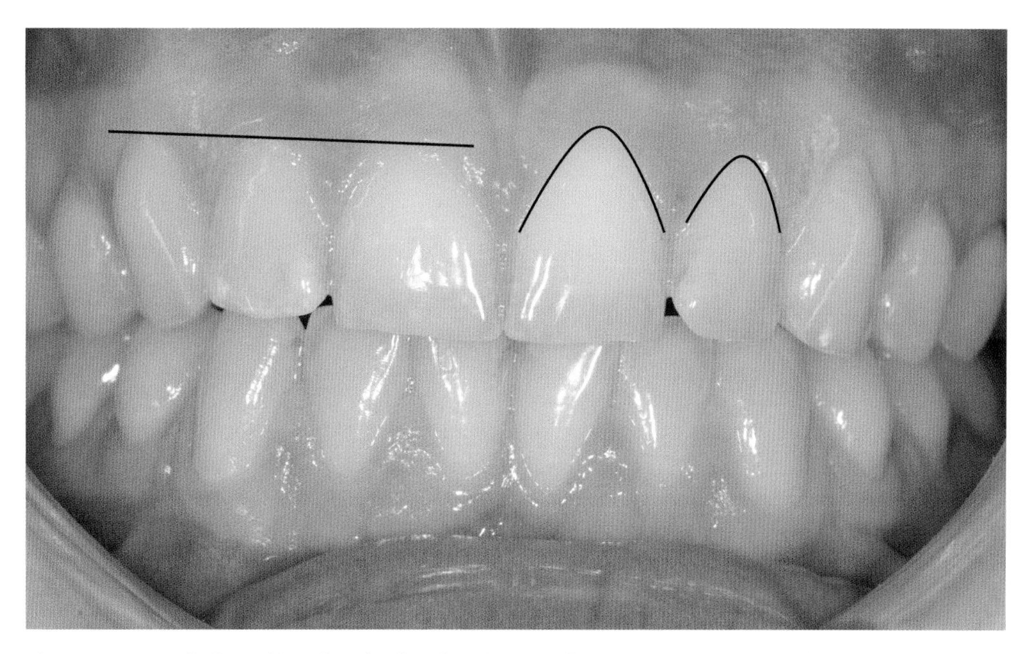

Fig. 6.5 Anatomical considerations in planning therapy. The UL12 appears to be a Miller class I recession defect but the cemento-enamel junction (CEJ) is at the correct level and the UR21 gingival levels are coronal to the CEJ.

procedures, a periosteal releasing incision is made to mobilize the flap. During the healing period, some shrinkage tends to occur. Studies have shown that the more coronal the flap is to the CEJ, the greater the probability of complete root coverage. It is therefore best to over-correct recession defects by at least 2 mm above the CEJ.[11]

WOUND STABILITY

The primary function of sutures is to stabilize the flap and allow the blood clot to adhere to the root surface during the healing process. This has been shown to be very important. Applying the correct suturing technique in mucogingival surgery is therefore fundamental to achieving complete root coverage. A combination of 5-0 and 6-0 monofilament sutures with a reverse cutting needle is best used in mucogingival surgery. There is evidence that larger needle sizes, such as 3-0, lead to more tissue breakage when compared to the use of 6-0- and 7-0-sized needles, which appear to reduce tissue trauma and flap tension.[12] A combination of a microsurgical technique and finer suture materials has been shown to improve revascularization of the connective tissue graft significantly during the healing phase.[13]

When suturing the buccal flap, a sling suture is employed to position and stabilize the flap at the correct level on the tooth. If flowable composite resin is placed between the contact areas as a temporary measure, a double-crossed suture can be placed (Fig. 6.6). This has been considered to help stabilize the flap by

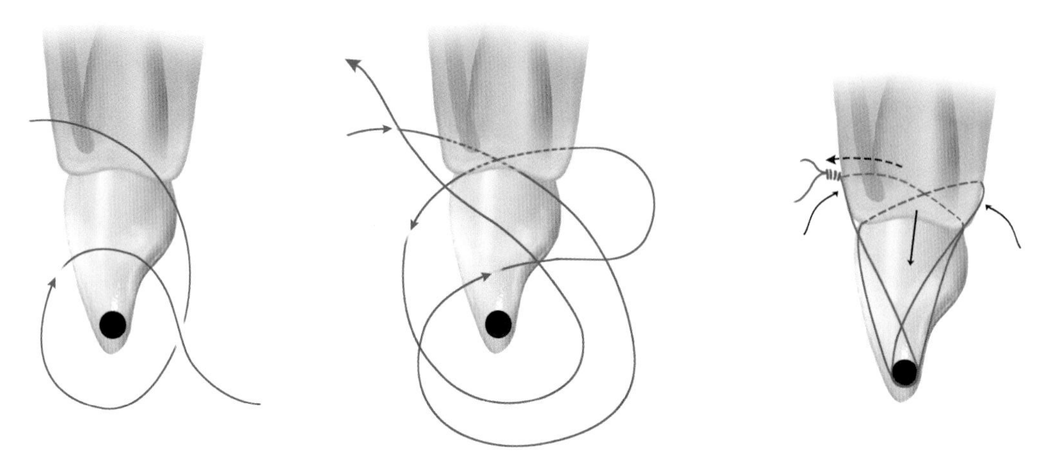

Fig. 6.6 The double-crossed suture.

adapting it more closely to the underlying tissues.[14] The crossed design of this anchorage suture compresses the flap on to the underlying tissues, enhancing the prospects of a successful outcome (see Fig. 6.6).

ROOT PREPARATION

Several studies have suggested that root surface preparation using ethylenediaminetetraacetic acid (EDTA), citric acid or tetracycline preparations may encourage greater attachment to the surface. The available evidence base does not, however, demonstrate that these preparations are superior to root surface instrumentation alone. Preparing the root surface using ultrasonic instrumentation, or curettes, while effective, may result in the flattening of prominent roots. It is essential in the use of such instrumentation to avoid damaging any connective tissue attachment embedded within the cementum. It is best, therefore, to prepare the root surface prior to raising the buccal flap. Research has shown that over-zealous root preparation can lead to external root resorption.

TREATMENT OF MUCOGINGIVAL RECESSION

Various mucogingival procedures have been described, including:

- free gingival grafts
- laterally positioned flaps
- semilunar coronally positioned flaps
- guided tissue regeneration (GTR)
- subepithelial connective tissue grafting.

Free gingival and subepithelial grafts can be harvested from the palate or edentulous ridge sites.

It has been shown that the use of a subepithelial connective tissue graft to cover treated carious root surfaces and non-carious cervical lesions is highly effective and predictable.[9] This approach resolves the problem biologically, rather than prosthetically.

The treatment of a gingival recession defect with a pedicle flap can result in the formation of a long junctional epithelial attachment,[15] whereas a free gingival graft may lead to some regeneration of cementum, bone and connective tissue attachment.[16] Free gingival grafts are no longer justified to cover recession defects in the esthetic zone, given the resulting mismatch in colour and postoperative discomfort from the denuded palatal donor site. New bone and cementum formation has been reported following the use of GTR, but studies have shown that this technique offers no superior clinical benefit over subepithelial connective tissue grafting.[17] Such grafting results in some periodontal regeneration,[18] offering the combined advantages of free gingival and pedicle flaps.

Careful anatomical assessment of the amount of keratinized tissue in relation to the gingival defect will allow the clinician to assess what type of surgical flap needs to be raised to achieve root coverage (Fig. 6.7). The width of the defect may also influence the amount of coverage that can be predictably achieved. Wide defects are less predictable for complete root coverage compared to long,

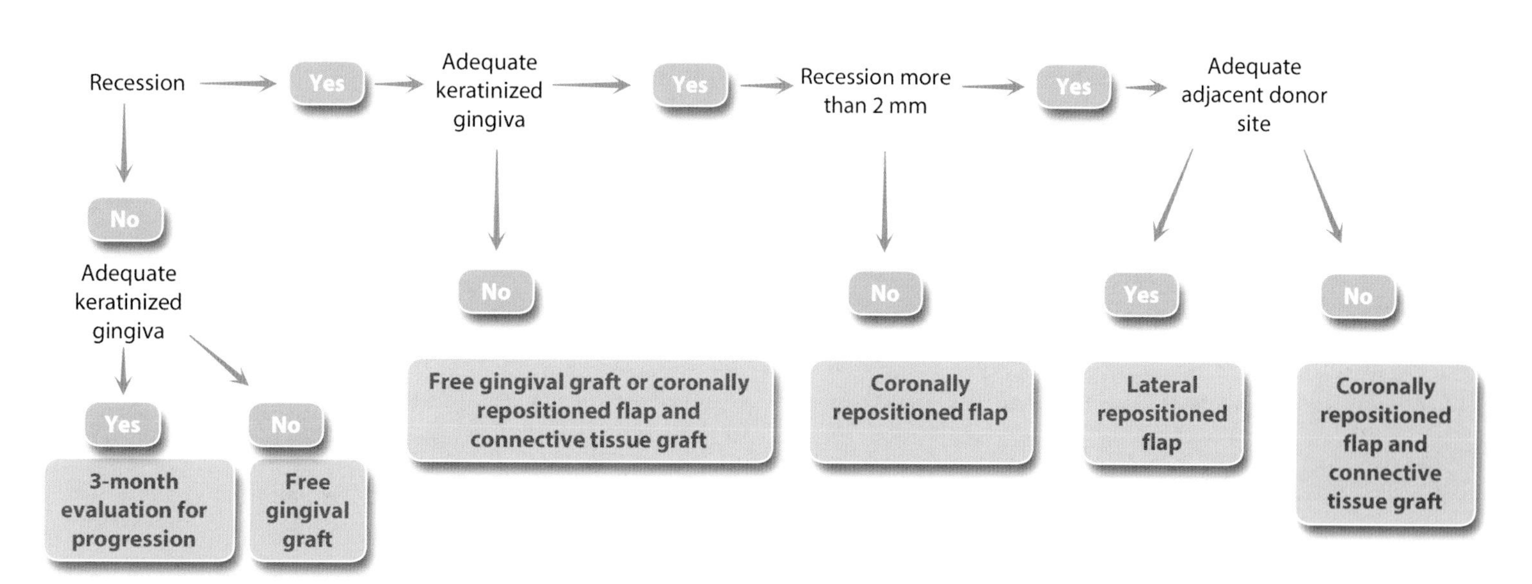

Fig. 6.7 Flow diagram to assess the type of surgical procedure required for root coverage.

narrow defects. Most importantly, the gingival tissues need to be healthy before any mucogingival surgery is performed.

Smoking is one of the major risk factors to be considered. It has been shown that less root coverage is achieved in smokers than in non-smokers, given the adverse effects of smoking on wound healing.[19]

An atraumatic surgical approach is essential when performing mucogingival surgery. The aims include achieving a tension-free flap and stabilization of any harvested graft. Excellent visualization of the operative site, aided by the use of LED-illuminated, 2.0–2.5x magnification loupes, is recommended. It has been suggested by some clinicians that the use of an operating microscope can improve predictability and esthetic outcomes in mucogingival surgery.[20] There is, however, no evidence to substantiate this claim.

SUBEPITHELIAL CONNECTIVE TISSUE GRAFTS

If the gingival tissues adjacent to the recession are thin, the biotype can be altered to a thicker one by placing a subepithelial connective tissue graft over the root. The subepithelial connective tissue is harvested from the palate using a trapdoor technique, being careful to avoid the greater palatine vessels, which are normally located mesial to the second permanent molar. It is important to make the initial incision at least 2 mm palatal to the gingival margin (Fig. 6.8). The scalpel is then run parallel to the palatal mucosa, leaving the connective tissue still attached to the bone. Incisions are then made to the bone to elevate the connective tissue. The graft is placed on gauze soaked in saline solution. It is important to keep the graft moist. Transfer to the recipient site should be achieved as soon as possible, to limit cell necrosis. Once the recipient site has been dealt with, the palatal flap is sutured using sling-criss-cross sutures. Good adaptation and stabilization of the clot are achieved by such sutures (Fig. 6.9).

CORONALLY REPOSITIONED FLAP

This technique relies on the presence of a certain amount of keratinized tissue apical to the recession defect. The buccal sulcus also needs to be of at least moderate depth. A buccal mucoperiosteal flap is raised and a periosteal relieving incision made to advance the flap coronally to achieve full root coverage.

A horizontal incision is made at the level of the CEJ (Figs 6.10–6.13). This begins with a split-thickness approach to the level of the apical extent of the recession defect; then two vertical incisions are made, extending beyond the mucogingival junction, creating a broad base to the flap. The horizontal

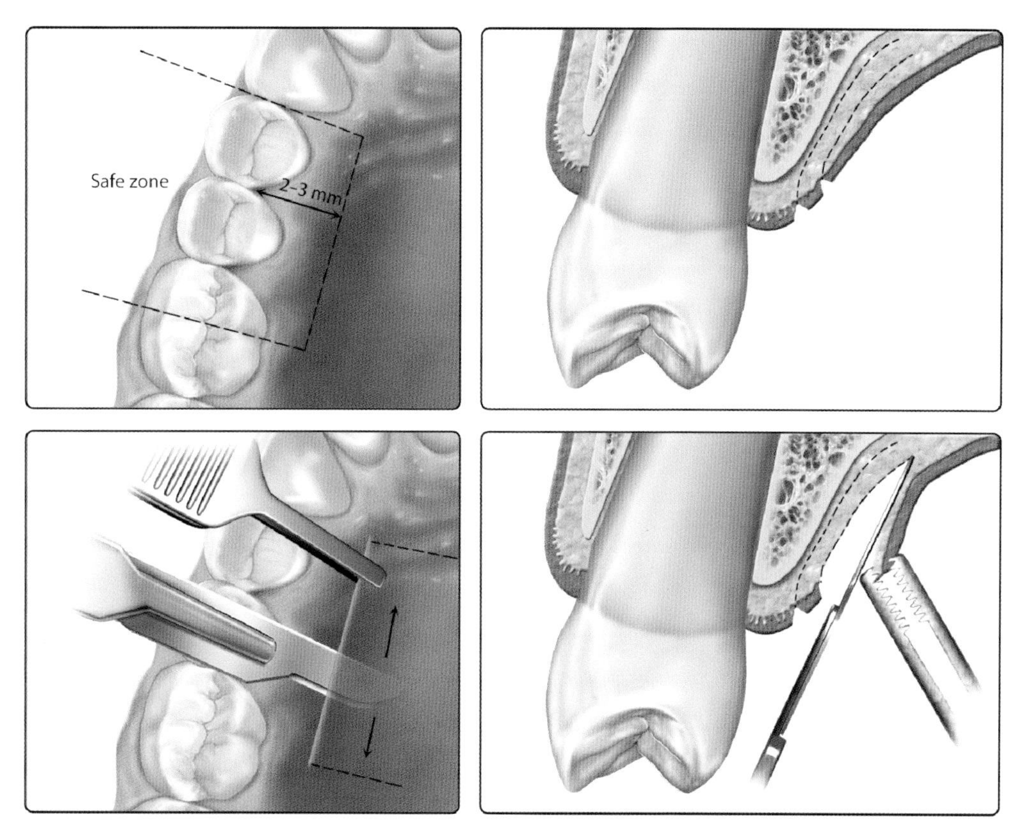

Fig. 6.8 Harvesting the subepithelial connective tissue graft.

incision becomes a full-thickness flap beyond the most apical portion of the recession. The incision is then extended beyond the mucogingival junction and once more becomes a split-thickness flap, where the periosteum is released to advance the flap coronally above the CEJ by at least 2 mm.[11] When making the periosteal releasing incision, it is important for a fresh blade to be used. The blade is positioned parallel to the buccal flap to avoid perforating the flap. The papillae need to be de-epithelialized, exposing the underlying connective tissue. The buccal flap can then be advanced over the de-epithelialized papilla to achieve primary closure. A 5-0–monofilament suture is used to create a sling of interrupted and double-crossed sutures.

LATERALLY REPOSITIONED FLAP

It is essential to assess the amount of keratinized tissue related to the adjacent teeth, so that a split-thickness flap can be rotated over the recession defect from the donor site. The gingival biotype should be thick to enable the raising of the split-thickness flap. The depth of the buccal sulcus does not affect this surgical technique, as the flap is being rotated. It is essential, however, to release the periosteum to achieve a tension-free flap closure.

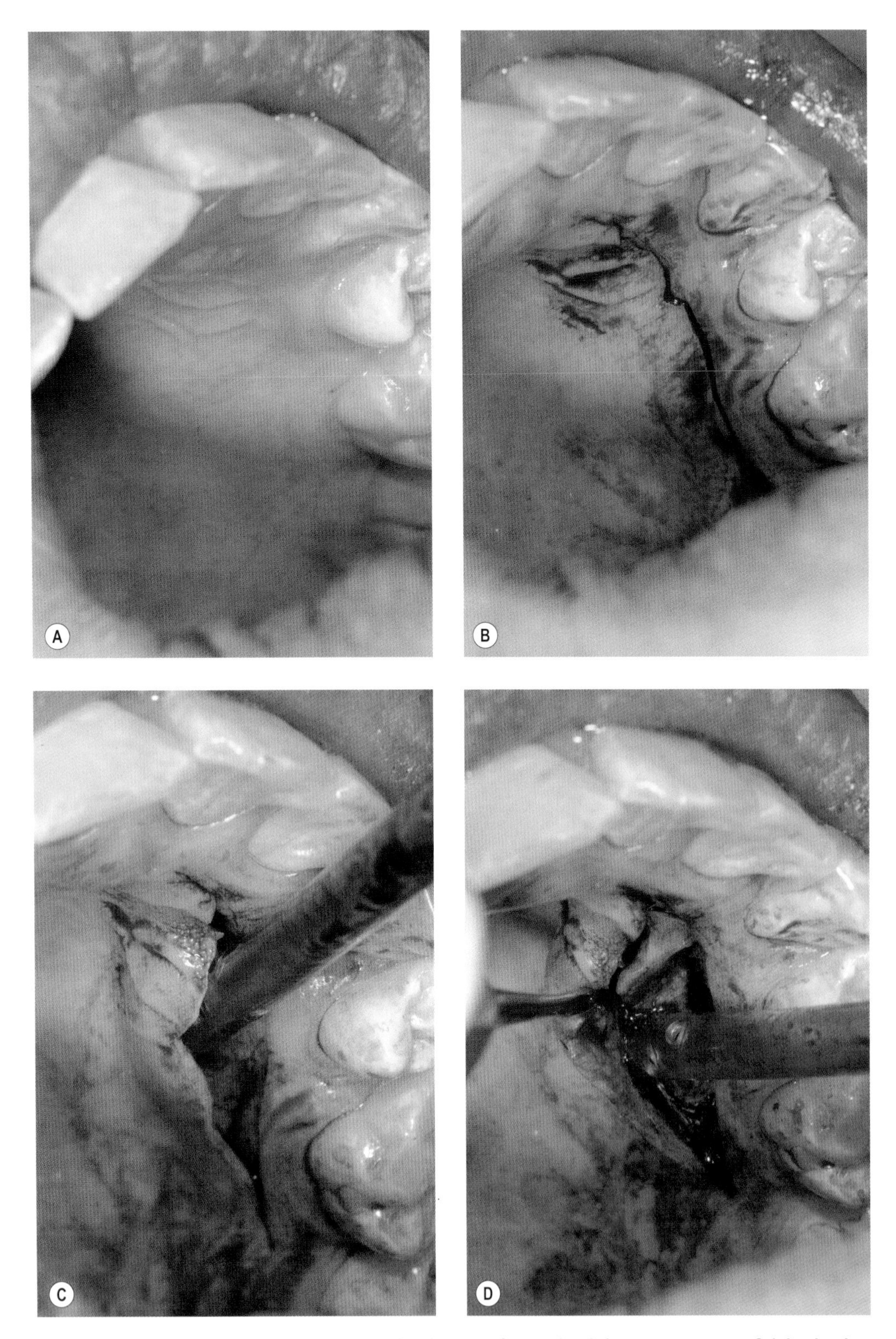

Fig. 6.9 Harvesting the subepithelial connective tissue graft. A. Palatal site UL346. B. Superficial palatal incision 2–3 mm below the gingival margin. C. Vertical incision running parallel to the palate splitting the palatal flap from the connective tissue. D. The connective tissue is raised off the periosteum.

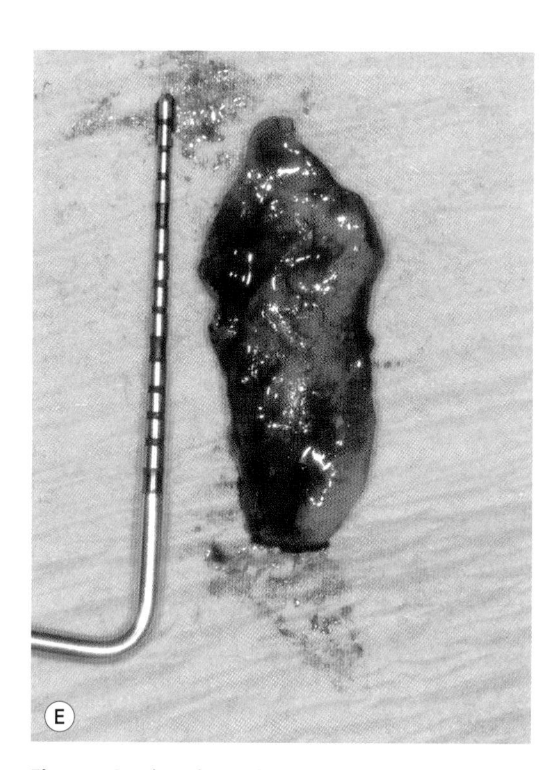

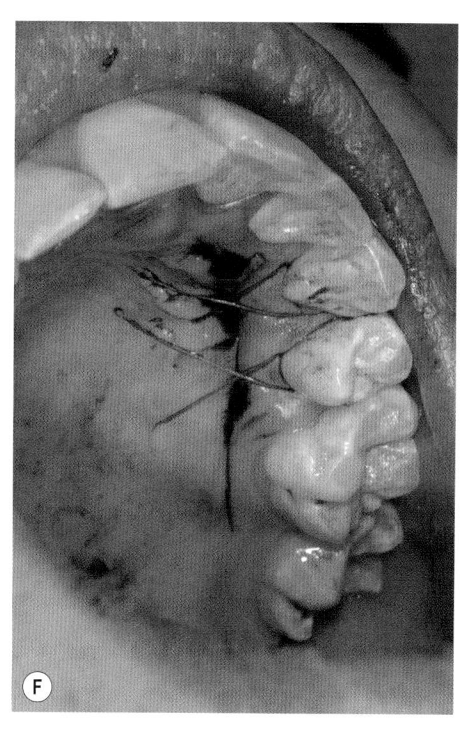

Fig. 6.9 ***Continued*** **E. The harvested connective tissue graft. F. Compressive sutures to stabilize the flap to the palate bone.**

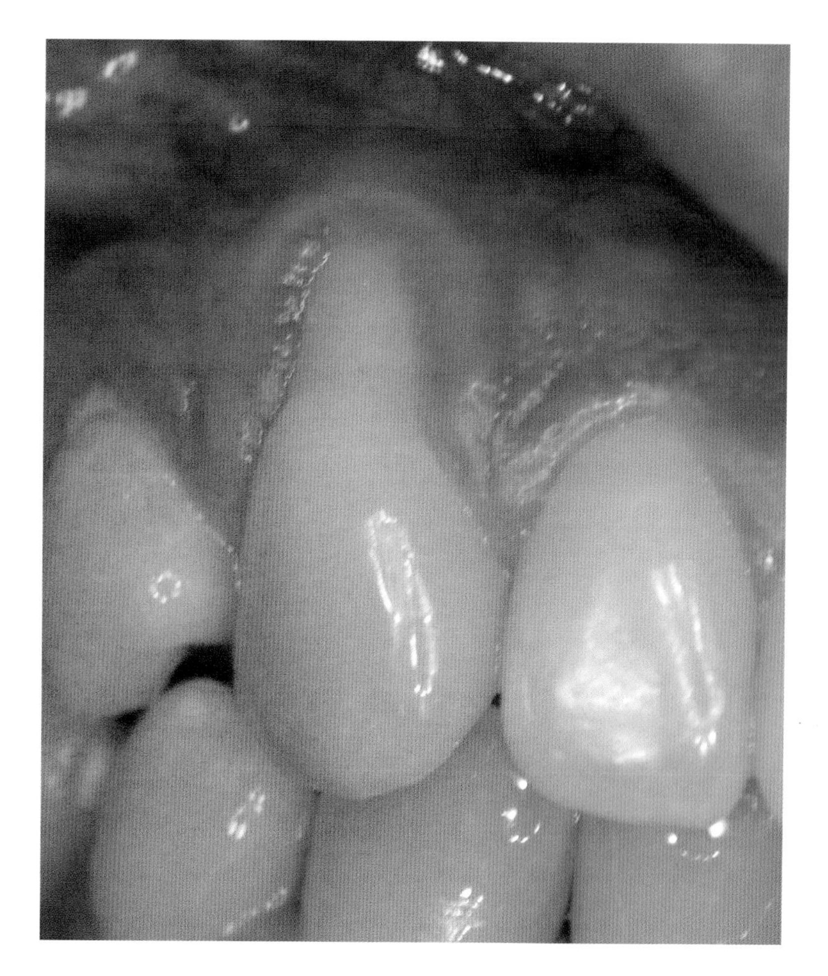

Fig. 6.10 Miller class I recession defect at UR3.

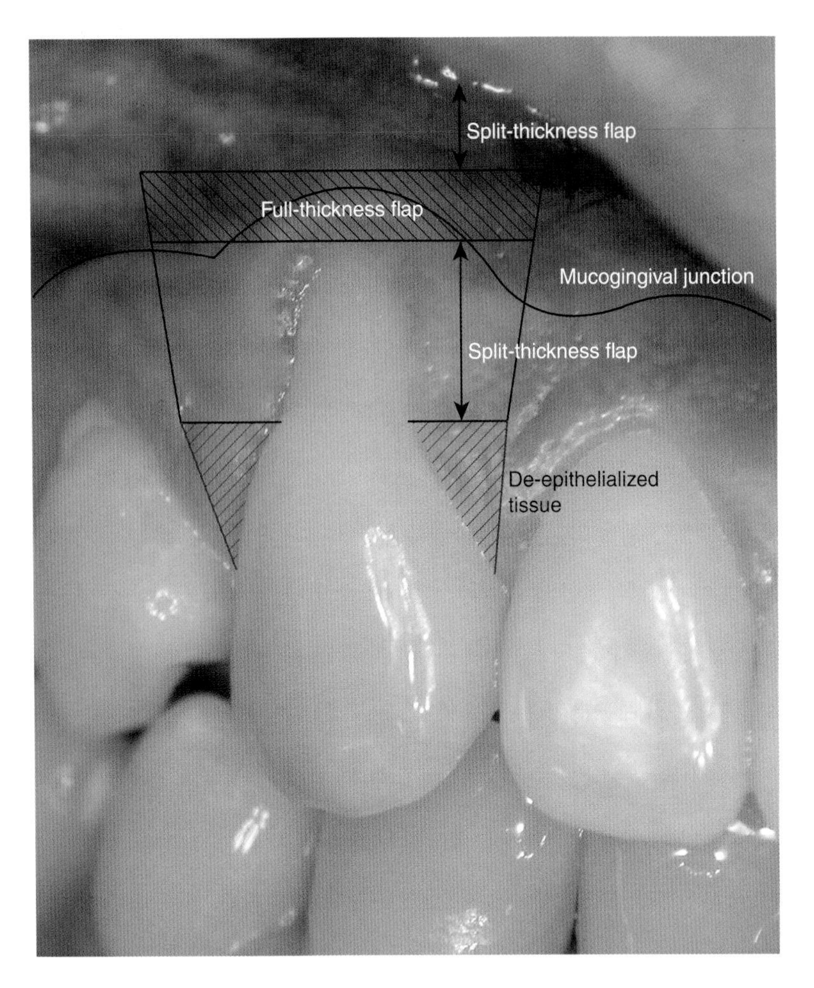

Fig. 6.11 **Coronally repositioned three-sided flap split-full-split raised. The red outline indicates excision of tissue.**

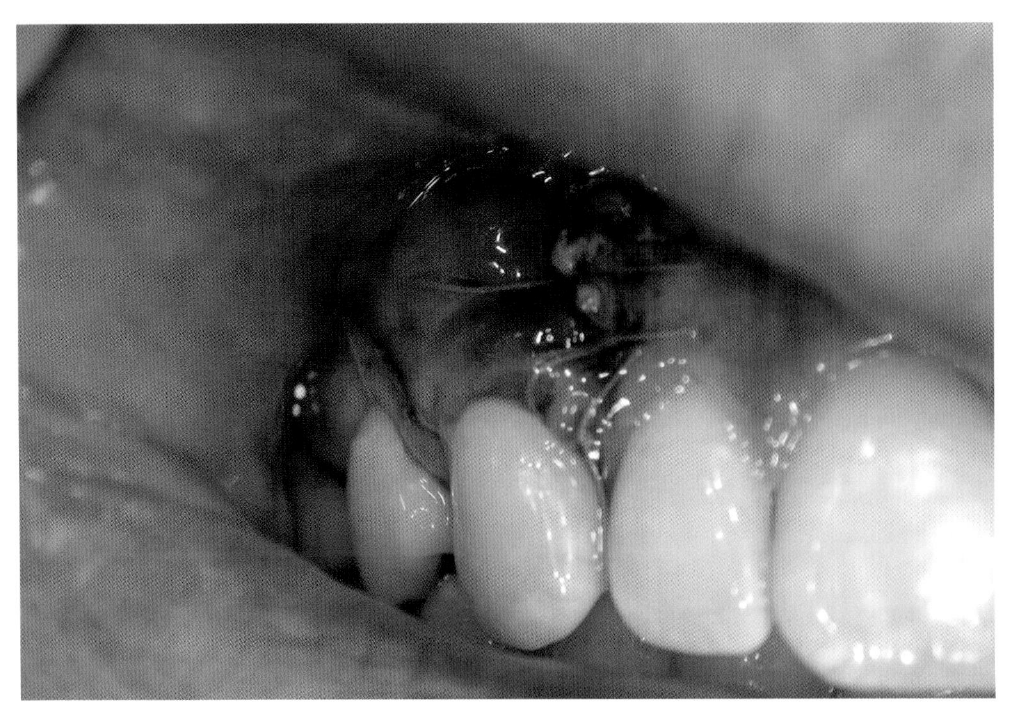

Fig. 6.12 **Coronal advancement of the buccal flap stabilized with 5-0 sutures.**

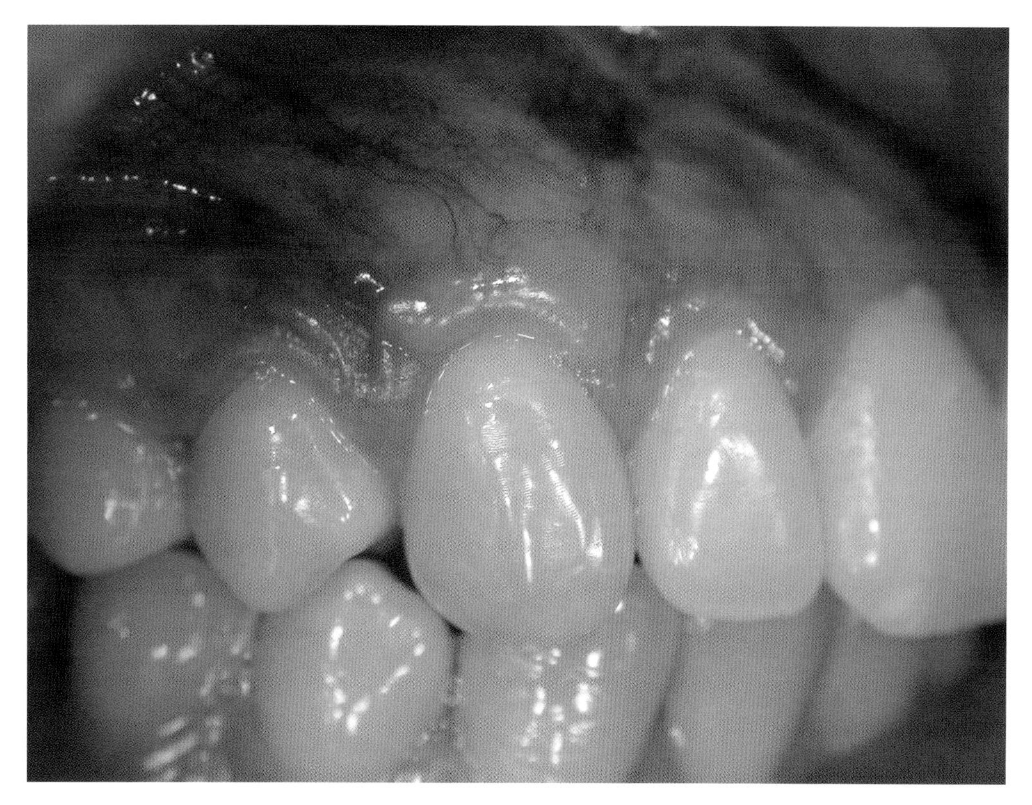

Fig. 6.13 Nine months postoperative.

A V-shaped wedge of gingiva surrounding the recession needs to be excised to the level of the CEJ. This will provide a vascular bed for the lateral flap to sit over the defect and to which it may adhere. Part of the wedge becomes one of the vertical incisions and the other is placed over the donor site (Figs 6.14–6.17). To prevent recession of the gingiva at the donor site, it has been suggested that an incision is made 1–2 mm below the gingival sulcus. A split-thickness flap is raised and becomes a full-thickness flap in the direction of the recession defect. Then a split-thickness flap is made beyond the mucogingival junction, thereby releasing the periosteum and the muscle attachments, allowing greater mobility of the flap to rotate over the recession defect. The gingiva of the recipient site is de-epithelialized, exposing the underlying collagen. The flap is sutured into place using a 5-0 suture to create a sling of double-crossed and interrupted sutures. The stages employed for a laterally repositioned flap, including 1-week and 1-, 3- and 6-month follow-up images are illustrated in Figure 6.18.

DOUBLE PAPILLA FLAP

The advantage of this technique is that it allows keratinized tissue to be sutured together to cover the root surface. The gingival biotype should be thick to

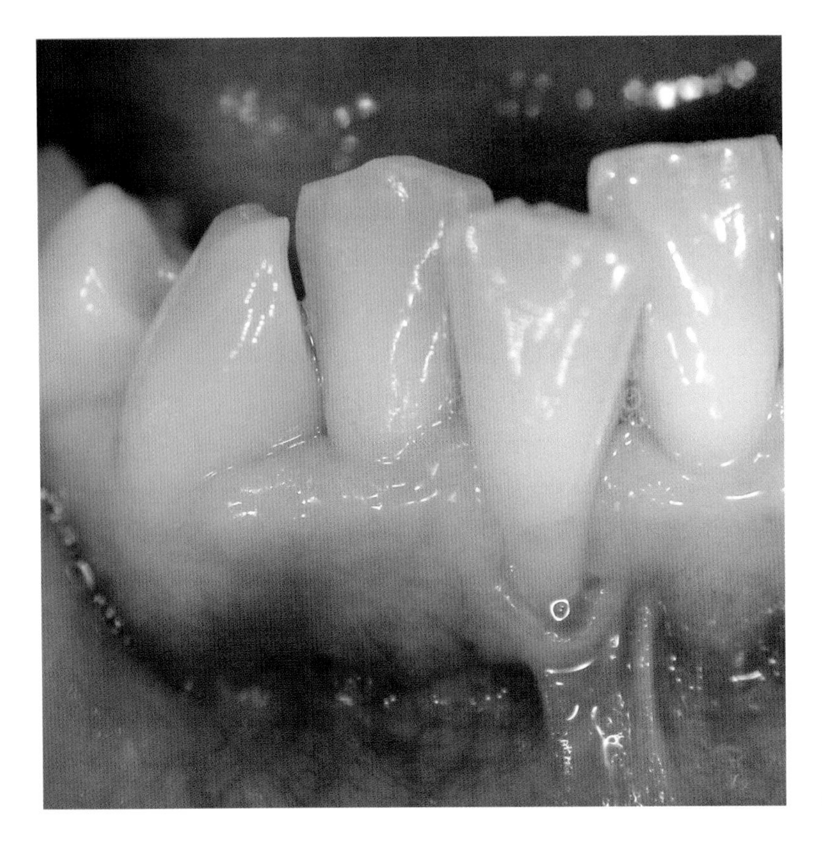

Fig. 6.14 Miller class I recession defect at LR1.

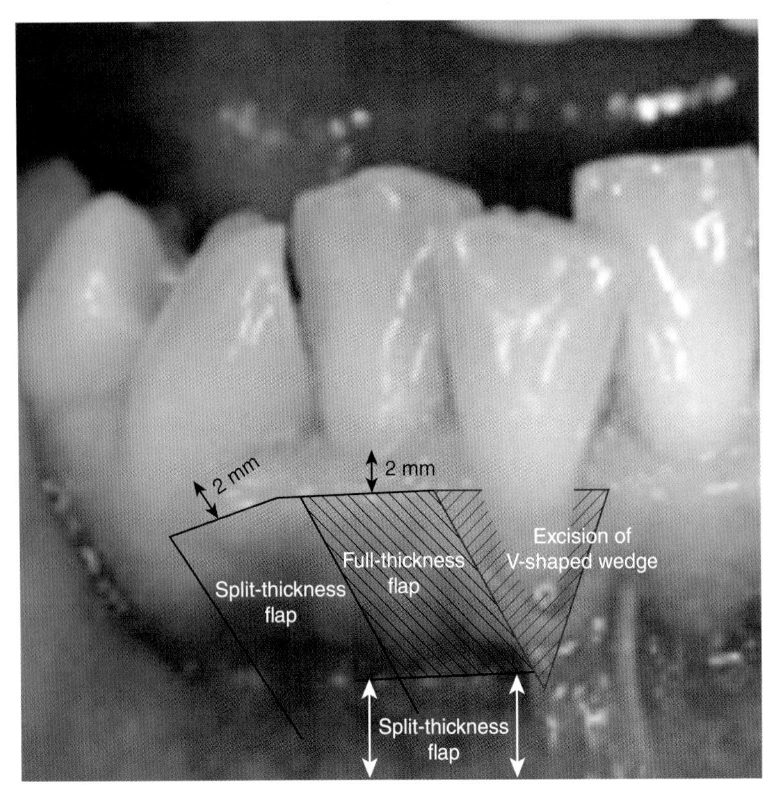

Fig. 6.15 Laterally repositioned 'split-full-split' flap. The red outline indicates excision of tissue.

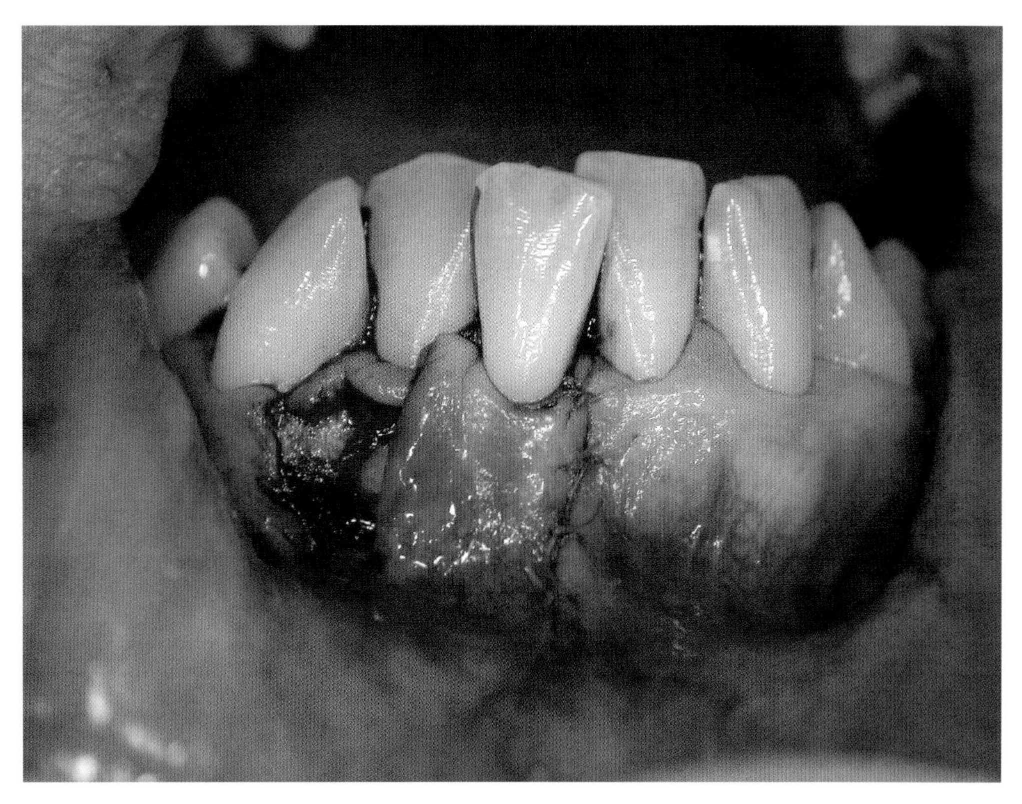

Fig. 6.16 **Mobilization of the lateral flap with periosteum left exposed. The flap is stabilized with 5-0 sutures.**

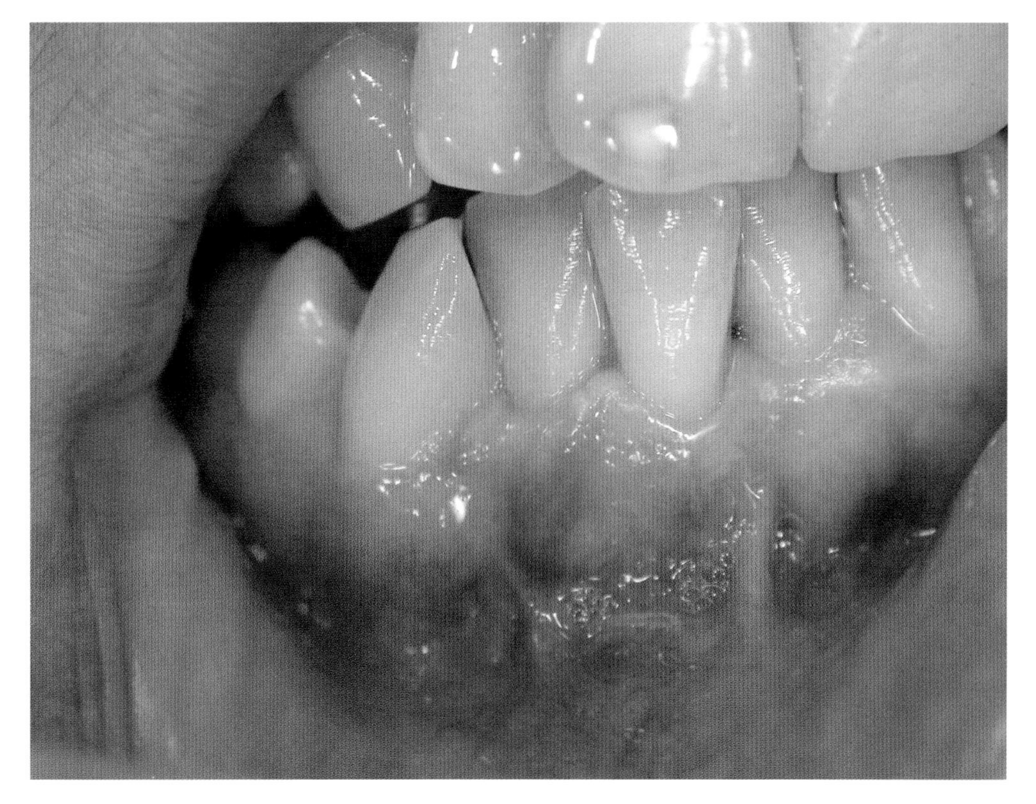

Fig. 6.17 **Three months postoperative.**

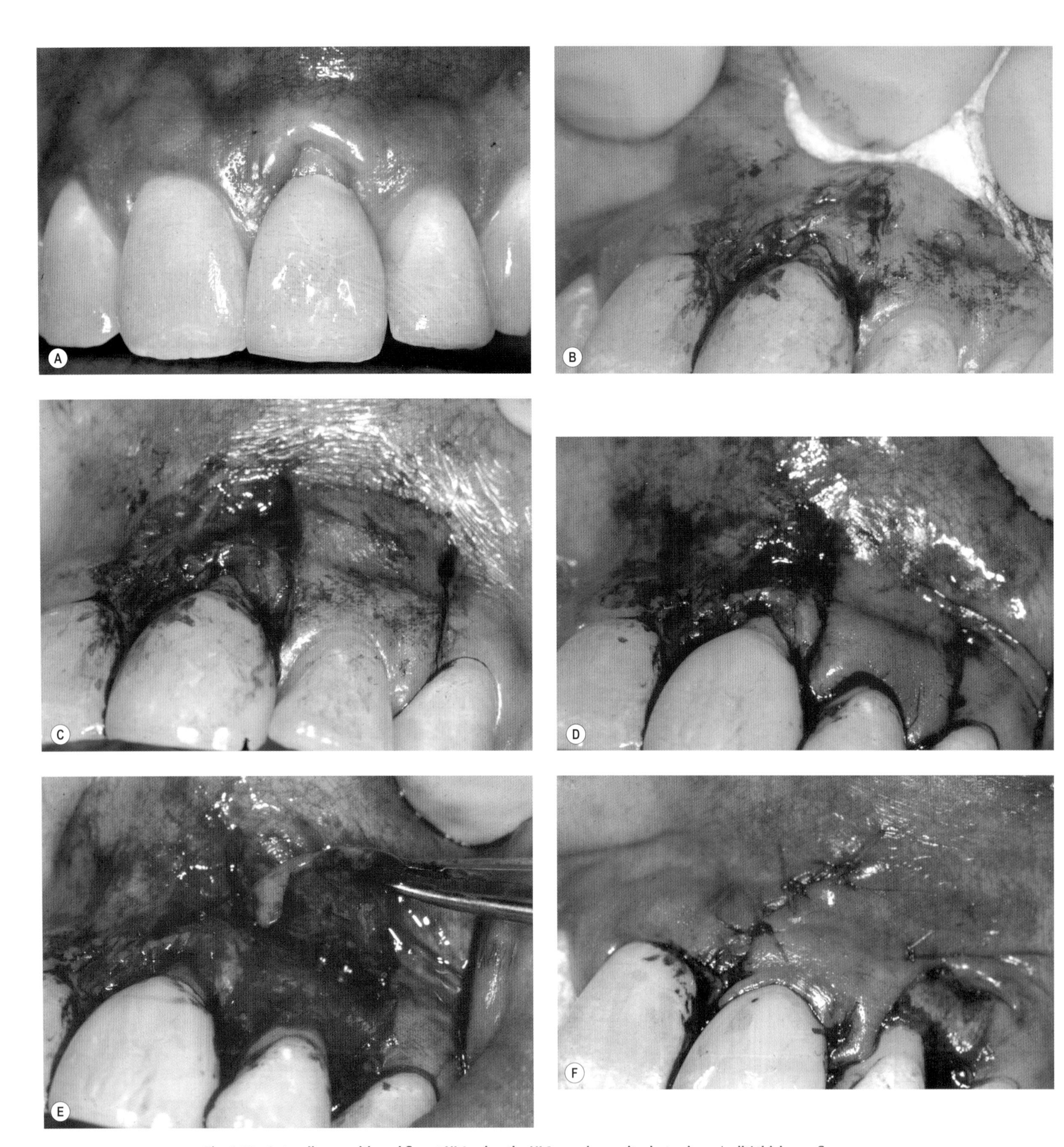

Fig. 6.18 Laterally repositioned flap at UL1 using the UL2 as a donor site, but using a 'split' thickness flap only and raising the papillae from the donor site. A. Defect pre-surgery. B. Excision of inflamed marginal tissue in 'V-shape'. C. Three-sided split thickness flap raised including donor papillae. D. Donor flap ready to mobilize. E. Flap mobilized. F. Flap rotated into position and sutured.

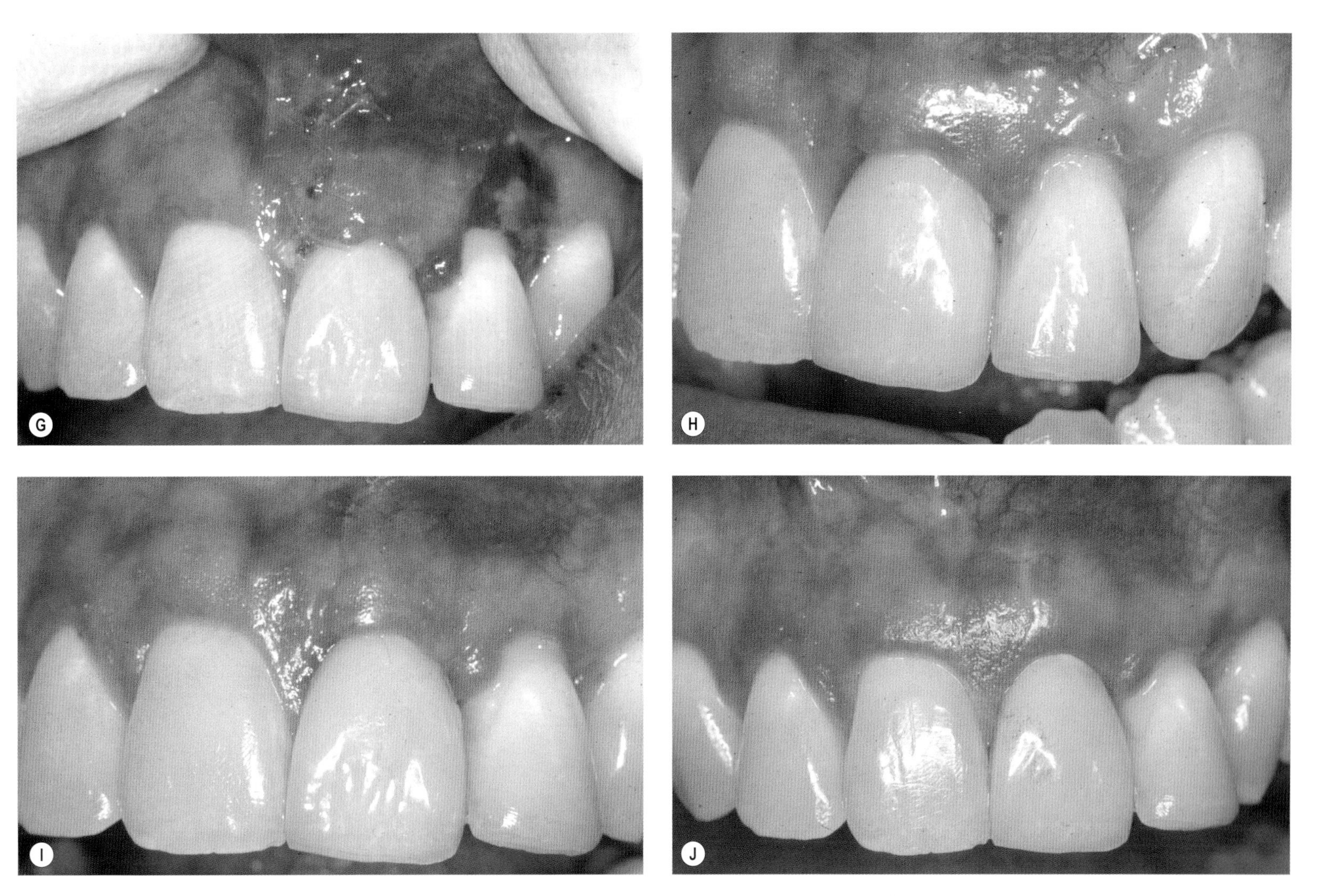

Fig. 6.18 ***Continued*** **G. Healing after 7 days. H. Healing after 14 days. I. Healing after 1 month. J. Healing after 3 months.**

moderate in order to perform this surgical technique. The sulcus depth does not affect the surgical technique, given the small displacement of the papillae flaps (Figs 6.19–6.22).

The surgical site is prepared by excising a V-shaped wedge of gingiva surrounding the recession defect, as described for the laterally repositioned flap. Horizontal incisions are made at the level of the CEJ (see Figs 6.19–6.22). This begins with a split-thickness approach. Then two vertical incisions are made, extending beyond the mucogingival junction with a broad base. The horizontal incision becomes a full-thickness flap beyond the most apical portion of the recession. The incision is then extended beyond the mucogingival junction and becomes a

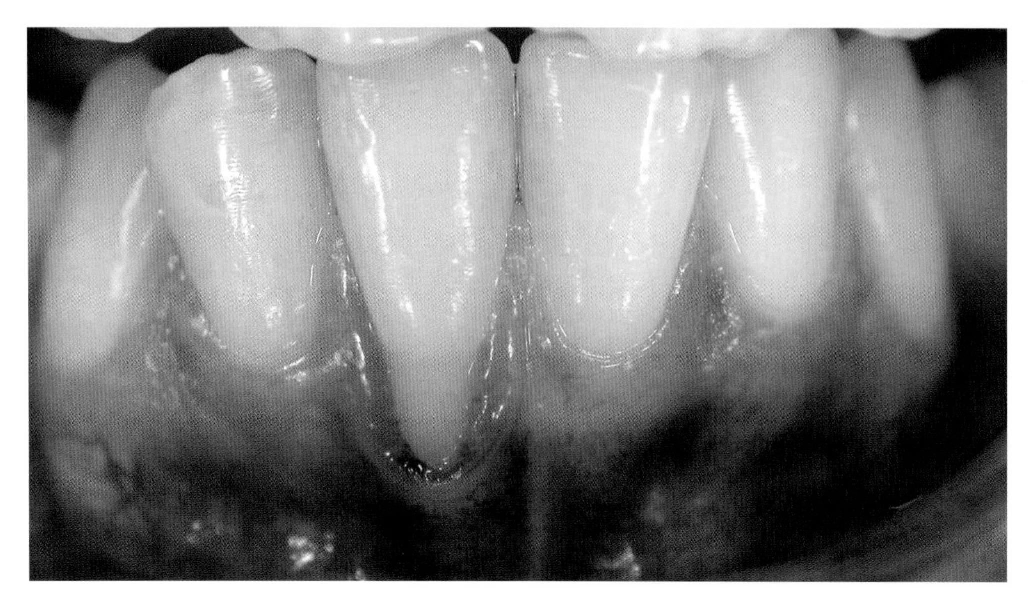

Fig. 6.19 Miller class I recession defect at LR1.

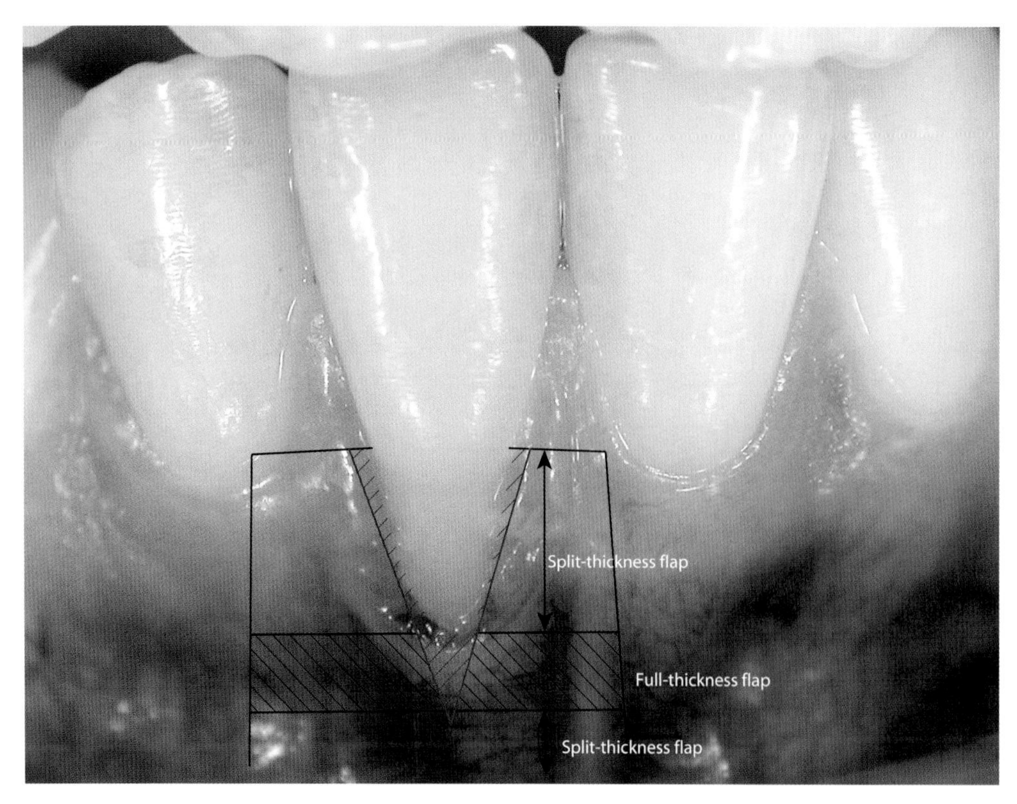

Fig. 6.20 Double papillae flaps raised. The red outline indicates excision of tissue.

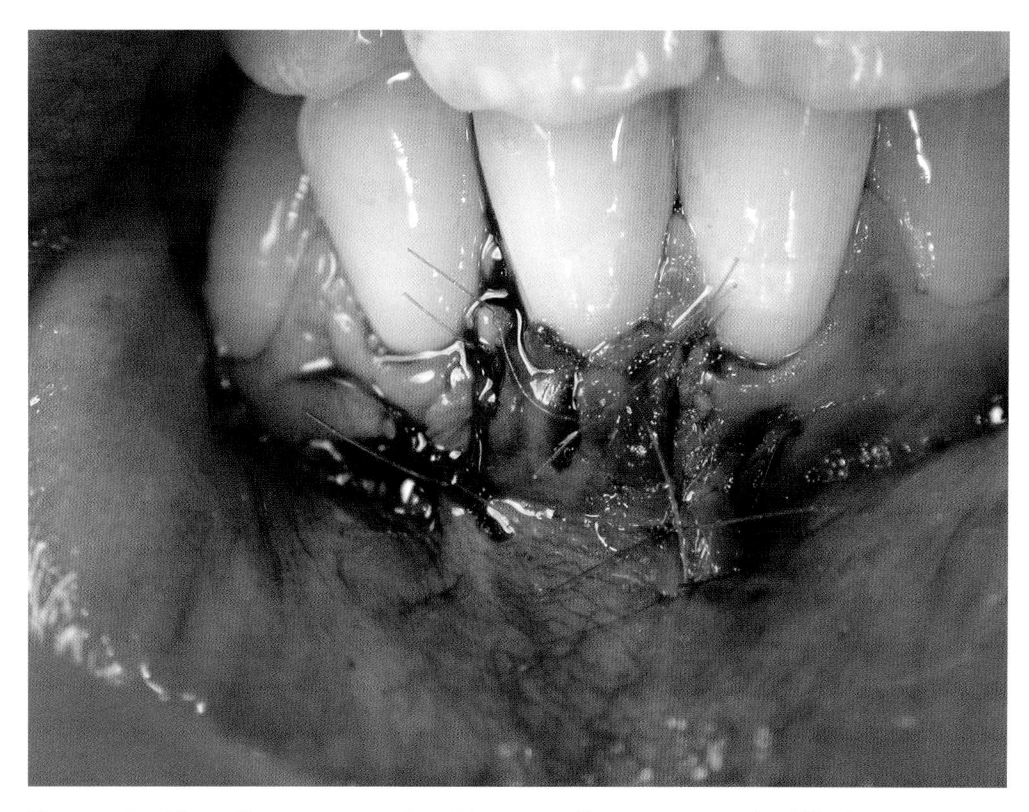

Fig. 6.21 Double papillae sutured together with 5-0 monofilament sutures and stabilized.

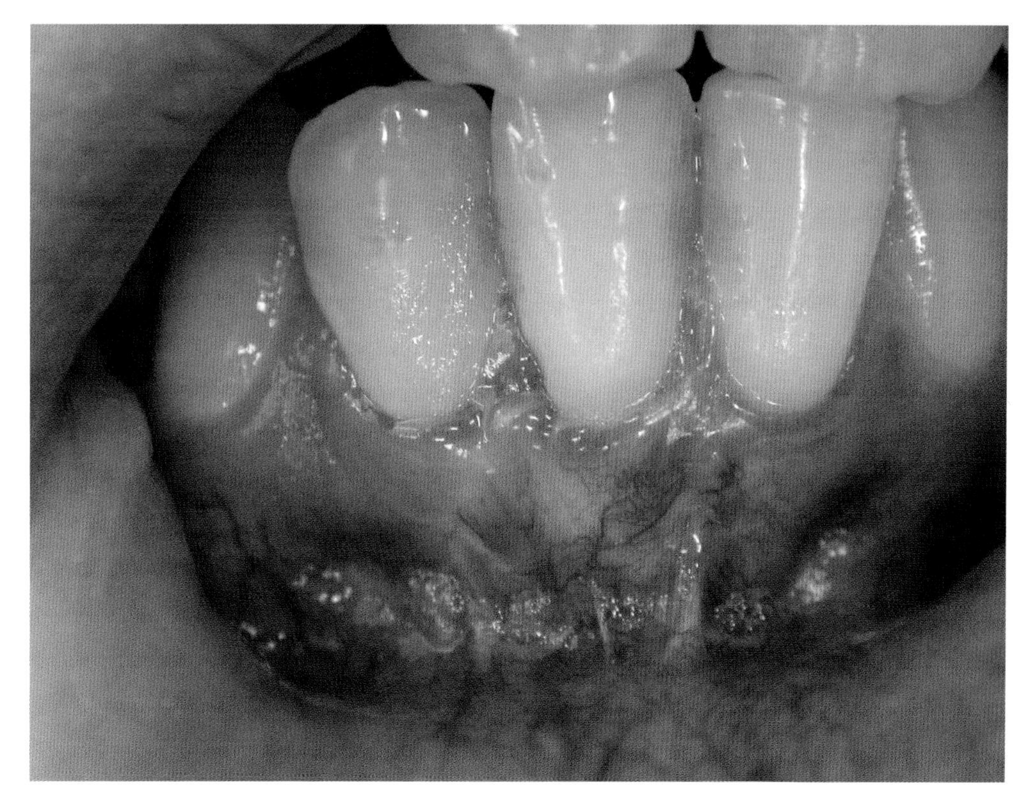

Fig. 6.22 Three months postoperative.

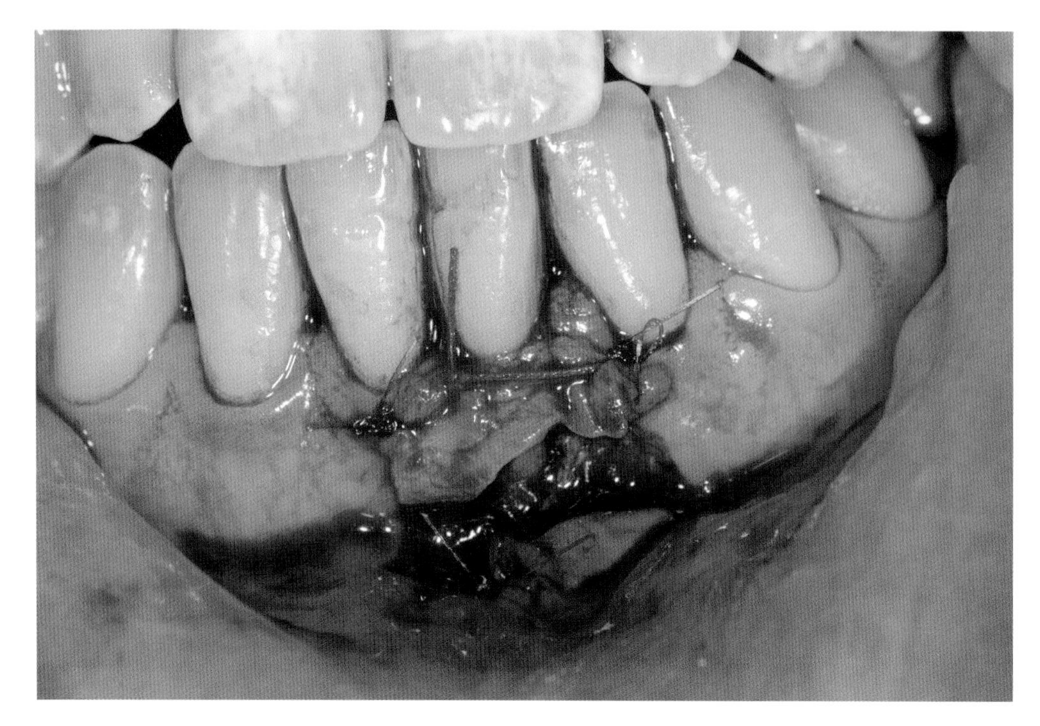

Fig. 6.23 Subepithelial connective tissue graft is not stable apically.

split-thickness flap where the periosteum is released to rotate the double papilla over the denuded root surface. The mobile portions of the papillae are sutured together using a 5-0–monofilament suture (see Fig. 6.21). This makes the buccal flap easier to manipulate when suturing. Sling, double-crossed and interrupted sutures are placed to achieve tension-free flap closure.

COMBINATION METHODS

Using a subepithelial connective tissue graft, as suggested in all the root coverage procedures discussed, ensures a thick biotype. It is essential for the graft to be stabilized, placing a resorbable fine (5-0) suture sling that compresses the graft to the recipient bed (Fig. 6.23). It may also be necessary to place a compressive suture into the periosteum (Fig. 6.24). If the biotype of the defect is thick and flat, the use of a graft may be contraindicated, as this can lead to scarring and a poor esthetic result. If scarring occurs, it may be addressed 4–6 months postoperatively by means of a gingivoplasty to even out and blend the tissues.

KEY POINT SUMMARY

Remember: it is important to take clinical photographs of recession defects before mucogingival surgery. These form part of the patient's clinical records and allow both the patient and the operator to evaluate the final result.

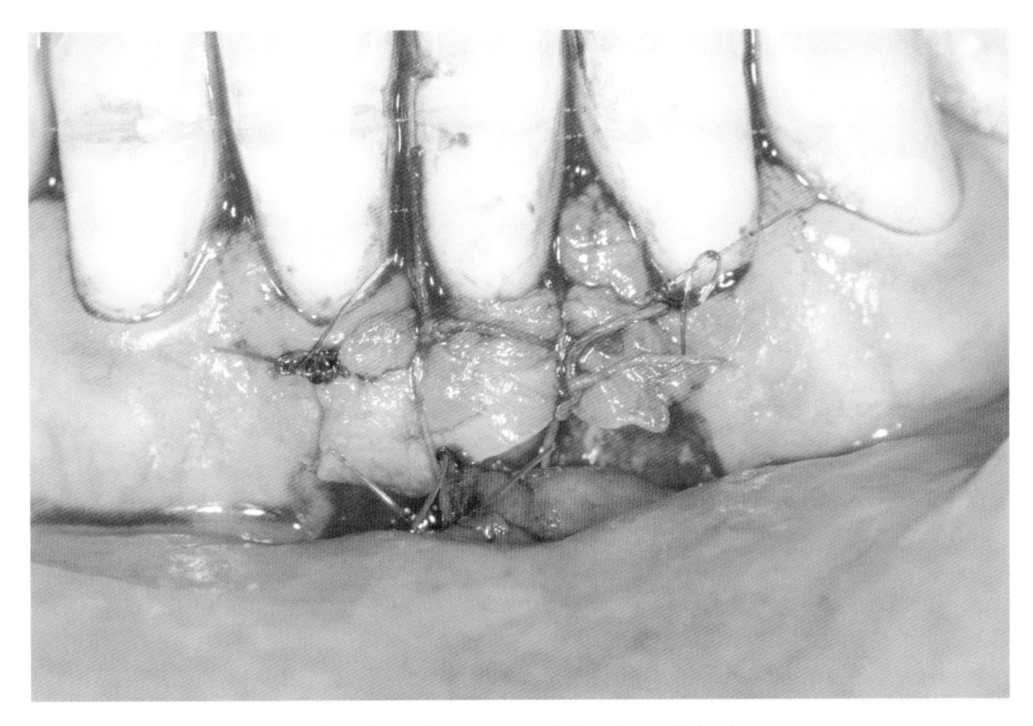

Fig. 6.24 Compressive suture into the periosteum to stabilize the graft further.

POSTOPERATIVE INSTRUCTIONS

Patients who have undergone mucogingival surgery need to be reviewed initially on a weekly basis, when professional mechanical cleaning of the area can be performed. This also allows the clinician to assess how well the tissues are healing.

If a subepithelial connective tissue graft has been harvested, the sutures are removed 1 week postoperatively. At week 2, the remaining monofilament sutures are removed at the primary surgical site. The surgical site is cleaned carefully using cotton wool pledgets soaked in 0.2% chlorhexidine gluconate, and the teeth are cleaned using fine curettes on a weekly basis for 4 weeks. The patient is then reviewed on a monthly basis for 3 months, assessing the sufficiency of the patient's oral hygiene technique at each visit.

PATIENT PROTOCOL

This comprises:

- Chlorhexidine gluconate (0.2%) used twice a day for 4 weeks. The chlorhexidine is held in the region of the surgical site. It is not used as a mouthwash, as this may displace the flap, particularly if it has been advanced significantly.

- Avoidance of the surgical site when brushing for 2 weeks, and then gentle brushing of the area with a soft toothbrush.
- Soft diet for 3–4 weeks to avoid the buccal flap being traumatized or displaced.

KEY POINT SUMMARY

The first step in the management of recession defects is improving oral hygiene and eliminating risk factors such as smoking. If you do not establish good habits beforehand, there is less chance of achieving acceptable oral hygiene levels afterwards, and therefore the procedure may well fail.

CONCLUDING REMARKS

The success of root coverage depends upon careful assessment of the gingival tissues, an atraumatic surgical approach, the preservation of the gingival blood supply to increase initial healing and the success of the mucogingival surgery. Studies have shown that mucogingival surgery is predictable and can lead to up to 100% root coverage. With good maintenance, the coverage achieved can be retained.[21]

REFERENCES

1. Loe H, Anerud A, Boysen H. The natural history of periodontal disease in man: prevalence, severity and extent of gingival recession. J Periodontol 1992;63:489–95.
2. Goldstein M, Nasatzky E, Goultschin J, et al. Coverage of previously carious roots is as predictable a procedure as coverage of intact roots. J Periodontol 2002;73:1419–26.
3. Lindhe J, Socransky SS, Nyman S, et al. Dimensional alteration of the periodontal tissues following therapy. Int J Periodontics Restorative Dent 1987;7:9–21.
4. Agudio G, Pini Prato G, Cortellini P, et al. Gingival lesions caused by improper oral hygiene measures. Int J Periodontics Restorative Dent 1987;7:52–65.
5. Lang NP, Loe H. The relationship between the width of keratinized gingiva and gingival health. J Periodontol 1972;43:623–7.
6. Miyasato M, Crigger M, Egelberg J. Gingival condition in areas of minimal and appreciable width of keratinized gingiva. J Clin Periodontol 1977;4:200–9.
7. Wennstrom JL, Lindhe J. The role of attached gingiva for maintenance of periodontal health. Healing following excisional and grafting procedures in dogs. J Clin Periodontol 1983;10:206–21.
8. Dorfman HS, Kennedy JE, Bird WC. Longitudinal evaluation of free autogenous gingival grafts. A four year report. J Periodontol 1982;53:349–52.
9. Miller PD. A classification of marginal tissue recession. Int J Periodontics Restorative Dent 1985;5:9–13.

10. Baldi C, Pini-Prato G, Pagliaro U. Coronally advanced flap procedure for root coverage. Is flap thickness a relevant predictor to achieve root coverage? A 19 case series. J Periodontol 1999;70:1077–84.

11. Pini-Prato G, Baldi C, Nieri M. Coronally advanced flap: the post-surgical position of the gingival margin is an important factor for achieving complete root coverage. J Periodontol 2005;76:713–22.

12. Burkhardt R, Preiss A, Joss A, et al. Influence of suture tension to the tearing characteristics of the soft tissue: an in vitro experiment. Clin Oral Implan Res 2008;19:314–19.

13. Burkhardt R, Lang NP. Coverage of localized gingival recessions: comparison of micro- and macrosurgical techniques. J Clin Periodontol 2005;32:287–93.

14. Zuhr O, Rebele SF, Thalmair T, et al. A modified suture technique for plastic periodontal and implant surgery – the double-crossed suture. Eur J Esthet Dent 2009;4:338–47.

15. Pasquinelli KL. The histology of new attachment utilizing a thick autogenous soft tissue graft in an area of deep recession: a case report. Int J Periodontics Restorative Dent 1995;15:248–57.

16. Caffesse RG, Kon S, Castelli WA, et al. Revascularization following the lateral sliding flap procedure. J Periodontol 1984;55:352–8.

17. Danesh-Meyer MJ, Wikesjo UM. Gingival recession defects and guided tissue regeneration: a review. J Periodontal Res 2001;36:341–54.

18. Harris RJ. Successful root coverage: a human histological evaluation of a case. Int J Periodontics Restorative Dent 1999;19:439–47.

19. Trombelli L, Scabbia A. Healing response of gingival recession defects following guided tissue regeneration procedures in smokers and non-smokers. J Clin Periodontol 1997;24:529–33.

20. Burkhardt R, Hurzeler MB. Utilization of the surgical microscope for advanced plastic periodontal surgery. Pract Periodontics Aesthet Dent 2000;12:171–80.

21. Lee YM, Kim JY, Seol YJ, et al. A 3yr longitudinal evaluation of subepithelial free connective tissue graft for gingival recession coverage. J Periodontol 2002;73:1412–18.

CHAPTER 7

Clinical Techniques: Assessment and Minimal Intervention

CHRISTOPHER HO

INTRODUCTION

Esthetic dentistry is the marriage between the 'art and science of dentistry'. The simultaneous application of technical and artistic skills enables a practitioner to achieve outstanding esthetic and functional results. The importance of diagnosis and treatment planning prior to any procedure cannot be overemphasized, remembering that oral health and function are integral to successful esthetic dentistry. To practise successful esthetic dentistry, the dental team must understand the relevant principles, notably those of smile design, and be aware of the different inter-disciplinary treatment modalities that are available. They should also possess an intimate knowledge of the different esthetic materials available, and their clinical indications, application and limitations in practice. Additionally, as discussed in other chapters in this book, effective communication within the dental team, with the dental technologist and, in particular, the patient is of paramount importance to ensure that the goals of esthetic dentistry are achieved, including patient satisfaction and the avoidance of unmet, possibly unrealistic, expectations. All these elements underpin and provide the foundations for successful esthetic dentistry.

This chapter focuses on the techniques and materials used in the practice of modern, minimal intervention (MI) esthetic dentistry.

ASSESSMENT TECHNIQUES

PHOTOGRAPHY

Photography is an essential diagnostic and communication tool for esthetic dentistry. The old adage, 'a picture paints a thousand words,' is often quoted. In esthetic dentistry, photographs help patients to understand the need for and the nature of proposed treatment while being an invaluable aid to the practitioner in treatment planning and subsequent procedures, including the communication of specific requirements to the dental technologist. Photographs also make an important contribution to clinical records.

The change from conventional to digital cameras, including the development of intraoral cameras, has given photography the chance to assume many different roles in esthetic dentistry. Photography with digital single lens reflex (SLR) cameras and easy-to-use prosumer high-performance compact cameras provides the opportunity to take a wide range of images, including portrait and intraoral shots, from whole arches to individual teeth, with excellent resolution and contrast.

The benefits of photography include:

- *Improved patient communication.* Being able to show patients what is in their mouths is hugely advantageous, compared to just describing their problems or drawing diagrams. This allows patients to co-examine, contribute to the assessment and diagnosis of their clinical issues, and understand the need for treatment.
- *Laboratory communication.* Good-quality clinical photographs can effectively communicate features of smiles and dentitions to the dental technology team, and can illustrate the relationships, anatomy, surface morphology, value, hue, translucency and chroma of individual teeth. Being able to access images at any time makes the task of producing esthetically pleasing indirect restorations and prostheses much easier, improving the clinical outcome of esthetic dentistry.
- *Diagnostic tool and treatment planning aid.* Being able to store and magnify clinical images enables practitioners to identify what they may have missed in their clinical examination. The benefit of photography is the ability to refine treatment planning from images of patients, together with records and diagnostic models after the patient has left the surgery.
- *Opportunity to create a marketing library.* Being able to show and discuss 'before' and 'after' photographs of patients who have undergone successful treatment is both a means of education and a powerful marketing tool, subject to patients giving consent to their photographs being used in this way.
- *Medico-legal considerations.* With increasing risks of litigation in respect of dental care, it is prudent to obtain photographic records of patients before, during and after treatment, including all critical stages of the various procedures involved. Such records may prove to be invaluable evidence of the care and attention exercised in the provision of treatment.
- *Self-improvement.* Documenting your cases photographically allows you to critique and audit your clinical results, and to reflect on ways in which to improve your techniques and outcomes.

Photographic series

The series of photographs that are useful in esthetic dentistry are outlined below. All images should exhibit little or no saliva and should be free of other distracting features: for example, fingers and noses. Consent should be sought from the patient to obtain and keep a photographic record, and should include specific provisions if the photographs might be used for any other purpose: for example, marketing, lectures and publications. A chapter in Volume 2 covers photography in further detail.

Full face

This image is shot straight on to the face. It should include the whole head. The inter-pupillary line and midline of the face are used to align the camera (Fig. 7.1).

Full smile

A non-retracted, natural smile should be recorded. The incisal plane of the maxillary teeth should be in the middle of the image. It is helpful to ask patients to make an 'eeeee' sound if they do not easily volunteer a smile (Fig. 7.2).

Full smile – right and left lateral view

This view shows the lips, as well as the teeth visible from this angle. The maxillary lateral incisor should be located in the centre of the shot. The contralateral central incisor should be visible, possibly together with the mesial surface of the lateral incisor (Fig. 7.3).

Frontal retracted view

The upper and lower teeth are parted, sufficient to see the incisal edges of the lower anterior teeth. The midline of the face and the occlusal plane should divide the image into quarters (Fig. 7.4). A second view is then taken with the teeth in occlusion to record the inter-cuspal relationship.

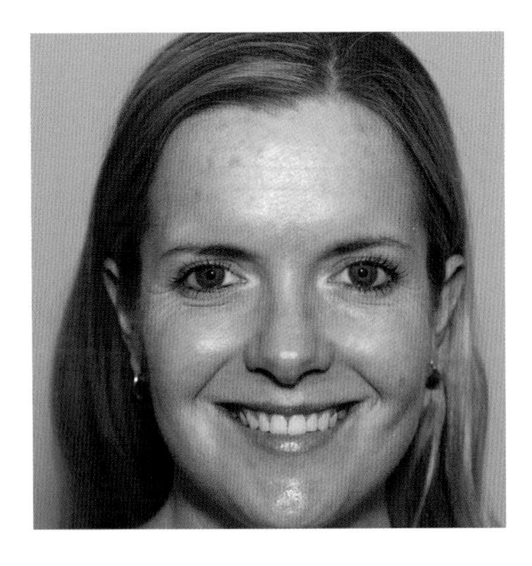

Fig. 7.1 Full-face photograph of a patient taken at the same level as the patient and covering the full head. The inter-pupillary line and horizontal plane are used to align the camera.

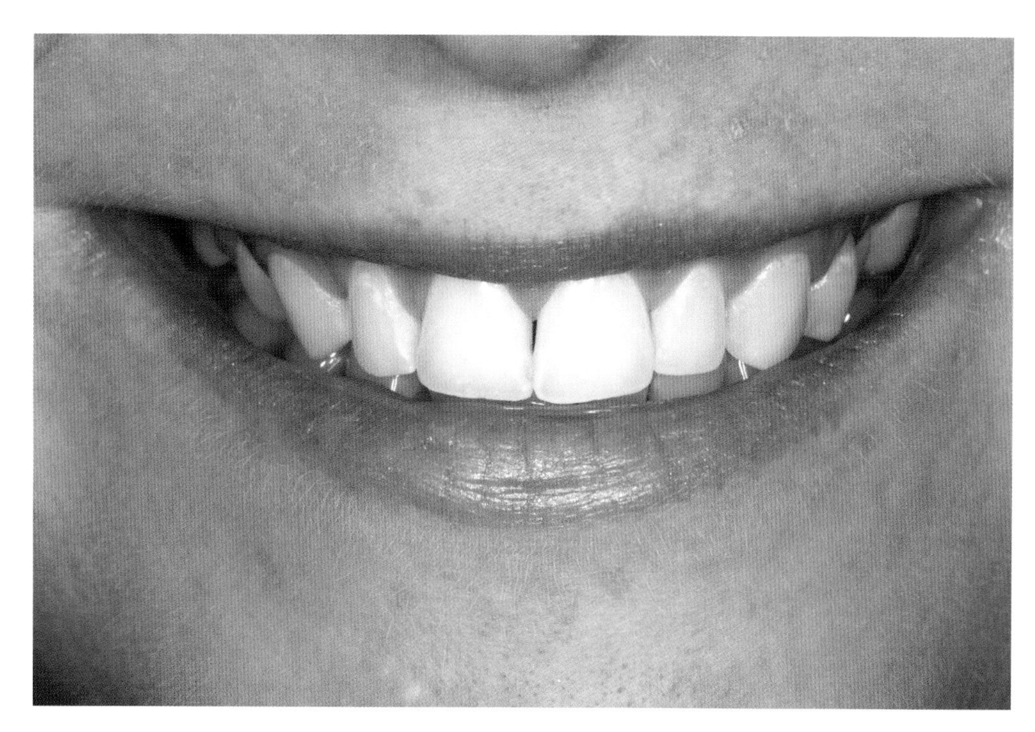

Fig. 7.2 Full-smile photograph. The incisal plane of the maxillary teeth should be located in the middle of the image.

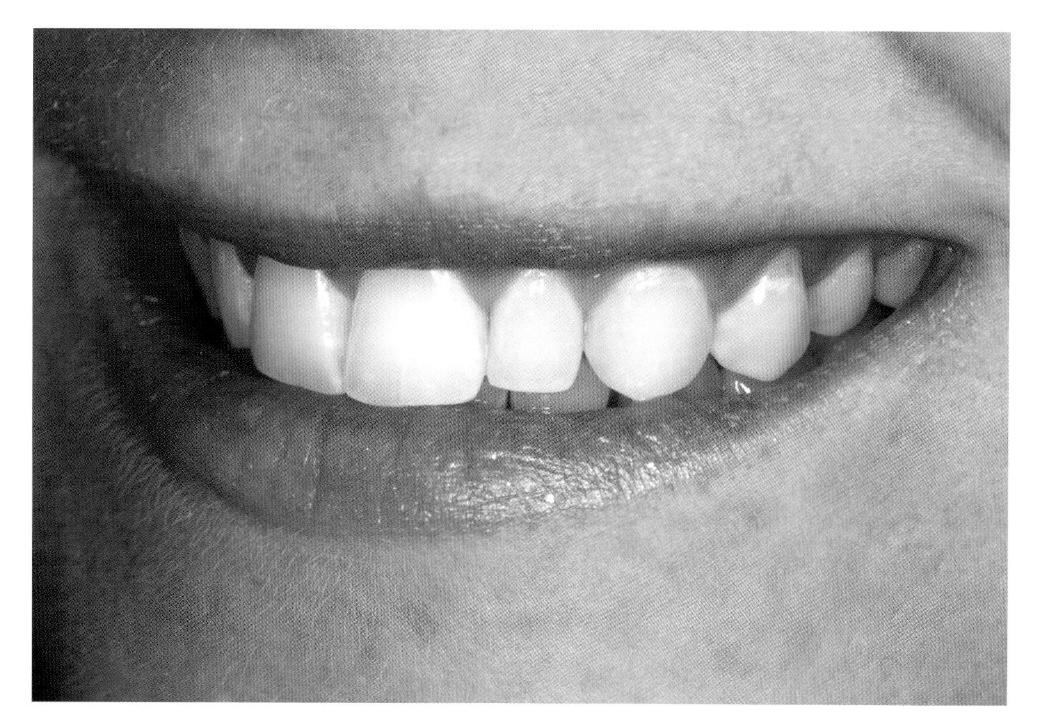

Fig. 7.3 Full-smile lateral view photograph.

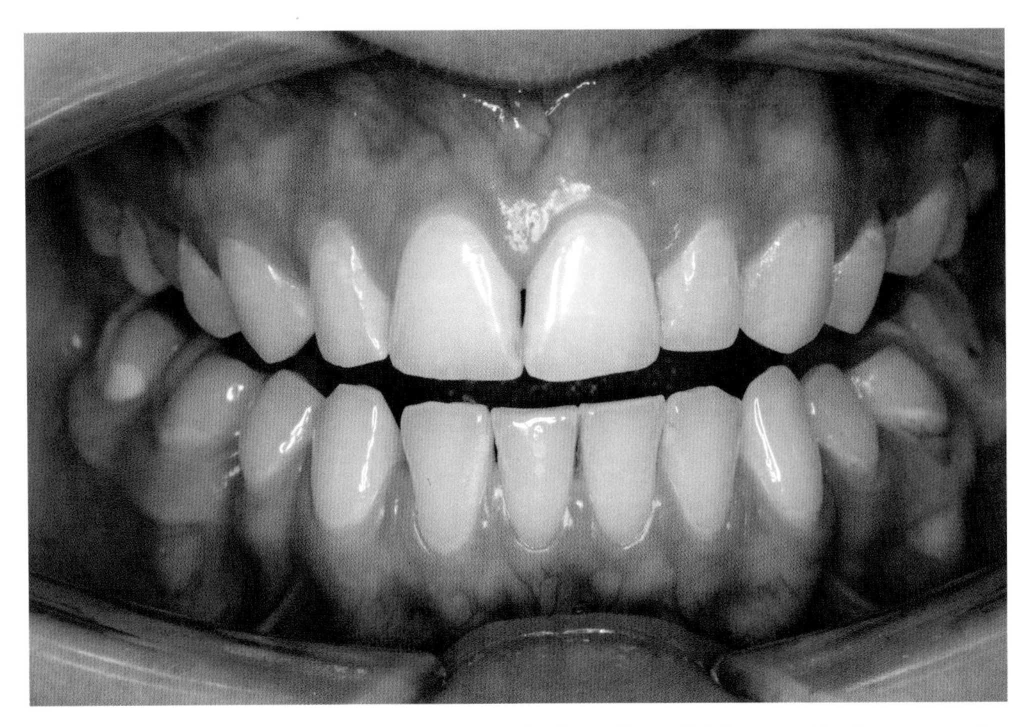

Fig. 7.4 Upper and lower frontal retracted photograph. The teeth are slightly apart, allowing capture of the incisal characteristics.

Upper and lower right and left lateral retracted views

These images are centred on the right or left maxillary lateral incisor. The retractor on the side the picture is being taken from is gently pulled back, while the contralateral retractor is allowed to slip forward (Fig. 7.5).

Upper arch occlusal retracted view (mirror)

This is a view taken in a high-quality mirror, to include as many teeth as possible. The mirror is kept clear of fogging by warming it prior to placement in the mouth, and by blowing air across its surface, using the three-in-one syringe, while in the mouth. The mouth should be opened as wide as possible to facilitate the positioning of the mirror (Fig. 7.6).

Lower arch occlusal retracted view (mirror)

This view is similar to the upper occlusal view. The patient needs to be asked to keep the tongue back; otherwise it will obscure the teeth and wet the surface of the mirror.

Repose

This is the rest position of the lips. It shows tooth display in the rest position and can be of great help in determining tooth length and incisal display. Asking patients to say 'mmm' or 'Emma' and then relax allows the position to be photographed (Fig. 7.7).

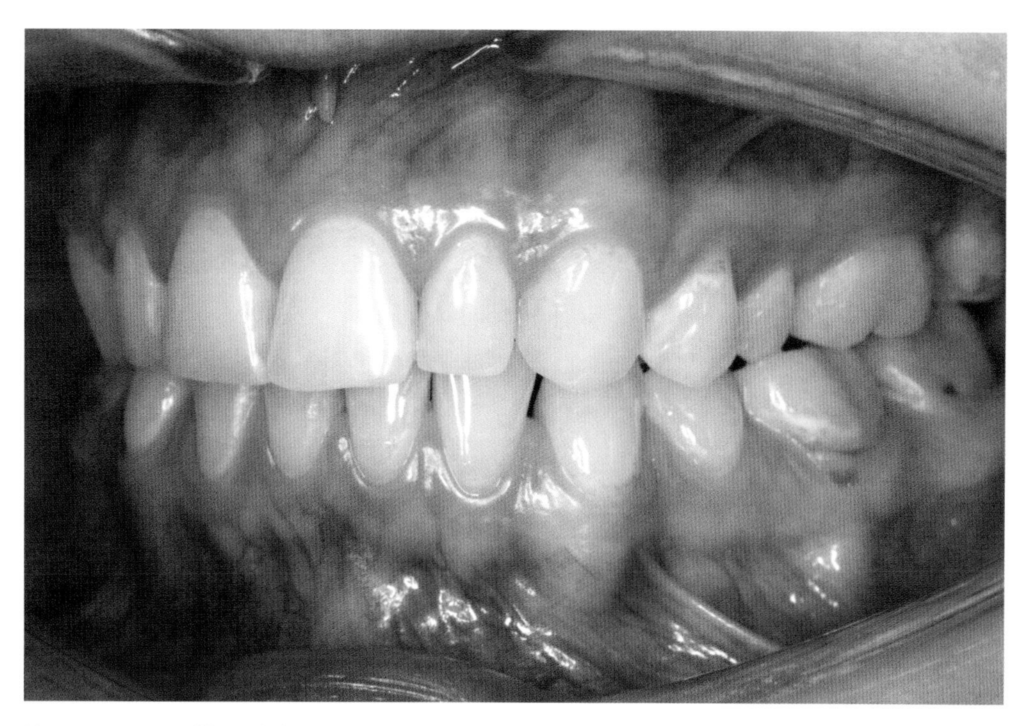

Fig. 7.5 Retracted lateral view photograph.

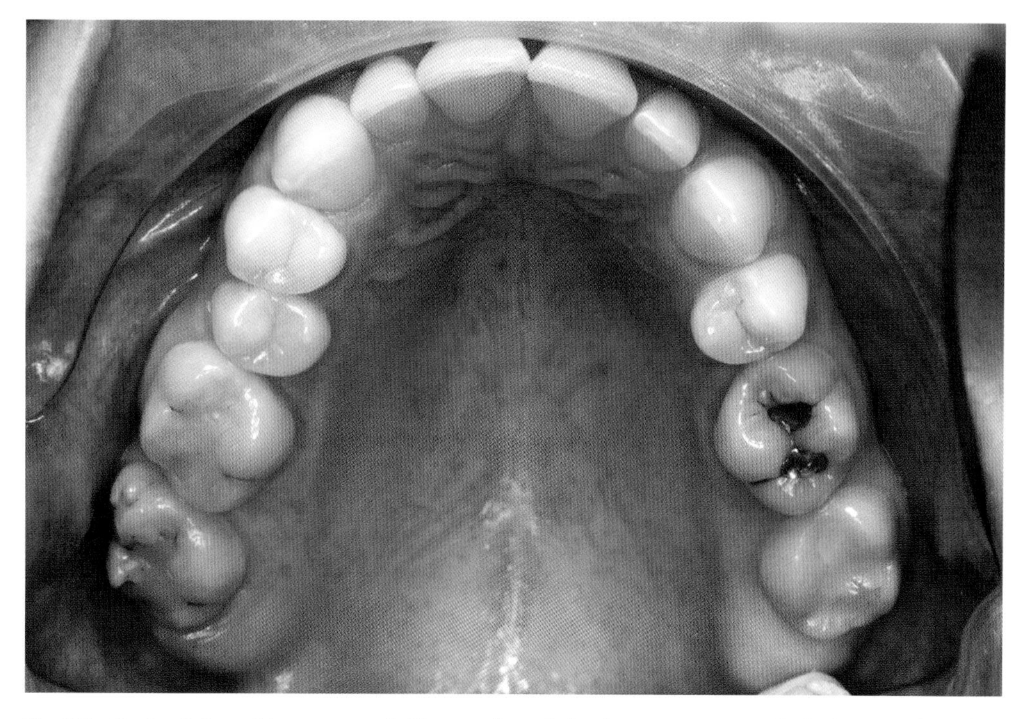

Fig. 7.6 Occlusal view of the upper arch. The use of specialized retractors may assist in the retraction of the teeth, as well as in placement of the mirror.

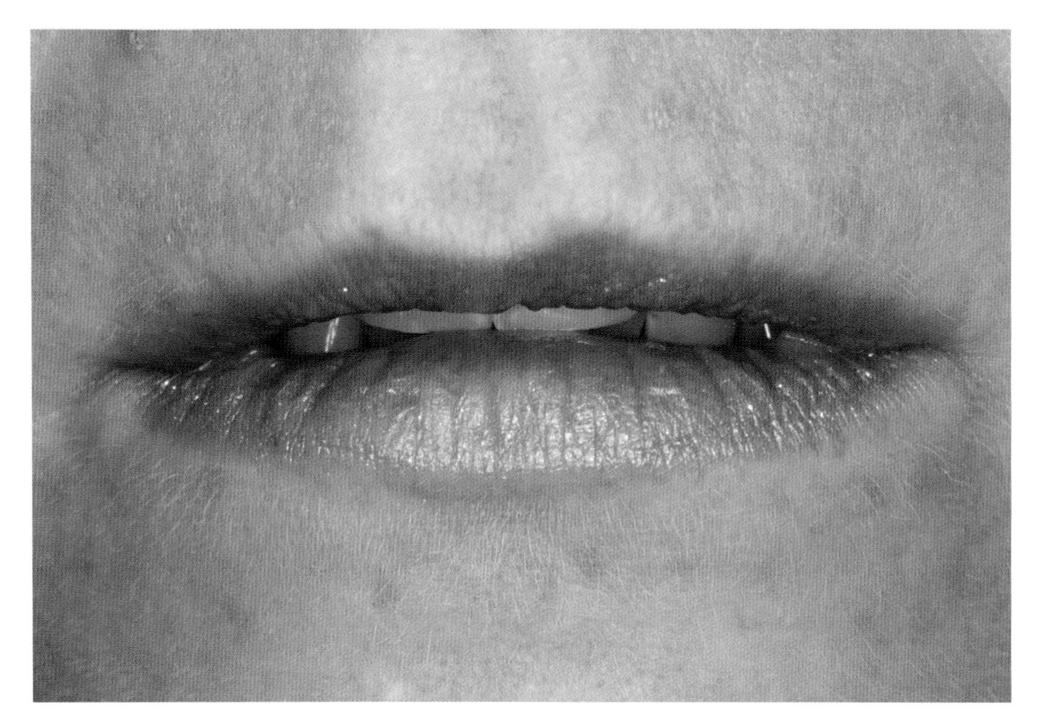

Fig. 7.7 The lips in repose position. This view may assist in the determination of tooth position.

CLINICAL TIP

In planning the length of the maxillary teeth, 1–2 mm of the maxillary central incisors should be displayed in the repose position, with the canines displaying 0–1 mm. This should be adjusted for lip dynamics when a patient smiles, in order to identify the correct length of the teeth. Additionally, this can be assessed with phonetic sounds like the 'f' or 'v' sounds, where the incisal edges of the teeth may just touch the wet/dry line of the lower lip. If the teeth are too long, then they will protrude into the lower lip and will need shortening.

COMPUTER IMAGING

Computer software allows the dental team to illustrate on screen what is planned. Different software is able to simulate the proposed improvement in appearance. The modified images can often be compared side by side with 'before' images. They may assist in discussions of the proposed treatment, and may help persuade patients to accept and give consent for it, especially when they are unable to visualize the final appearance. Clinicians using these software programs should always explain to the patient that there is no guarantee that the final result will exactly match the simulated image.

MINIMAL INTERVENTION TECHNIQUES

BLEACHING

Bleaching to whiten teeth remains the most conservative form of treatment to improve dental esthetics. The media have helped raise awareness of how an

BOX 7.1
CAUSES OF TOOTH DISCOLORATION

Extrinsic staining

- Dietary sources, including coffee, wine, tea
- Nicotine and tobacco tars
- Mouth rinses, e.g. chlorhexidine
- Stained plaque and calculus
- Iron supplements

Intrinsic staining

Systemic causes

- Genetic, e.g. amelogenesis imperfecta
- Drug-related, e.g. tetracycline
- Metabolic, e.g. fluorosis

Local causes

- Non-vital pulp
- Ageing
- Pulpal calcification
- Restorative and endodontic materials
- Root resorption

attractive smile impacts on a person's image and self-confidence. This has led to an increasing consumer demand for dental bleaching.

A comprehensive examination and history is essential to diagnose the source or causation of the discoloration (Box 7.1). This may determine the success of the bleaching procedure. Extrinsic, superficial discolorations are typically caused by the staining effects of various products and foods, including tobacco, tea, coffee, red wine and iron supplements. Extrinsic stains can usually be readily removed and are therefore best managed by professional hygiene treatment. In contrast, intrinsic stains require the use of peroxides for chemical reduction and solubilization of the chromogens responsible for the discoloration. Discoloured teeth should be examined radiographically, especially if the discoloration is limited to one tooth, as this may be indicative of loss of vitality or of calcified pulpal canals. The presence of existing restorations may complicate the treatment, as bleaching does not lighten restorations. As a consequence, the restorations may need to be replaced subsequent to bleaching.

Bleaching can be divided into one of four types:

1. *External bleaching – nightguard vital bleaching or tray bleaching.* This involves the provision of custom-made soft trays to apply a bleaching

solution of carbamide peroxide (<10%) nightly while the patient sleeps. Alternatively, a hydrogen peroxide gel (normally 7.5%, but limited to 6% in the UK) may be used during the day for about 1 hour at a time. These trays are normally worn for a period of days, or possibly weeks, depending on the nature and extent of the discoloration present and the patient's goals.

2. *In-office (chairside) bleaching.* This involves the isolation of teeth with a traditional rubber dam or a paint-on dam and the application of a 25–38% solution of hydrogen peroxide for approximately 60 minutes. The use of lights and heat has been claimed to help activate the gels and speed up the chemical action of whitening.

3. *Over-the-counter (OTC) products.* These contain relatively low concentrations of hydrogen peroxide. They comprise strips, wraps or pens used for 30 minutes once or twice a day. As the carrier component of the OTCs is not customized to the patient, they do not provide an ideal vehicle for the application of peroxide gels. As a consequence, OTCs may take some time to achieve the desired result, or may not provide uniform bleaching.

4. *Internal (non-vital) bleaching.* This involves the placement of a bleaching agent within the pulp chamber of a discoloured, endodontically treated tooth. This can be achieved by means of the walking bleach technique, which involves the placement of a mixture of sodium perborate and hydrogen peroxide directly over a cement base sealing the obturated root canal. This is left in place for approximately 1 week, and the process repeated until the desired shade is obtained. Other techniques include the thermocatalytic technique and intra-radicular in-office external bleaching techniques, using high concentrations of hydrogen peroxide and carbamide peroxide. The thermocatalytic method, which involves heating of the hydrogen peroxide solution, is not recommended, as this procedure increases the risk of external cervical resorption.[1]

There has been controversy over whether the use of lights as part of in-office procedures accelerates and enhances bleaching. Recent literature suggests that the use of a light does not make a difference to the final outcome.[2,3] The initial whitening effect in such procedures is caused by dehydration. There may, therefore, be significant relapse after in-office bleaching. Patients may require multiple in-office procedures to achieve the desired effect. It is therefore recommended that in-office bleaching is best carried out as a combination of a single in-office treatment followed by subsequent tray bleaching. This approach may lead to a more predictable outcome.

CLINICAL TIP

Transient mild to moderate tooth sensitivity can occur in some patients during stages of bleaching treatment. Use of potassium nitrate-containing toothpaste before bleaching and throughout the bleaching therapy can help minimize tooth sensitivity. Other options may include the application of topical fluoride, casein phosphopeptide–amorphous calcium phosphate, or the use of non-steroidal anti-inflammatory drugs (NSAIDs).

Alternatively, the use of a different bleaching concentration or reduction of wear time and intervals of application may also assist in lessening teeth sensitivity.

Existing anterior restorations may not lighten, leading to a subsequent mismatch between the lightened teeth and the restorations. Patients should be informed of the possible requirement to replace these restorations once the other teeth lighten.

Tetracycline-stained teeth may be difficult to whiten successfully. This may require repeated whitening of up to 2–6 months and may not yield ideal results.

Bleaching and restorative dentistry

Restorative treatment should be delayed for at least 2 weeks following the completion of bleaching. This is necessary for a number of reasons,[4,5] including:

- *Shade stabilization*. On completion of bleaching, the shade may relapse, becoming about one shade darker over 1–2 weeks. Hence, the selection of a shade for a restorative procedure should be delayed until this has occurred.
- *Reduced adhesion*. Bleaching reduces bond strengths to both dentine and enamel. This is caused by residual oxygen in the teeth, which can inhibit the polymerization of resins. Two weeks should be allowed for the leaching of peroxide from the teeth prior to adhesive procedures.

MICROABRASION

This chemical and micromechanical method is often used to treat fluorosis affecting the superficial enamel. It involves applying a paste comprising acid and pumice. The teeth must first be isolated with a rubber dam to protect the soft tissues from the acid. The pumice–acid slurry is then applied to the tooth or teeth and moved around and worked across the affected surfaces. This is done either manually, or using a very slow, rotating polishing cup to avoid splatter of the acidic paste, which may cause tissue burns and damage clothing. This removes the outermost, limiting layer of enamel containing the imperfections and discoloration. The procedure is continued until the desired result is obtained, or the patient begins to experience sensitivity. Great care is required with this technique, especially in situations in which the enamel is very thin.

ESTHETIC CONTOURING

Selective contouring of teeth can be used to enhance the appearance of imbricated, chipped or atypically shaped teeth (Fig. 7.8). It is helpful to mark the teeth prior to performing the procedure to help guide the contouring (Fig. 7.9). This allows patient and practitioner to visualize the intended improvement in appearance. Discs or burs may be used to sculpt the tooth artfully to the desired shape. Use of this technique is limited to the management of minor intra-enamel discrepancies only. The aim is to enhance symmetry and alignment during the contouring process.

SHADE SELECTION

The ability to select shades accurately and reliably (Fig. 7.10) is critical to successful clinical outcomes in esthetic dentistry. Restoration needs to blend in harmoniously with the patient's existing dentition. This requires a knowledge of colour science and an understanding of the optical properties of teeth. The perception of colour is dependent on the ambient light and on the way light is reflected by the teeth and observed by the eyes.

The colour of an object can change, depending on the illuminant – colour rendition. For example, tungsten light may cast a yellow colour compared to daylight. Within any dental practice there are normally several different light sources,

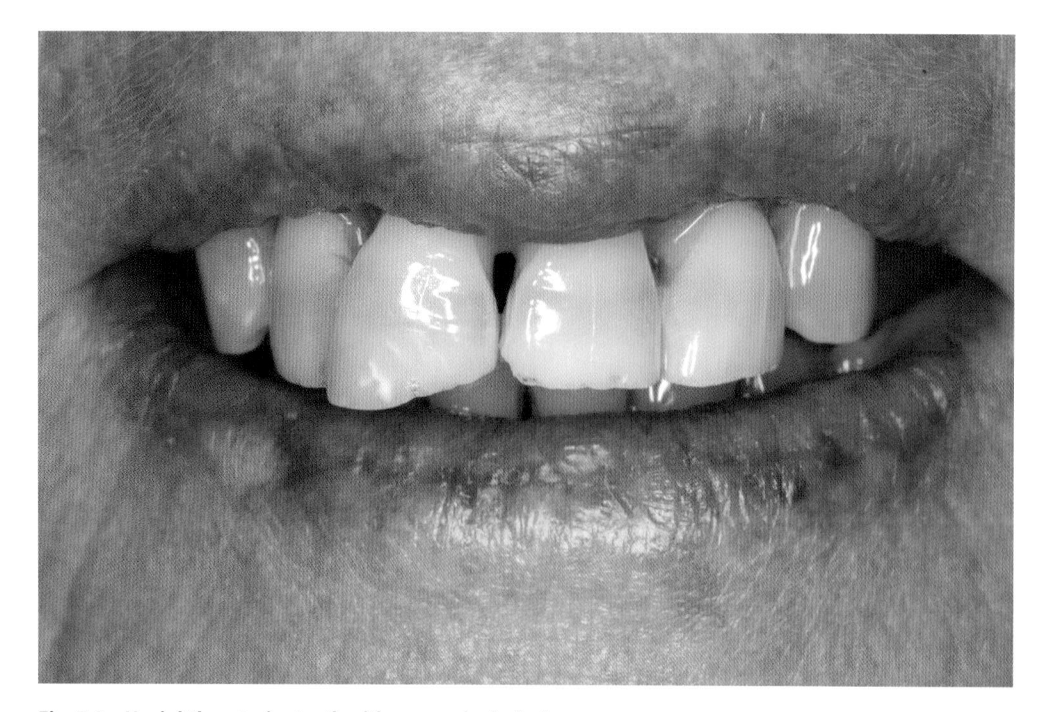

Fig. 7.8 Unsightly anterior teeth with uneven incisal edges.

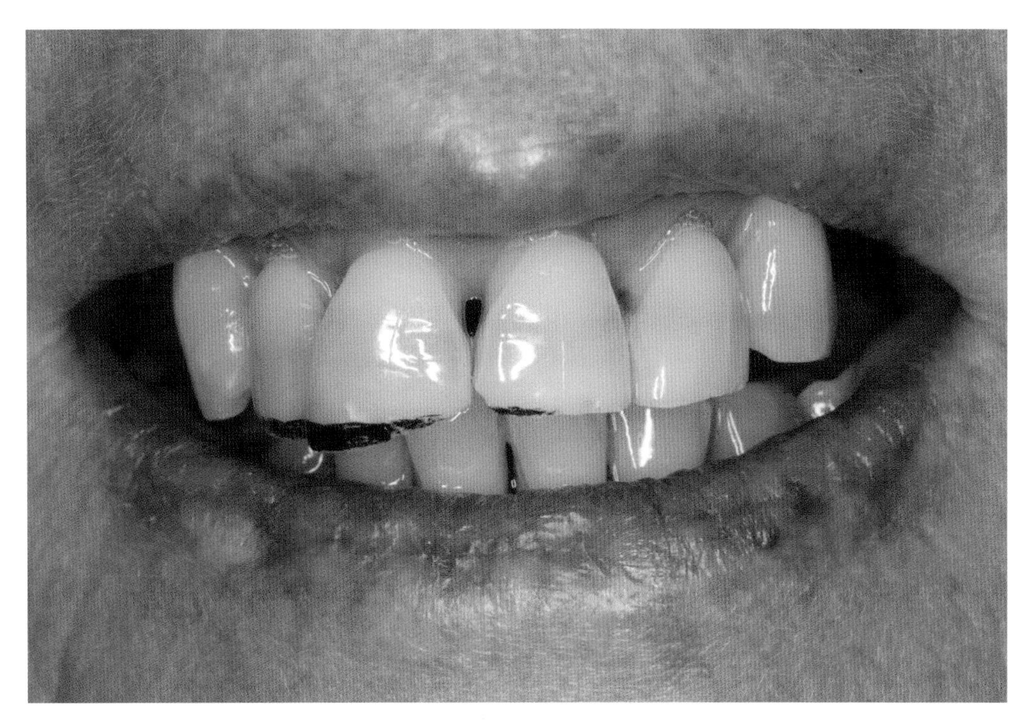

Fig. 7.9 **Areas marked on the teeth to guide esthetic contouring.**

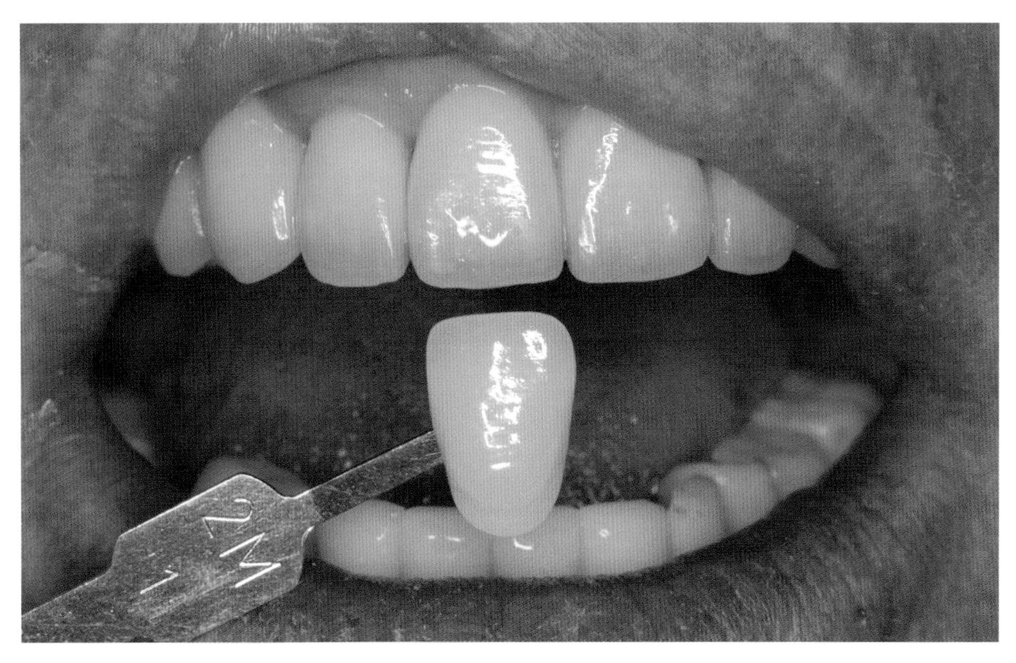

Fig. 7.10 **Shade matching. The shade tab should be placed in the same vertical plane as the tooth. Note that the incisal edge is placed towards the tooth, as the gingival portion is stained with colourants and is not a true reflection of the shade. It may also be helpful to take photographs at slightly different angles to avoid flash reflections that may obscure areas of the tooth.**

including natural, incandescent and fluorescent sources of different qualities. Natural sunlight is variable, with light appearing blue at noon, when the sun has reduced atmosphere to penetrate, and red/orange during the morning and evening. Incandescent lighting is predominantly red/yellow and lacking in blue, while fluorescent lighting is high in blue tones and low in red. Initial shade selection should be made using colour-corrected lights, with a colour temperature of 5500 K. The shade is then matched under different lights to avoid metamerism – the phenomenon that occurs when shades appear to match under one lighting condition and not another.

Shade selection is dependent on the clinician's aptitude to interpret a multilayered structure of varying thicknesses, opacities and optical surface characteristics. The basic hue of a tooth is determined by the colour of the underlying dentine, while value is a quality of the enamel overlay. Chroma is the saturation of colour in the dentine, but is influenced by the value and thickness of the enamel. Teeth are often termed 'polychromatic'. They have variations in hue, value and chroma, giving three-dimensional depth and characteristics. The dentition of a young patient is characterized by opaque, high-value enamel, which blocks underlying dentine. As teeth age, the enamel becomes more translucent and dull (low-value), revealing the underlying dentine, which may yellow as secondary dentine is laid down. This layering can make reading of tooth colour difficult since the value of enamel and surface lustre often complicates colour evaluation of the underlying dentine.

Shade selection sequence

Environment

- Ensure that the surgery surroundings are of neutral colour, so that there is no colour cast.
- Have the patient remove any lipstick.
- If the patient is wearing bright clothing or any item that may distract the eye, it should be covered with a bib.
- Make sure that teeth are clean and free of stains before attempting shade selection.

Chairside

- Perform shade selection before any procedure is undertaken, as teeth can become dehydrated when dried or otherwise operated on, resulting in a higher value.
- The patient should be in an upright position, at a level similar to the operator.

- Observations should be made quickly (5 seconds) to avoid eye fatigue.
- Use colour-corrected light illumination, which should be of a diffuse nature.
- Choose the basic shade to match the centre of the tooth.
- Look at the other parts of the teeth, dividing the teeth into nine sections from apical to incisal, and mesial to distal.
- Necks of shade tabs should be removed or not taken into account, as they include a great deal of colourant that may introduce errors.
- Examine the tooth or teeth for translucency and any other features, including cracks, hypocalcifications and other defining anomalies.
- Create a shade/chromatic map to ensure correct placement of different effects, characterizations and shades.
- Take a photograph of the teeth with a shade tab held adjacent to them. This needs to be on the same vertical plane and should include details of the shade tab, to allow the ceramist to check any variation in the photographic reproduction of the tooth and selected shade (Fig. 7.11).

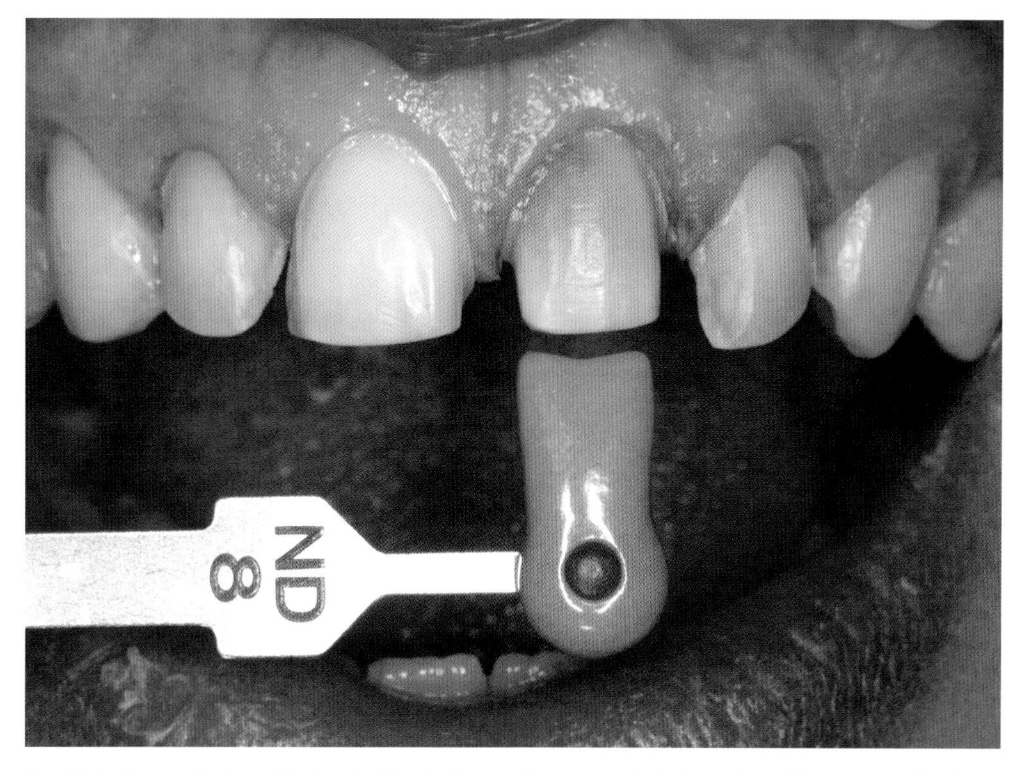

Fig. 7.11 Stump shade guide (Ivoclar Vivadent), used to communicate the colour of the prepared tooth.

Stump shade

With the increasing use of all-ceramic restorations, it is important to communicate the prepared tooth or 'stump' shade, as the colour of the underlying tooth substrate influences the shade of the final restoration. It is essential for the practitioner to communicate the stump shade to the ceramist, especially when there are requirements to mask the remaining darkened tooth tissues. Photographs of the prepared tooth, including the selected stump shade, can be useful. These enable the dental team to select the most appropriate material for each indication. The use of opaque polycrystalline materials, such as zirconia and alumina, allows better masking of underlying teeth than silica-based restorations – feldspathic porcelains and glass ceramics. More recently, the introduction of lithium disilicate materials with different opacities – high translucency (HT), lower translucency (LT), medium opacity (MO) and high opacity (HO) – has allowed the dental team to customize restorations for specific circumstances. The use of opaque ingots permits the masking of dark stumps or metallic posts, while translucent shades are used for teeth that have a stump shade within the normal range.

Instrumental assessment

Visual shade assessment is based on a subjective interpretation of colour and can vary at different times of the day. There is also variation from one clinician to another. The use of digital shade selection devices, developed to evaluate shades objectively, may eliminate human subjectivity, allowing a more reliable and reproducible shade assessment. The available devices include electronic colorimeters, spectrophotometers and digital image analysis instrumentation. When using such devices, it may, in certain cases, be prudent to check the selected shade using a conventional shade guide.

OCCLUSAL CONSIDERATIONS

Mounted diagnostic models are an essential diagnostic and communication tool, allowing an unobscured, three-dimensional assessment of the teeth, the jaw relationship and functional movements. Historically, the mounting of diagnostic models has been based on functional requirements. The occlusion is translated to an articulator using a facebow, which orientates the maxillary casts to the condylar hinge axis of the jaw. This permits detailed study of the occlusion and greatly facilitates treatment planning, but is of relatively little use when considering esthetic aspects, particularly in complex cases. The esthetic display of teeth is based on the incisal plane of the teeth, which, when examined, should generally be parallel to the floor for reference with other landmarks, including the inter-pupillary, ophraic (eyebrow) and commissural lines. This imparts an

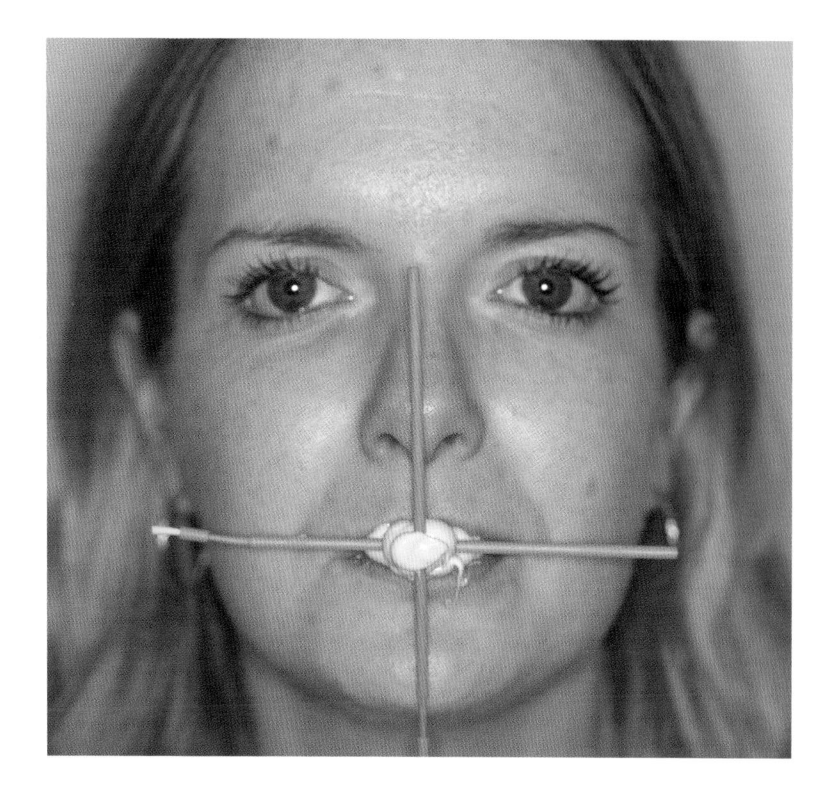

Fig. 7.12 Stick bite to orientate the incisal plane to the horizontal.

overall harmony and horizontal perspective to the face. The inter-pupillary line may not be aligned with the inter-condylar axis, as a consequence of natural asymmetries. Hence, the functional and esthetic planes may not coincide. If these planes do not coincide, restorations may not be esthetically pleasing, with the teeth having a canted incisal plane and possibly a deviated midline.

For esthetic cases, dental technologists require esthetic display information, so that they can orient the models and place the incisal plane correctly, allowing the teeth to sit esthetically in the face. The transfer of information can be achieved by use of a symmetry bite (stick bite – Fig. 7.12) or a facial plane analyser, which enables the transfer of the relationship between the occlusal plane and the inter-pupillary line or horizontal plane.

DIAGNOSTIC MOCK-UP

A mock-up can be used at the chairside to demonstrate to a patient the anticipated results of a clinical procedure, greatly enhancing understanding of the proposed treatment. It allows patients to see their 'trial smile'. Alternatively, composite resin may be temporarily applied, with no etching or bonding. In cases involving an additive approach, putty keys of the wax-ups can be filled with temporary materials and applied to the teeth, providing a quick and simple means of allowing patients a preview of the planned outcomes of treatment.

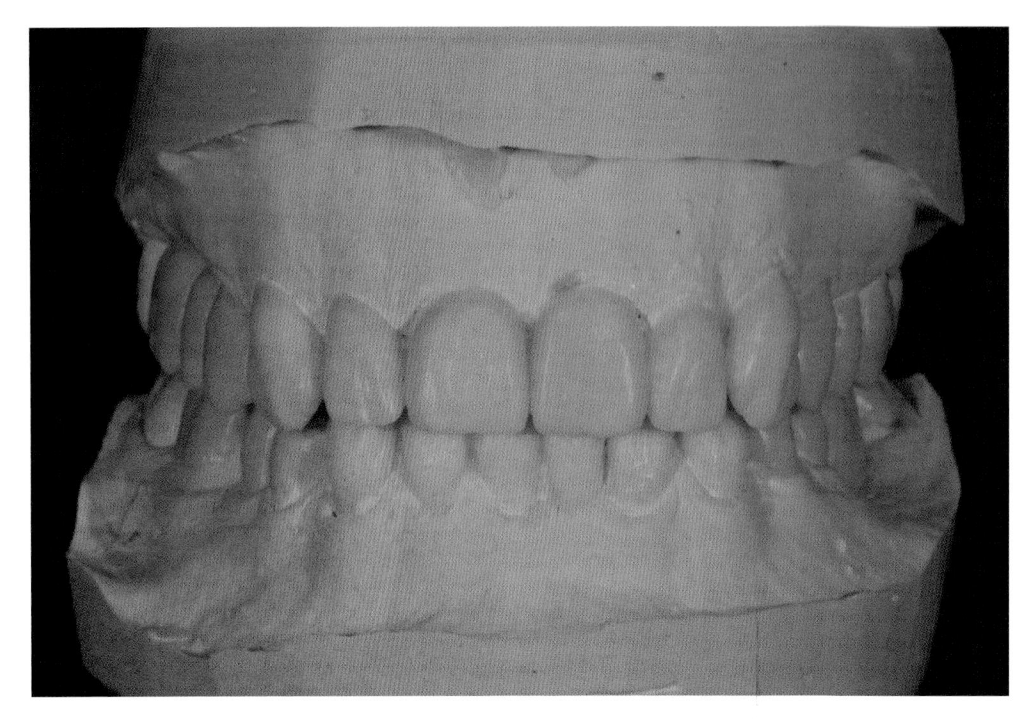

Fig. 7.13 Diagnostic wax-up.

Diagnostic wax-up

It is important to have a clear idea of the treatment objectives. The use of a wax-up (Fig. 7.13) can help plan the desired esthetic appearance. This should incorporate the patient's expectations and requirements, as expressed in the initial treatment planning discussions; examples could include increasing the length of incisors, changing the shape and alignment of teeth, and closing the diastema.

The diagnostic wax-up provides a blueprint of the final restorations. The wax-up also allows the manufacture of putty keys for the provision of temporary restorations and reduction guides for tooth preparation.

The contours and form of the proposed restorations can be transferred from the completed wax-up to the provisionals, allowing patients to preview their planned appearance and reconfirm that they are happy with the proposed changes. It is advantageous for a patient to be able to view planned changes prior to the construction of, for example, veneers, given the cost implications of remaking restorations if the patient is not satisfied. The use of provisional restorations also allows evaluation of occlusion and phonetics. Once the provisional restorations are considered satisfactory by both practitioner and patient, an impression can be made to communicate the size, shape, length and form of the required restorations to the laboratory.

PERIODONTAL PROCEDURES

The primary objective of periodontal therapy is optimal soft-tissue health and stability. This is vitally important to ensure successful clinical outcomes in restorative and esthetic treatments. Inadequate management of unhealthy soft tissues may lead to poor clinical outcomes and subsequent unstable soft-tissue relationships. In esthetic treatment planning, the importance of 'pink esthetics' to the final esthetic outcome cannot be over-emphasized. The correction of gingival anomalies is an essential step, given that the soft tissues act as a frame for the teeth. The soft tissues should be symmetrical, with pleasing, harmonious contours and dimensions. Tjan et al.[6] reported that 80% of patients have an average to high smile line, emphasizing the importance of periodontal health and harmonious gingival architecture in esthetic cases, particularly in patients with a broad smile.

Common gingival esthetic problems include:

- excessive gingival display
- uneven, asymmetrical gingival contours
- loss of papillae
- exposure of root surfaces.

KEY POINT SUMMARY

Periodontal techniques to correct soft-tissue esthetics include:

- resective techniques, including gingivectomy and crown lengthening
- root coverage
- ridge preservation
- site development

Excessive gingival display

The patient's smile line is determined by the position of the lips during a smile. The upper lip helps determine the length of the maxillary teeth and the position of the gingival margins.

Excessive gingival display, commonly called 'gummy smile', may be a result of:

- *A short upper lip.*
- *Vertical maxillary excess.* There is an overgrowth in the maxillary skeletal base. In such cases, treatment modalities range from orthodontic intrusion

alone, through to complex treatments involving orthognathic surgery, orthodontics, restorative treatment and periodontal plastic surgery.

- *'Hypermobile' lip*. This occurs when there is increased activity of the elevator muscles of the upper lip in smiling. Lip-repositioning surgery[7] has been suggested as a technique for managing the hypermobile lip. In this technique, the internal connection of the upper lip is severed, tissue is removed and the lip sutured back above the free gingival margin. This procedure of reconnection restricts upper lip elevation during the smile, limiting the amount of gingival display. Recently, Polo[8] has suggested the use of botulinum toxin (Botox) injections as a non-surgical method for treating excessive gingival display. The toxin is injected into the area of the upper lip to decrease the elevator muscle activity, aimed, in particular, at the levator labii superioris muscle. The major disadvantage of this technique is the short-term effect of the toxin, which lasts 3–6 months only. Consequently, this procedure needs to be repeated on a regular basis to maintain the clinical outcome.
- *Over-erupted anterior teeth with the associated dento-gingival complex*.
- *Altered passive eruption*. Passive eruption is a normal process in which the gingival margins recede apically to the level of the cement-enamel junction (CEJ) after the tooth has fully erupted. Altered or delayed passive eruption (Fig. 7.14) occurs when the gingival margins fail to recede to the level of the CEJ, and subsequently the teeth appear short. A resective surgical

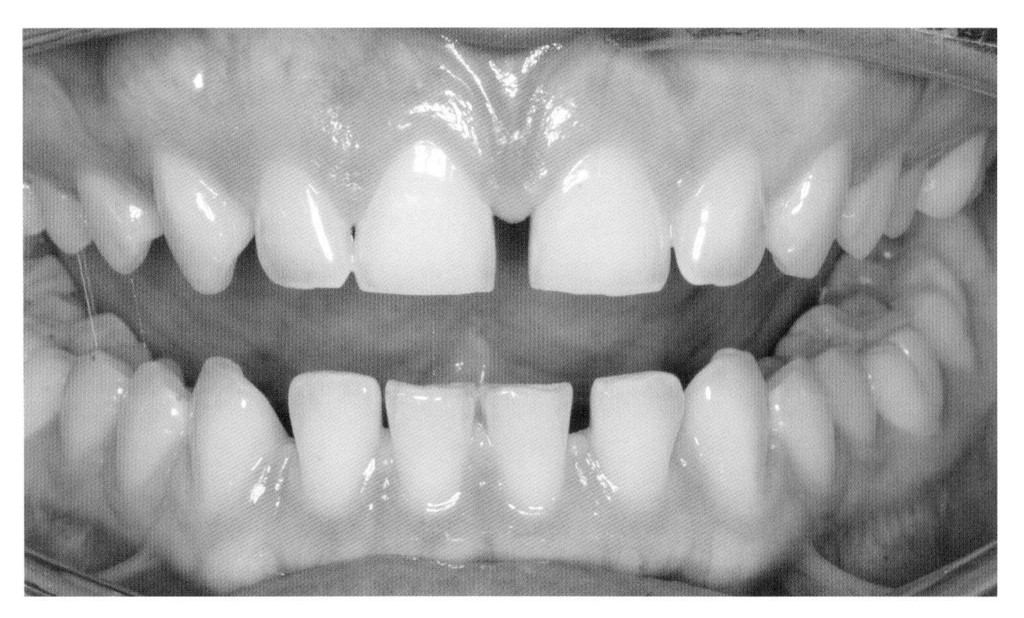

Fig. 7.14 Altered passive eruption. The patient displays short teeth and diastema.

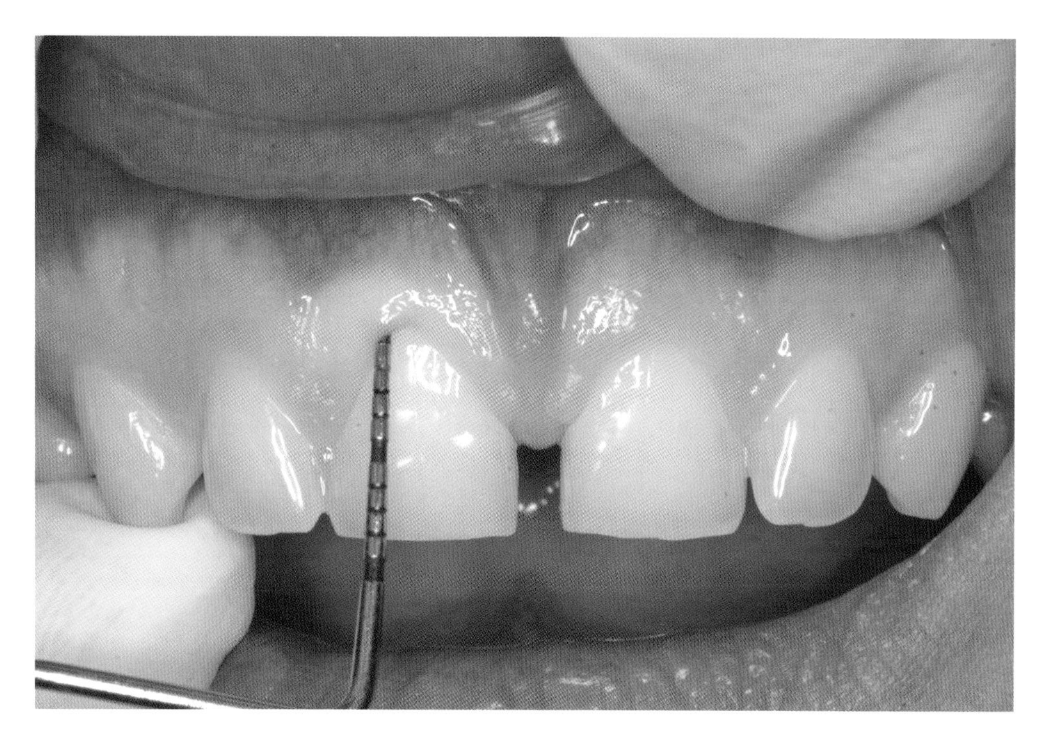

Fig. 7.15 Bone-sounding with a periodontal probe to assess biological width prior to a gingivectomy (resective) procedure.

exposure may be performed to correct gingival profile (Fig. 7.15). Selective osseous recontouring can be achieved by performing submarginal incisions to the desired height of the clinical crown. A biological width of at least 2 mm between the alveolar crest and the CEJ should be retained to ensure the health of the attachment gingiva. The maintenance of a zone of attached gingiva is important for long-term gingival health (Fig. 7.16).

Gingival asymmetries

Gingival asymmetries (Fig. 7.17) are common in the esthetic zone. In managing these asymmetries, it is critically important to achieve symmetry first between the central incisors, and then between the central and lateral incisors, followed by the canines. As the maxillary central incisors are the most dominant teeth and in the centre of the smile, their gingival symmetry is of paramount importance. Uneven gingival contours can be corrected surgically, using either crown-lengthening and root-coverage procedures. Alternatively, correction may be achieved by means of orthodontic extrusion or intrusion. When teeth are orthodontically moved, the accompanying hard and soft tissues will follow; however, as the root is extruded, the diameter becomes narrower, leading to other esthetic challenges with emergence profiles.

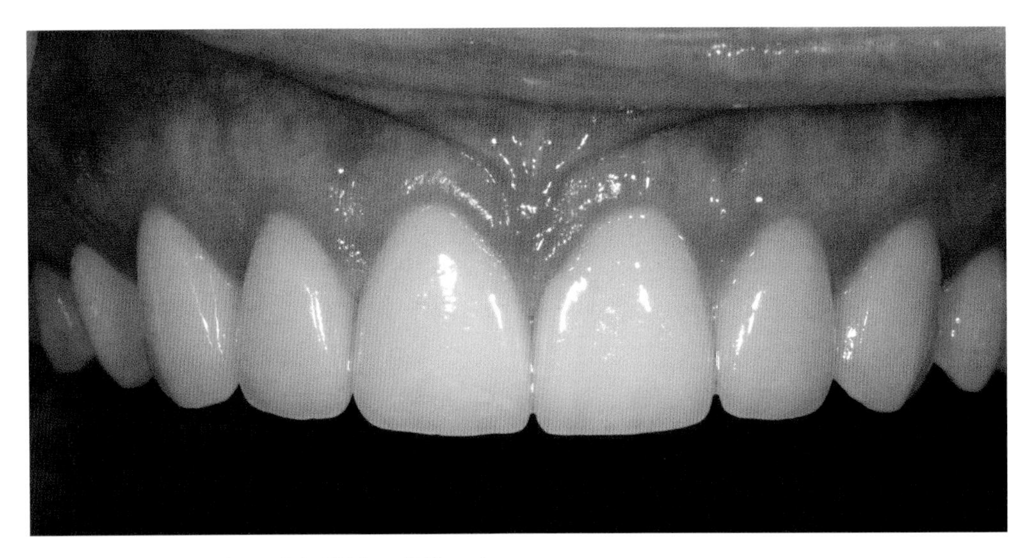

Fig. 7.16 Completed porcelain (lithium disilicate) veneers.

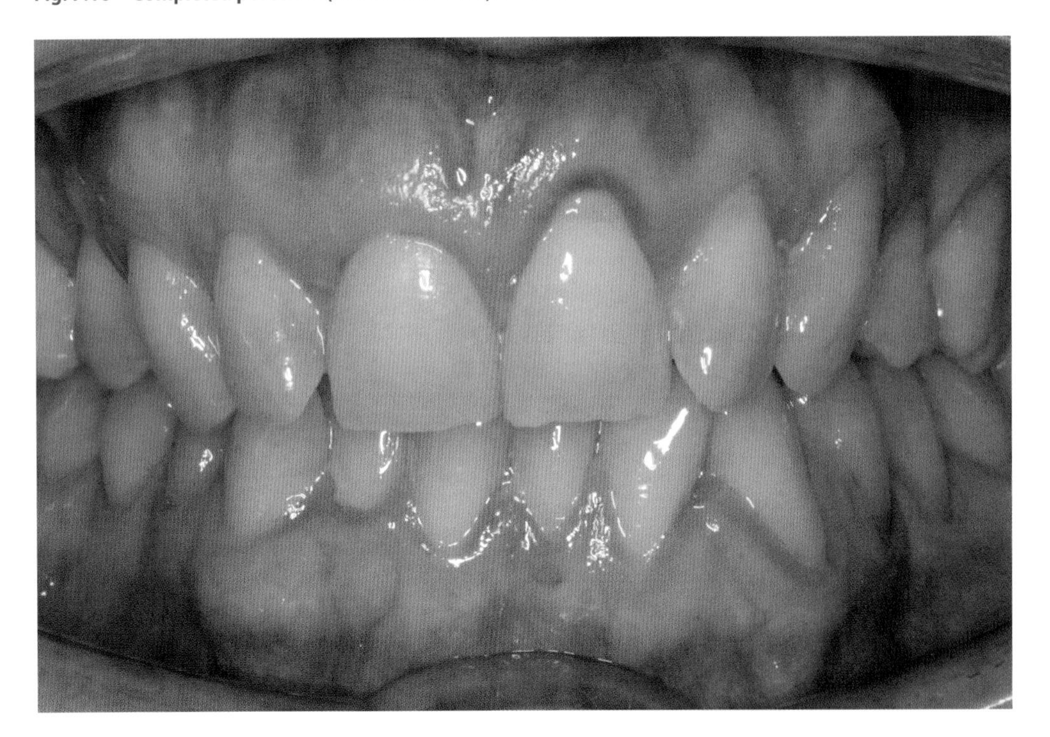

Fig. 7.17 Unilateral gingival recession.

KEY POINT SUMMARY

Treatment for uneven gingival contours includes:

- crown-lengthening procedures
- root coverage procedures
- orthodontic extrusion
- orthodontic intrusion

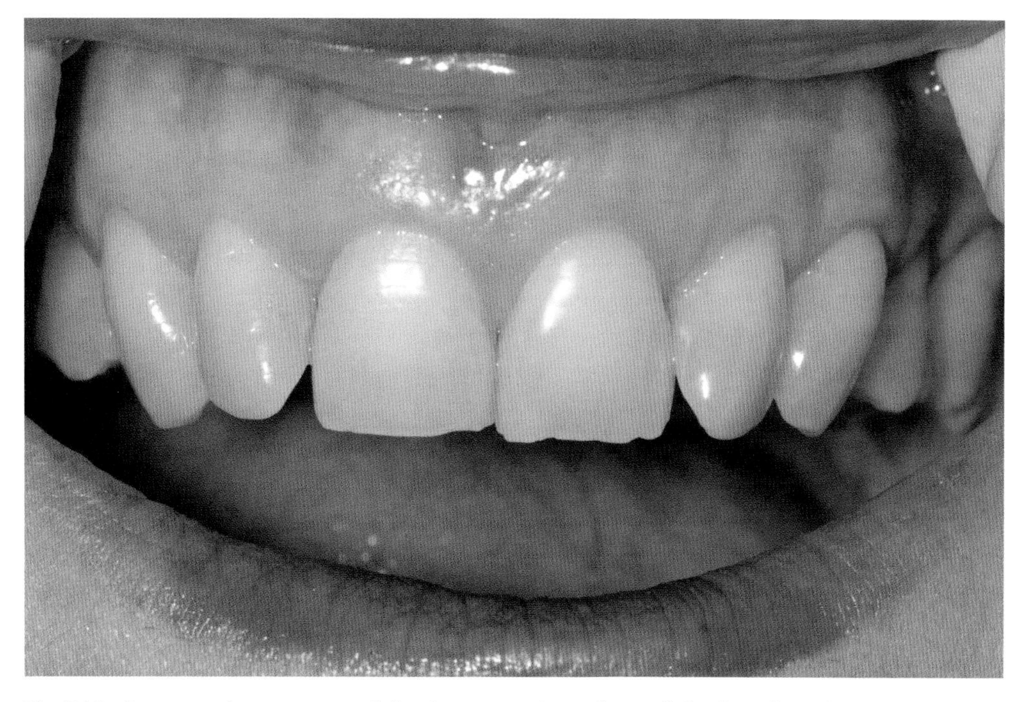

Fig. 7.18 Postoperative appearance following a procedure using acellular dermal matrix. (Courtesy of Dr Kevin Todes.)

Root coverage procedures

Numerous surgical techniques have been described to correct labial–gingival recession defects (Fig 7.18). These have been discussed in Chapter 6.

Loss of papillae

Patients with a history of periodontal disease and recession may present with the loss of inter-dental papillae, producing so-called black triangular defects. This is esthetically displeasing, may cause phonetic issues and leads to food entrapment.

Tarnow et al[9] reported on the effect of the distance between the contact area and the most coronal portion of the bone crest on the level of vertical loss of the inter-dental papilla. They showed that when the distance between the contact area and the crest of bone was 5 mm or less, the papilla was typically present; when the distance was 6 mm, the papilla was present 56% of the time; and when the distance was 7 mm or more, the papilla was present only 27% of the time or less.

Management of black triangle defects is one of the most challenging gingival esthetic procedures. Rather than subjecting a patient to multiple surgical

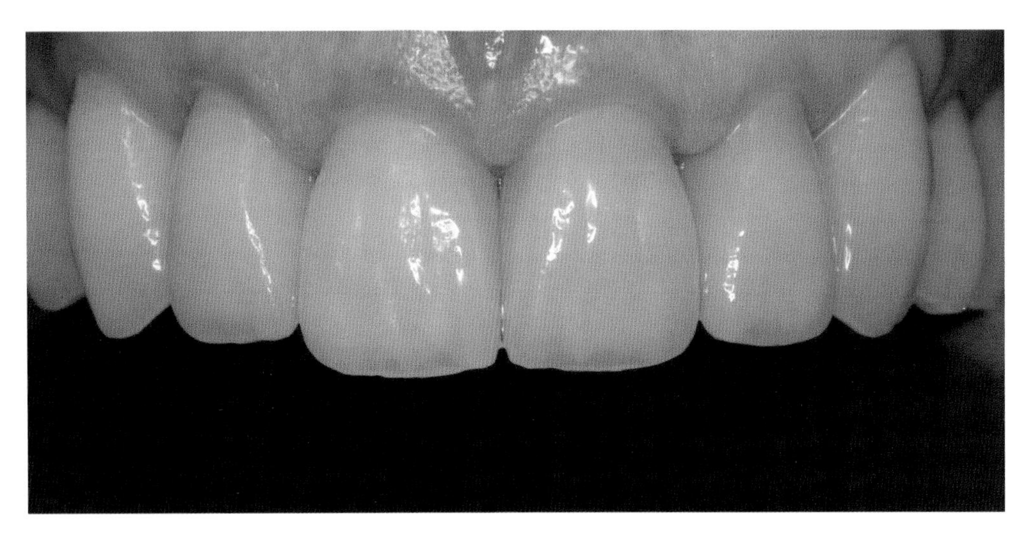

Fig. 7.19 All-ceramic crowns on the anterior teeth. Closure of black triangular defects is demonstrated, with the application of porcelain and inter-proximal staining.

interventions, with an unpredictable outcome, it may be preferable to treat the condition by means of one of the following approaches:

- *Orthodontic treatment*. The teeth are stripped, the enamel reduced inter-proximally, and the dental arches collapsed to bring the roots closer together. As this occurs, the inter-dental papillae are compressed, helping to fill the inter-dental spaces.
- *Microsurgery papilla regeneration procedures*. Surgical reconstruction of the dental papilla is extremely difficult and has varying degrees of success.
- *Restorative treatments*. Direct restorations, porcelain veneers and crowns can be used to reduce black triangular defects (Fig. 7.19). In partially edentulous cases, it may be possible to use prosthetic gingivae to mask the defects. Encroachment of restorations into the inter-dental spaces does, however, bring with it certain disadvantages, including reduced access for oral hygiene procedures and, in turn, the risk of adverse gingival response.

Site development

In edentulous saddles, where teeth have been missing for many years, there may have been significant atrophy of the tissues, and augmentation may be required. Augmentation procedures with bone and connective tissue grafts may assist in bulking up the tissues for site development. The objective of site development is to provide adequate bone and soft tissues for implant placement, or prior to conventional bridgework to provide a soft-tissue bed for an ovate pontic. As its name indicates, the profile of an ovate pontic is egg-shaped, giving the illusion that the tooth appears to emerge from the soft tissues in an esthetically pleasing manner. The shape should be carefully contoured to facilitate effective cleansing by means of normal oral hygiene aids.

ORTHODONTIC TREATMENT

Orthodontic treatment is often a conservative means of bringing teeth, lips and jaws into proper alignment. It may aid in achieving facial balance without the biological cost of tooth preparation and the consequential ongoing maintenance of replacing restorations. This form of therapy may be used to correct esthetic concerns, or may be used as an adjunct to various forms of restorative treatment. Orthodontic therapy prior to restorative treatment often leads to a better long-term overall esthetic result, given improved symmetry and spacing. Also, it typically results in more conservative tooth preparation during any subsequent restorative procedures.

Techniques

- *Fixed appliances* with orthodontic brackets, bands and wires.
- *Removable appliances and aligners*, e.g. Invisalign®, and expansion appliances. These appliances are not able to correct alignment to the same degree as fixed appliances. In particular, the bodily movement of teeth and torquing movements are limited. These effects are better managed with fixed appliances. A further disadvantage is that these removable appliances rely heavily on the compliance of patients, which can be limited given the impact on speech and the need to remove the appliance to eat and drink. Patients undertaking this form of therapy should be carefully monitored.
- *Orthognathic surgery*. In patients with severe skeletal malocclusions, it may be necessary to carry out surgical correction in combination with conventional orthodontics.

Invisalign® treatment begins with an initial detailed assessment and examination, which should be fully documented. Digital models are reconstructed from polyvinyl siloxane impressions to yield accurate models, which are then scanned. The data are collated into proprietary software that allows the teeth to be replicated on-screen as a three-dimensional model.

The practitioner has the opportunity to view the 'virtual' models from presentation through to correction using a program called ClinCheck®. The patient's treatment can be reviewed aligner by aligner, and corrections made before the treatment plan is validated. Changes are made through the ClinCheck® system to the satisfaction of the practitioner. Following final approval, the aligners are made and dispatched.

Invisalign® is a useful treatment alternative, especially in adults seeking an orthodontic correction by means other than fixed appliances.

ADJUNCTIVE TOOTH MOVEMENT

Forced eruption

The use of forced eruption may be adopted as an adjunctive technique in esthetic dentistry. The technique for tooth movement is relatively simple.

The indications for the use of forced eruption include[10]:

- *Treatment of isolated intra-bony defects.* This is used to level intra-bony defects.
- *Salvage of a non-restorable tooth.* In clinical situations where caries, trauma or pathology has resulted in non-restorable subgingival margins, the options for restoration encompass either the performance of crown-lengthening procedures or orthodontic eruption of the tooth to expose sound tooth structures for restoration.
- *Alteration of free gingival margins.* The harmonious symmetry and positioning of gingival margins are important for a good esthetic outcome, particularly in patients with a smile line that exposes the free gingival margins. The relocation of gingival margins may be effectively performed with both the extrusion and the intrusion of teeth.
- *Implant site development.* Orthodontically extruding teeth allows the underlying bone and soft tissue to be vertically augmented since the dento-gingival complex follows the tooth as it is extruded.

CONCLUDING REMARKS

KEY POINT SUMMARY

Clinicians today have a whole range of techniques at their disposal. While this is of benefit to the patient, it places increased demand on the clinician to be aware of and competent in a broad range of techniques. Many of these will not have been taught at dental school and will need to be acquired through a range of continuing professional development programmes or formal postgraduate training.

Clinical techniques in esthetic dentistry continue to be developed at an ever-increasing rate. To keep up to date with these techniques, practitioners active in the field of esthetic dentistry need to be proactively engaged in relevant continuing professional development. Clinicians need to be aware of a broad range of treatment modalities that may need to be brought together to treat an individual case. Applying an MI approach to esthetics will challenge traditional thinking and techniques.

REFERENCES

1. Trope M. Cervical root resorption. J Am Dent Assoc 1997;128(SI):56–9.
2. Marson FC, Sensi LG, Vieira LCC, et al. Clinical evaluation of in-office dental bleaching treatments with and without the use of light-activation sources. Op Dent 2008;33:15–22.
3. Matis BA, Cochran MA, Eckert GJ. Review of the effectiveness of various tooth whitening systems. Op Dent 2009;34:230–5.
4. Spyrides GM, Perdigao J, Pagani C, et al. Effect of whitening agents on dentine bonding. J Esthet Dent 2000;12:264–70.
5. Haywood VB. Achieving, maintaining and recovering successful tooth bleaching. J Esthet Dent 1996;8:31–8.
6. Tjan AHL, Miller GD, Josephine GP. Some esthetic factors in a smile. J Prosthet Dent 1984;51:24–8.
7. Rosenblatt A, Simon Z. Lip repositioning for reduction of excessive gingival display: a clinical report. Int J Period Rest Dent 2006;26:433–7.
8. Polo M. Botulinum toxin type A in the treatment of excessive gingival display. Am J Orthodont Dentofac 2005;127:214–18.
9. Tarnow DP, Magner AW, Fletcher P. The effect of the distance from the contact point to the crest of bone on the presence or absence of the interproximal dental papilla. J Periodontol 1992;63:995–6.
10. Celenza F. The development of forced eruption as a modality for implant site enhancement. Alpha Omega 1997;90:40–3.

CHAPTER 8

Clinical Techniques: Composites and Indirect Methods

CHRISTOPHER HO

INTRODUCTION

Restorative treatments are often used to enhance dental esthetics. Historically, full-coverage crowns were commonly used to improve dental attractiveness. The invasive nature of full-coverage preparations, especially on intact teeth, involves the considerable biological cost of substantial tooth structure removal. There are also the financial costs of treatment, both initial and over time with maintenance and, when required, replacement of failed or failing restorations. It was not until 1955, with the introduction of bonding by Buonocore, that esthetic techniques began to become more conservative in nature. Adhesive dentistry has been made possible by the introduction of adhesive techniques, together with developments in resins through to indirect, bonded, all-ceramic restorations.

It is critical for restorative treatment decisions to be based on a comprehensive assessment, comprising a detailed history and clinical examination. Control of any active disease and prevention are first priorities. The planning of esthetic treatments follows thereafter.

The esthetic treatment planning process begins with:

1. A thorough medical and dental history, along with discussion in respect of the patient's expectations and wishes, and the treatments available to achieve the desired outcomes.
2. Initial assessment, comprising a thorough hard- and soft-tissue examination, as discussed in Chapter 3. A systematic approach should be adopted, documenting all clinical findings, including periodontal findings, existing restorations, occlusion and any other relevant information. Radiographic examinations and study models should be included in this initial examination. A photographic series of the patient, including extraoral photographs of the full smile and lateral smiles, as well as intraoral photographs, as discussed in Chapter 7, should be part of the documentation process.
3. Informed consent, discussion of which will be facilitated by the information collected as part of the history, assessment and examination procedures. The patient should be fully appraised of the 'pros' and 'cons' of the possible treatment options. This should be done in a simple manner, detailing the proposed treatment steps and limitations. Care must be exercised not to exaggerate the anticipated final outcome, and to ascertain whether the patient is expecting unachievable results.

Proper treatment planning is based on the principle of 'primum non nocere' – 'first, do no harm'. If a patient can be treated by minimal intervention (MI) approaches, such as orthodontics, bleaching or alternative non-invasive treatment, then this should be recommended to the patients as the preferred choice.

COMPOSITE RESIN

The introduction of composite resins and adhesive systems, together with subsequent improvements in the longevity, clinical performance and colour compatibility of bonded restorations, have allowed the ever-increasing application of direct tooth-coloured restorative systems in both anterior and posterior regions of the mouth.

Composite resins offer excellent esthetic potential, with the availability of multiple shades, in different opacities. Composite restorations demonstrate good clinical longevity, if placed with due care and technical expertise. Composite resins can be used to improve the appearance of misshapen, chipped or discoloured teeth, and to replace unsightly restorations. In addition, composite resins can be used for veneers and diastema closure, and to increase tooth length (Fig. 8.1).

Composite restorations can be applied by different means:

- *Direct* composite is applied and polymerized directly to the teeth to be treated, allowing typically one-visit outcomes.
- *Semi-direct* techniques are normally completed in a single appointment. They combine direct additions and the contouring and finishing of restoration produced in part in the laboratory, or away from the chairside and then luted using an adhesive resin cement. For one-visit indirect procedures, it is necessary to adopt a technique to produce a die at the chairside. Pre-formed, laboratory-cured composite labial surfaces have recently become available to speed up the shaping and finishing process.
- *Indirect* techniques require an impression to allow the restoration to be made in a laboratory and cemented at a subsequent visit. The use of indirect procedures may provide the opportunity for more complete polymerization, thus giving the restoration better physical and mechanical properties. Indirect techniques are especially helpful when it is anticipated that it will be difficult to produce the required contours and contact areas using a direct approach.

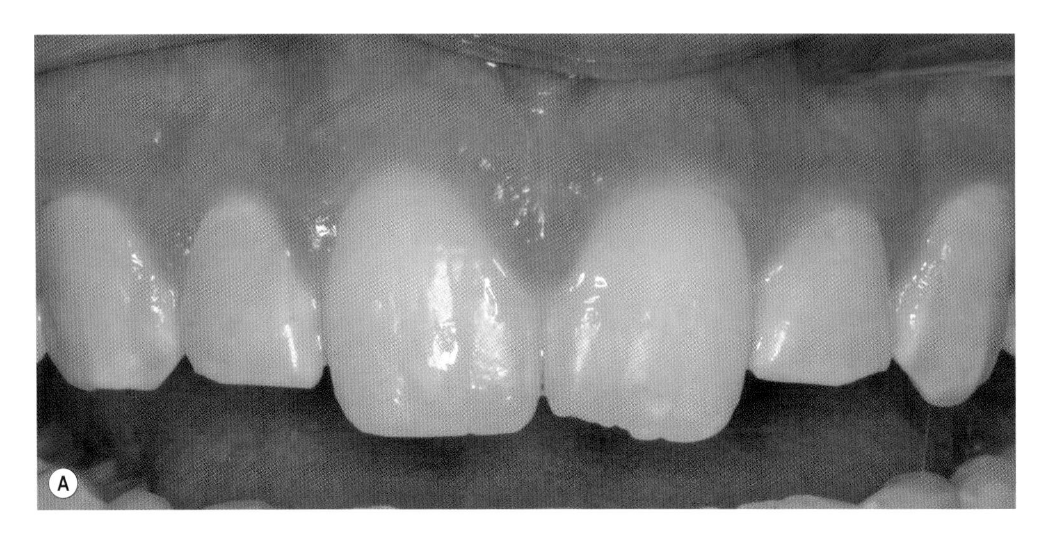

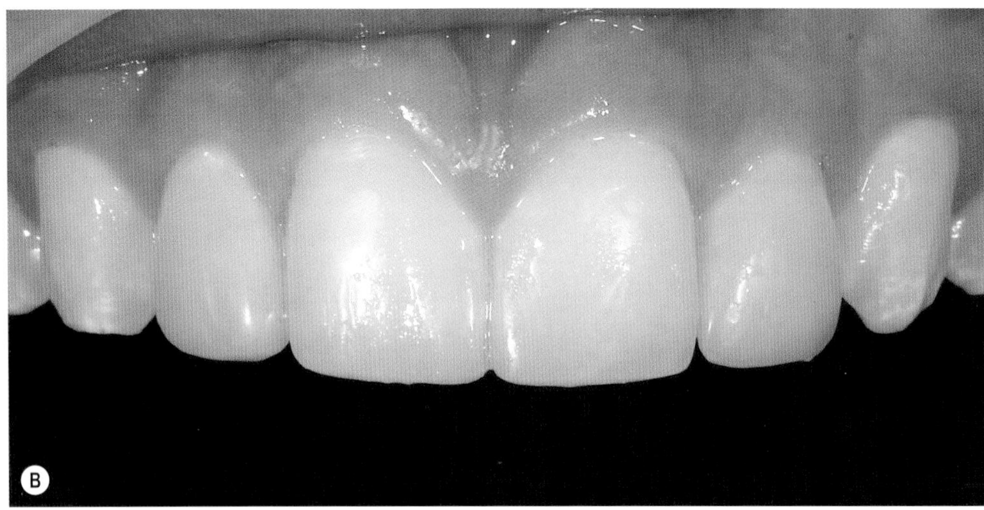

Fig. 8.1 Composite resins. A. Preoperative photograph of a young patient with uneven incisal edges. B. Postoperative photograph of the same patient with direct composite resin placed on the maxillary incisors, improving esthetic alignment and symmetry. The restorations were completed using an additive approach, demonstrating the conservative nature of the procedure.

The use of direct resin approaches is a popular treatment option for patients and practitioners, given the relatively low cost and single-visit convenience. Direct approaches with composite resins are considered conservative because they involve minimal, if any, preparation of the teeth to be treated. Advantages and disadvantages can be seen in Table 8.1. The availability of materials with different opacities, translucencies, natural fluorescence and opalescence allows practitioners to adopt a layering approach in the application of composite resin to create outstanding natural esthetic appearances. This allows the practitioner to replicate nature with the use of translucent shades to replace enamel and more opaque shades as a replacement for dentine. This anatomical approach allows the build-up of successive layers of dentine, enamel and incisal

TABLE 8.1 ADVANTAGES AND DISADVANTAGES OF DIRECT COMPOSITE RESIN RESTORATION

Advantages	Disadvantages
Immediate esthetic result	May be technically demanding
Conservative procedure	Time taken to place
Relatively low cost	Requires meticulous attention to detail to create esthetically pleasing outcomes
Controlled by operator	Longevity largely dependent on skill and relevant knowledge of operator
Good potential for repair	Reliant on patient to maintain good oral hygiene
Single appointment	
Bonded resins may enhance the strength of the restored tooth	

TABLE 8.2 PHYSICAL AND OPTICAL PROPERTIES IN SELECTING A COMPOSITE RESIN

Physical properties	Colour and optical properties
Fracture toughness	Opalescence
Wear resistance	Fluorescence
Sculptability	Translucency (enamel shades)
Polishability	Opacity (dentine shades)
Colour stability	

composites, allowing light to be reflected, absorbed and transmitted naturally, giving the lifelike esthetics necessary for dental attractiveness (see Table 8.2 for composite resin properties).

PLACEMENT OF COMPOSITE RESIN

Isolation

The placement of composite resin restorations is technique-sensitive. The operating field needs to be kept clean and dry. It is essential to secure good moisture control, preventing contamination with water, saliva and blood. Contamination can lead to compromised esthetics, postoperative sensitivity, leakage and secondary caries. Therefore, placement of a rubber dam is highly recommended. Additionally, a well-placed rubber dam assists in retracting the oral tissues for better access, simplifies the operative procedures, and enhances the appreciation of the qualities and features of the teeth to be treated.

Composite resin selection

The evolution of composite resins has led to numerous improvements over the years, including enhanced mechanical and physical properties, as well as reduced polymerization shrinkage. The properties have been improved mainly by changing the filler type and content. Contemporary resin materials are divided into micro-filled, microhybrid and nano-filled/nanohybrid materials. Micro-filled composites have particle sizes of approximately 0.04 microns, resulting in excellent polishability and lustre retention. However, micro-filled composites have inadequate mechanical properties for high-stress areas, typically limiting their application to enamel additions in the anterior zone. Hybrid composites, in particular nanoparticle-containing materials, have a high filler load. They have the advantages of excellent mechanical properties and exceptional surface polish and retention of lustre. This has resulted in hybrid composites enjoying universal use for both anterior and posterior indications.

Preparation

This involves the removal of failed restorations and caries through to minimal preparations for composite additions and facings. The use of bevelled margins in anterior teeth increases the surface area for bonding, improves retention and reduces leakage. It also allows for a chameleon-like blending of the resin to the tooth surface.

Adhesive bonding

Careful and meticulous adhesive procedures are followed to achieve bonding to both dentine and enamel. Sealing exposed dentine by effective hybridizing of exposed collagen matrix provides retention to the dentine, resistance to leakage and elimination of sensitivity. Rubber dam isolation can greatly increase the likelihood of optimizing adhesive bonding.

Placement

Incremental layering is the technique of choice to minimize stresses from polymerization shrinkage. Marginal gaps will develop when adhesion is insufficient to resist the forces of polymerization shrinkage. This may lead to postoperative sensitivity, leakage and recurrent caries under the restoration. Composite resins should be placed incrementally in layers 1.5–2 mm thick to control stresses and optimize the light curing. In addition, layering allows the development of a lifelike, natural-looking restoration. Teeth are polychromatic, having a three-dimensional effect, which can be simulated by layering composite resin restorations to give the appearance of natural tooth structure. Successive layers of dentine, enamel, and translucent and other composite shades create a restoration with lifelike optical properties similar to those of natural teeth.

Matrix systems

Posterior restorations

It can be a challenge to create tight inter-proximal contacts in occluso-proximal restorations of composite. Open contacts can lead to food impaction and subsequent periodontal problems. The establishment of a correct inter-proximal contact requires a well-contoured matrix that is stabilized and adapted gingivally with a wedge. The Tofflemire or universal matrix band, although versatile, is not capable of giving a proper contour to composite resin restorations. The circumferential matrix often causes the band to flatten inter-proximally when tightened. The flat inter-proximal contour leads to the contact point migrating from the upper middle third of the tooth to the marginal ridge. This may result in an open contact when adjusting the restoration, and can also lead to marginal ridge fracture caused by lack of support. There are other methods to create tight inter-proximal contacts, including pre-wedging, which gives initial separation of the teeth, as well as protection of the gingival tissues during preparation. Packable composite resins have also been developed but their use has not been found to make a major improvement in contact management. The use of special instruments, such as the Contact Pro II (Clinicians Choice) or Optracontact (Ivoclar Vivadent), may help restore the contact area during light polymerization, and is especially useful when the preparation is wide proximally. The use of pre-contoured matrices and separation rings has provided the most reliable means of restoring contact areas in recent times. Examples include the Composi-Tight 3D (Garrison Dental) and Triodent V4 system (Triodent). The use of contoured matrices allows the development of broad, well-contoured contact areas, along with the rings that provide separation of the teeth while stabilizing the band.

Anterior restorations

The use of clear Mylar strips or Teflon tape to separate the restoration from adjacent teeth prevents inadvertent contact-area bonding. It also facilitates the contouring of the restoration and allows simultaneous curing (Fig. 8.2). Customized crown formers can be used for the more extensive restorations. Where a matrix cannot be applied, an alternative is to coat adjacent teeth with a lubricant or isolate with polytetrafluoroethylene (PTFE) tape and freehand-sculpt the material. Another technique involves the use of a putty matrix, possibly from a diagnostic wax-up (Figs 8.3–8.6). The matrix provides a lingual key, and may be especially useful in incisal-proximal restorations and incisal build-ups in esthetic and tooth-wear cases. The aim is to create a lingual shell with the putty matrix. A thin layer of composite resin is closely adapted to the internal contours of the matrix and then cured. The palatal, proximal wall and also the incisal edge can be reproduced exactly as in the mock-up, so minimal adjustments are required when the next layer of composite is added.

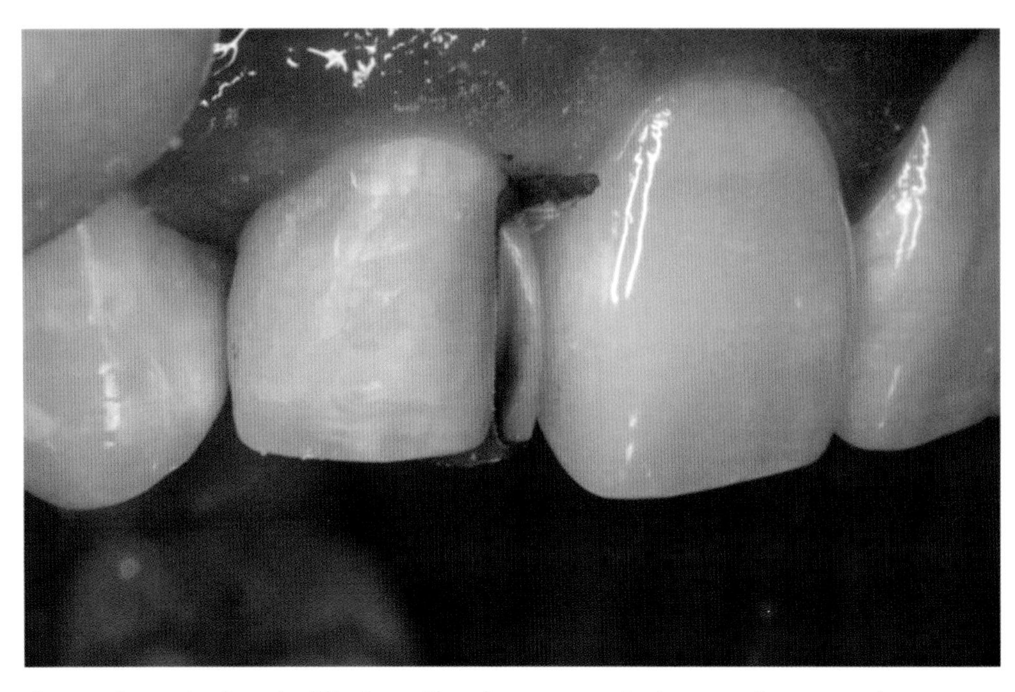

Fig. 8.2 Contouring. It can be difficult to achieve the correct proximal contour of upper anterior restorations with the use of strips and matrices, as they often lead to a flat and unnatural contour. The use of contoured metal or clear sectional matrices may allow the proper shape to be sculpted.

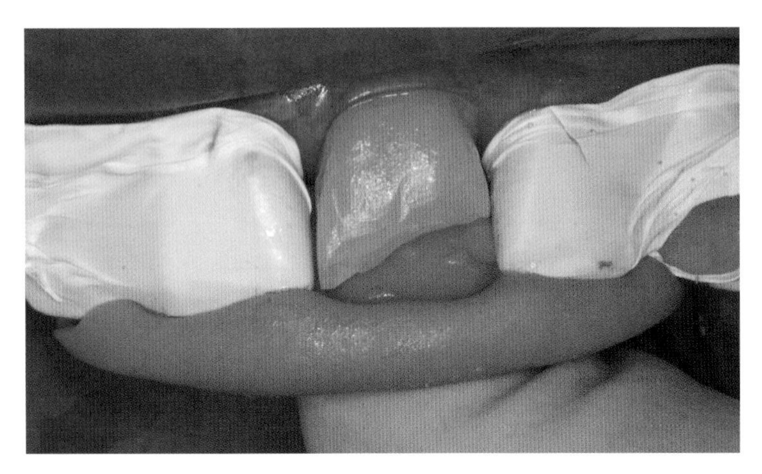

Fig. 8.3 Anterior incisal-proximal restoration of direct composite resin. The patient sustained trauma from a fall, resulting in an oblique fracture of the incisal edge. A putty matrix can be constructed from previous study models or a wax-up to form the lingual contour. The adjacent teeth have been isolated with Teflon tape.

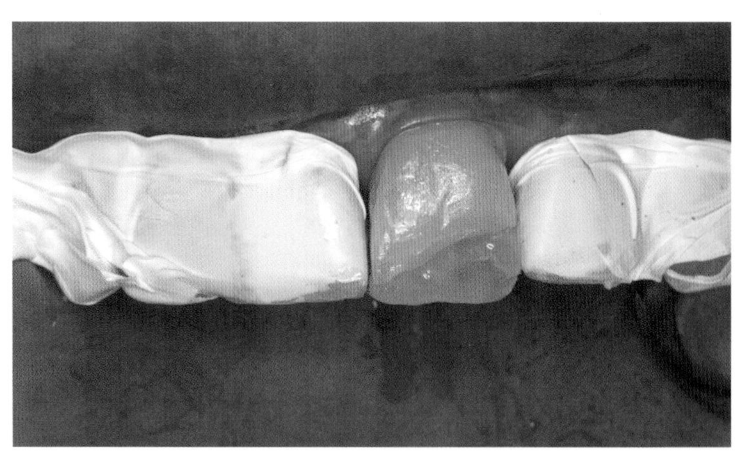

Fig. 8.4 Use of putty matrix. This has allowed a thin lingual shell of enamel composite to facilitate the anatomical incremental build-up of resin.

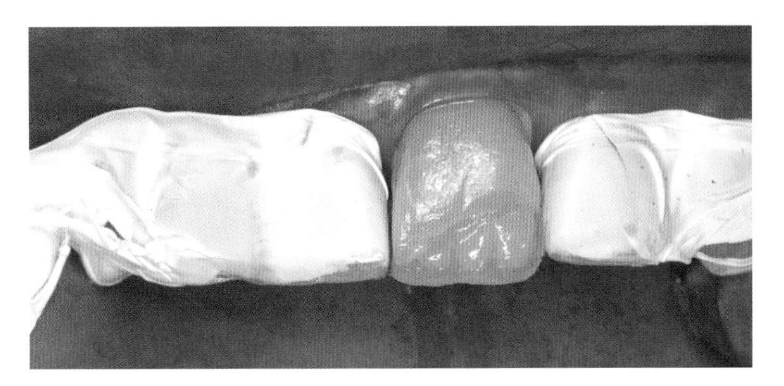

Fig. 8.5 Anatomical, incremental layering of direct resin with the placement of dentine composite. This simulates the more opaque nature of dentine.

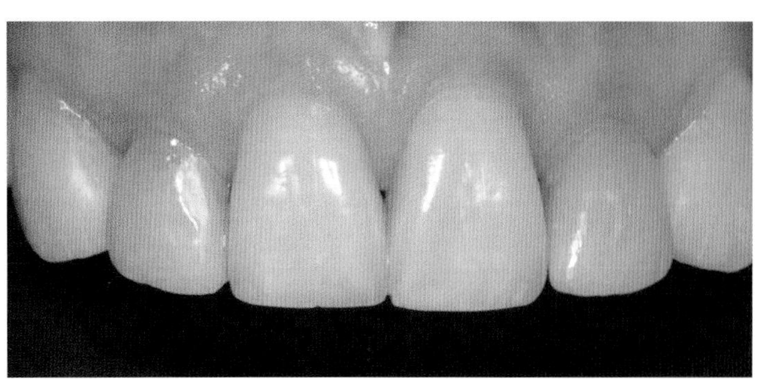

Fig. 8.6 Completed direct resin restoration with anatomical layering of dentine, enamel and incisal composite resins.

Finishing and polishing

Contouring and shaping of the restoration complete the primary anatomy. Polishing produces a smooth, light-reflective surface. This prevents plaque accumulation, resists stains and improves marginal adaptation, enhancing longevity and esthetics. To contour the primary anatomy and finish margins, multi-fluted carbide and diamond burs may be used, followed by abrasive and polishing devices including discs, strips and pastes. These comprise aluminium oxide particles, silicon carbide particles and silicon dioxide, and are used sequentially from larger to smaller particles to ensure a smooth, highly reflective surface. The over-use of polishing discs can lead to a flat profile of the final restoration. The judicious use of rotary burs and discs along the line angles of the tooth and copying of the convex (three-plane) labial contour of teeth will allow a natural tooth surface that reflects light correctly and has the correct form (Fig. 8.7).

INDIRECT RESTORATIONS

Direct esthetic restorations require careful and meticulous technique combined with creative and artistic skills. This involves considerable chairside time. Indirect techniques, using laboratory-manufactured restorations, outsource the skills required to provide an esthetic restoration, and may improve the long-term esthetics and performance.

Traditional metal–ceramic restorations have predictable strength and a history of long-term success, but typically less-than-ideal esthetics. The increasing demand from patients for improved esthetics has driven the development of all-ceramic systems. These systems have grown exponentially with the

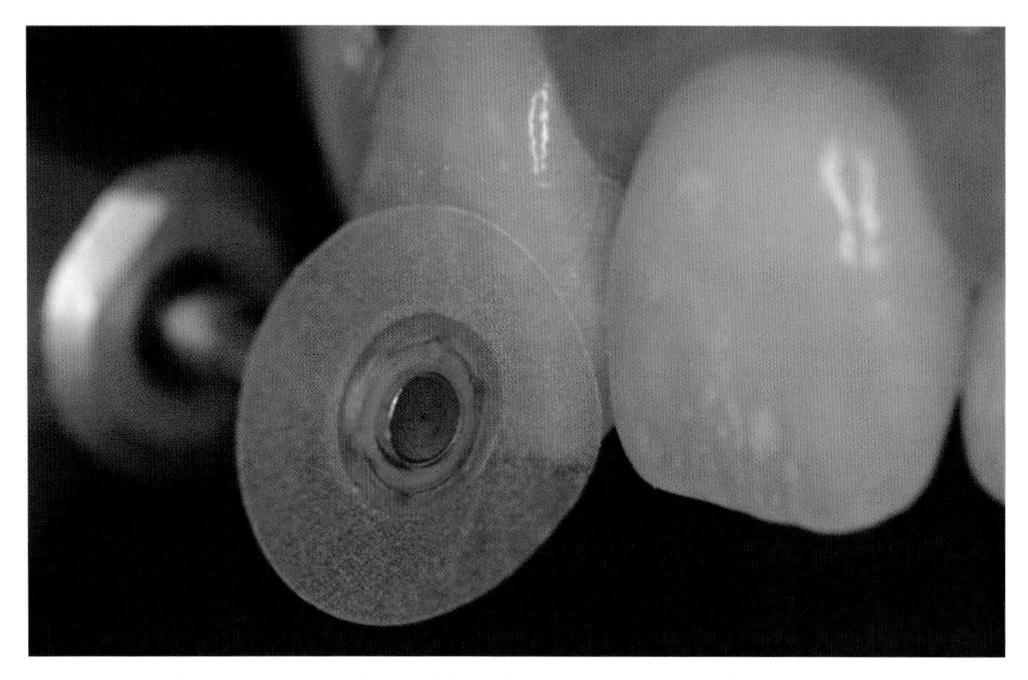

Fig. 8.7 The judicious use of rotary burs and discs allows a natural tooth surface.

development of esthetic and biocompatible ceramics. The absence of metal allows a natural transmission of light through the restoration. In addition, it improves the appearance of the gingival tissues where the transmission of light through a metal–ceramic restoration often leads to tissues looking discoloured, or to a dark line running circumferentially around the cervical margin.

In comparison to direct procedures, indirect approaches traditionally require more tooth preparation to create the space required for the necessary thickness of material, and to prevent over-contouring. There is also the added cost of these restorations, given the need for at least two appointments, temporary restorations and the laboratory fee. See Table 8.3 for the advantages and disadvantages of indirect restorations.

CLASSIFICATION OF CERAMIC SYSTEMS (Box 8.1)

Silica-based ceramics have a high glass content and provide the best optical and esthetic properties. They are used for porcelain veneers, inlays, onlays and crowns. These materials are etched with hydrofluoric acid and silanated to provide a micromechanical bond to remaining tooth structures, increasing the strength of the restored tooth unit. They are brittle, with low fracture toughness, and gain the majority of their physical properties by bonding either to teeth or to a coping. Polycrystalline ceramics, including alumina and zirconia, have higher flexural strengths

TABLE 8.3 ADVANTAGES AND DISADVANTAGES OF INDIRECT RESTORATIONS

Advantages	Disadvantages
Superior esthetic result	Abrasiveness to antagonists, especially if not polished
Excellent wear resistance	Complex techniques required in construction
Biocompatibility with soft tissues	Cost
Dimensional stability	Difficulty to adjust/polish intraorally
Excellent colour stability	Increase in number of appointments often
Inertness	Difficulty to repair
	Preparation required

BOX 8.1 CLASSIFICATION OF CERAMIC MATERIALS

Silica-based (etchable) ceramics

- Feldspathic porcelain
- Leucite-containing ceramics (Empress Esthetic; Ivoclar)
- Lithium disilicate (e.max; Ivoclar)

High-strength (non-etchable) polycrystalline ceramics

- In-ceram (Vita)
- Alumina-based ceramics, e.g. Procera (Nobel Biocare)
- Zirconia-based ceramics, e.g. Lava (3M), Procera Zircon (Nobel Biocare), Cercon (Dentsply)

and high fracture toughness. They are silica-free and cannot be prepared by traditional surface treatments such as hydrofluoric acid etching. These ceramics have inherent strength and, as a consequence, can be cemented conventionally or adhesively. See Table 8.4 for the different properties of ceramic materials.

PRODUCTION OF CERAMIC RESTORATIONS

Ceramic restorations produced by different methods have different properties that affect clinical performance – strength, translucency/opacity and accuracy of fit. The methods of production include:

- *Powder condensation.* This is the traditional method of building ceramic. Moist porcelain powder is applied with a brush, and moisture is then removed to

TABLE 8.4 PROPERTIES OF CERAMIC MATERIALS

Material	Translucency	Masking ability	Strength Flexural strength (approx. MPa)
Feldspathic	High	Low	Low 70–100 MPa
Leucite ceramics	Variable from highly translucent to opaque	Variable	Medium 170 MPa
Lithium disilicate-containing ceramics	Variable from highly translucent to opaque	Variable	Medium 360–400 MPa
Alumina	Medium	Good	Medium–high 600 MPa
Zirconia	Low	Good	High 1100 MPa

compact the powder particles. The porcelain is then fired in a vacuum, which allows compaction of the porcelain, by viscous flow of the glassy components.

- *Slip casting*. This method of manufacture is limited to the In-Ceram system. The procedure involves the use of fine-particle, high-alumina powder mixed with liquid to form slurry, which is applied as a slip material to a die. The moisture is absorbed into the stone, condensing the particles to form a dense layer. The material is then sintered and infiltrated with glass to give a final crystalline structure.
- *Hot pressing*. This method utilizes the lost wax technique. Molten material, from ingots of material formed of crystalline particles within a glassy matrix, is forced into the casting under pressure.
- *Computer-aided design/computer-aided manufacturing (CAD/CAM)*. Preparations are scanned and the restorations designed by computer (CAD) and then milled by computer (CAM).

PREPARATION FOR ALL-CERAMIC RESTORATIONS

To achieve the best clinical outcome, it is critical to conceptualize what is required in an all-ceramic restoration preparation, and to be clear on the depth in axial and occlusal/incisal planes, and on the location of the margins.

A key to success with all-ceramic restorations is meticulous tooth preparation. The aims of tooth preparation are to provide:

- sufficient thickness of the porcelain to ensure the necessary fracture resistance, without over-contouring of the final restoration
- a margin, so that the ceramist has a definite finishing line, allowing a normal emergence profile from the gingival margin
- a finished preparation that, in addition to supporting and retaining the restoration, is smooth and free of any sharp line-angles, which may cause stress concentrations within the ceramic.

The use of depth grooves and reduction guides (Fig. 8.8) may assist in obtaining the necessary reduction in an objective manner. It is important to remember that the tooth reduction required is based on the definitive wax-up–planned outcome and not on the position and shape of the original tooth. Failure to do this may result in excessive and unnecessary removal of tooth structures (Box 8.2).

There are situations where insufficient preparation by a clinician can lead to a poorly contoured or unesthetic crown due to the ceramist having to over-contour

BOX 8.2
TECHNIQUES FOR ATTAINING ADEQUATE REDUCTION

- Visual inspection
- Use of silicone putty reduction guides
- Depth grooves
- Use of burs of known dimension
- Bite tabs/wax
- Measurement of temporaries

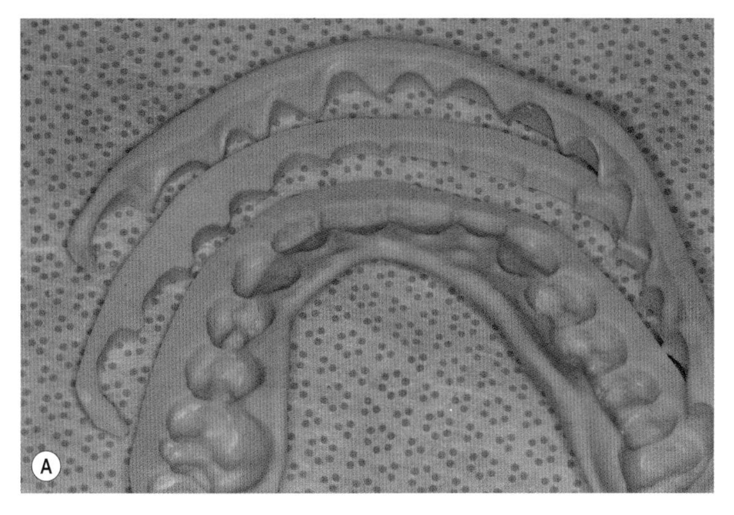

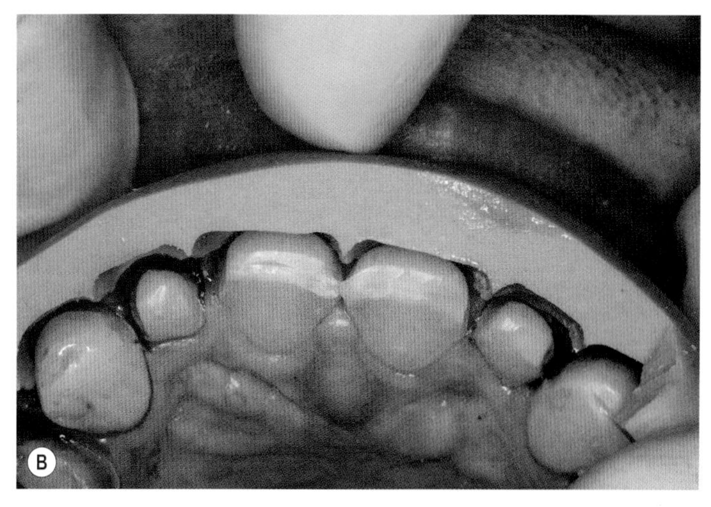

Fig. 8.8 Reduction guides. A. Use of silicone putty guides allows objective monitoring of reduction during preparation. B. Silicone reduction guide demonstrating the sufficiency of the reduction in preparation.

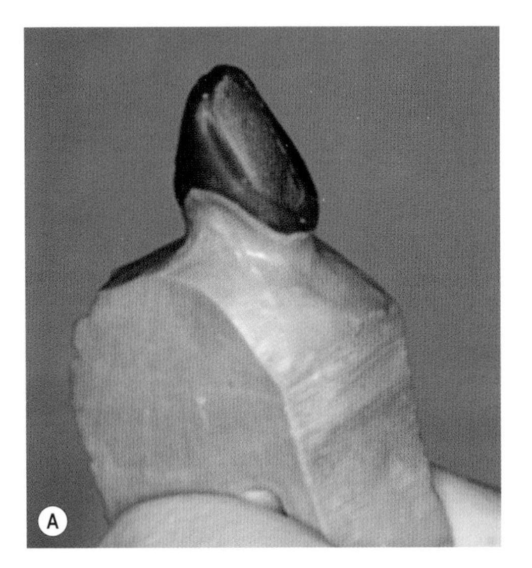

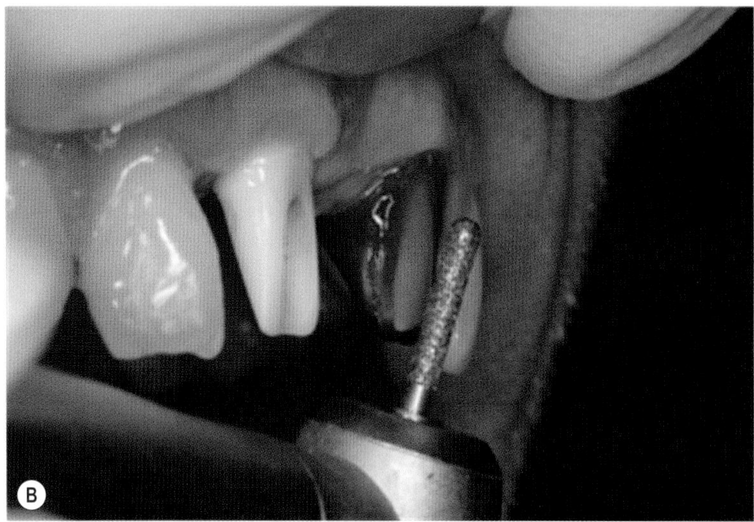

Fig. 8.9 Managing an insufficient preparation leading to a poorly contoured or unesthetic crown. A. Coping on prepared die with adjustment made as indicated by adjusted area. B. Coping transferred to preparation with adjustment made to the area as marked by coping.

the crown for adequate strength and esthetics. Rather than re-preparing and having to take a new impression, the clinician may use an adjustment coping to allow the ceramist to communicate the areas that need to be modified prior to seating the final crown, constructed from the original impression (Fig. 8.9).

MARGIN LOCATION

As the esthetic potential of all-ceramic restorations is superior to that of metal–ceramic restorations, it is often possible to place the margins of all-ceramic restorations supragingivally or equigingivally. This location of the margin simplifies the preparation, with the added benefit of ease of impression-taking and better periodontal health. Furthermore, emergence profiles are less likely to be over-contoured, as is common in metal–ceramic restorations. The use of highly translucent materials, such as glass-based ceramics, may allow margins to be located supragingivally, as there is little evidence of the margins of restorations made from such materials once they are adhesively bonded and carefully finished. The use of a translucent material allows a chameleon or 'contact lens' effect, where the margin becomes almost imperceptible.

Subgingival margins may be necessary for:

- extension beyond extensive restorations and caries
- sufficient crown length for retention
- ferrule effects
- esthetic reasons – to mask discoloured tooth tissue and metallic posts.

The more opaque high-strength polycrystalline materials may require margins to be placed subgingivally, given their opacity; however, the restorations made from these materials are still superior to metal–ceramic restorations in terms of esthetic qualities.

FULL-COVERAGE ALL-CERAMIC CROWN PREPARATION

It is recommended that a reduction of 0.8–1.0 mm axially and 2.0 mm occlusally be made as esthetic materials are brittle in thin sections. These materials have specific thickness requirements to withstand masticatory and parafunctional stresses. Chamfered or rounded shoulders are needed to provide sufficient bulk at the margins, and allow the transference of load and stress.

To minimize stress concentration within the restoration, all line angles should be rounded. Boxes, grooves and 'butt'-type shoulders are contraindicated.

REQUIREMENTS FOR ALL-CERAMIC CROWNS (Fig. 8.10)

- Chamfer preparation or rounded shoulder margins.
- Buccal/labial reduction of 0.8–1.0 mm.

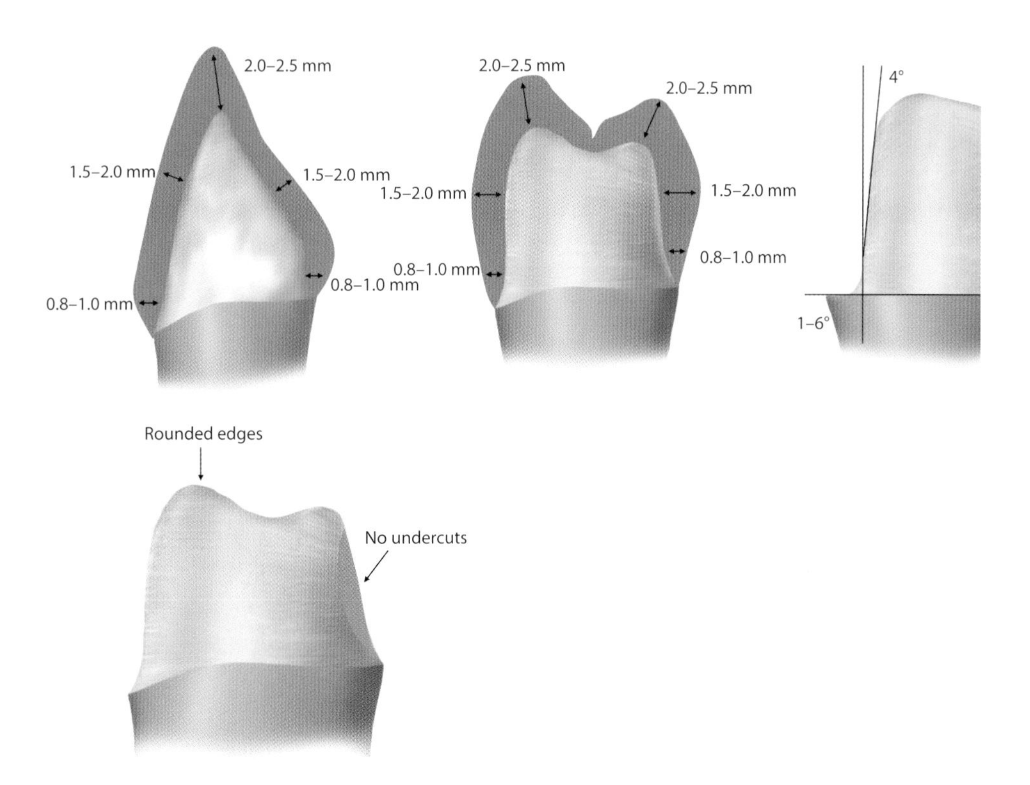

Fig. 8.10 All-ceramic crown preparation requirements.

- Adequate occlusal reduction of 2 mm and incisal reduction of 1.5–2 mm.
- Rounded internal angles, with no sharp transitions on line angles.
- Taper of about 6 degrees with no undercuts.

With recent developments in pure zirconium crown systems, whose esthetics are sufficient for at least posterior teeth, there is the prospect of less interventive preparation for all-ceramic crowns.

PORCELAIN LAMINATE VENEERS

Porcelain laminate veneers (PLVs) are a conservative treatment option, relative to crowns, to improve anterior esthetics. They have a long history of documented success. Preparations (Fig. 8.11) for PLVs should be based on the final smile design, with the shade and position of the margin of the restorations being taken into consideration. All efforts should be made to contain the preparation within enamel, as this provides the opportunity for a reliable and durable bond between restoration and remaining tooth tissue. Preparation into dentine should be avoided because of the less reliable bond to dentine, and the difference in elastic modulus and flexibility between dentine and porcelain. This puts the porcelain at risk of fracture when placed under tensile loading. In a 12-year study of 583 veneers, 7.2% or 42 veneers failed. Those veneers bonded to dentine and teeth with preparation margins in dentine were approximately 10 times more likely to fail than those bonded to enamel.[1]

LABIAL REDUCTION

Preparation of the convex labial surface of incisors needs to be addressed in three planes: incisal, middle third and cervical. Preparation requires a minimum

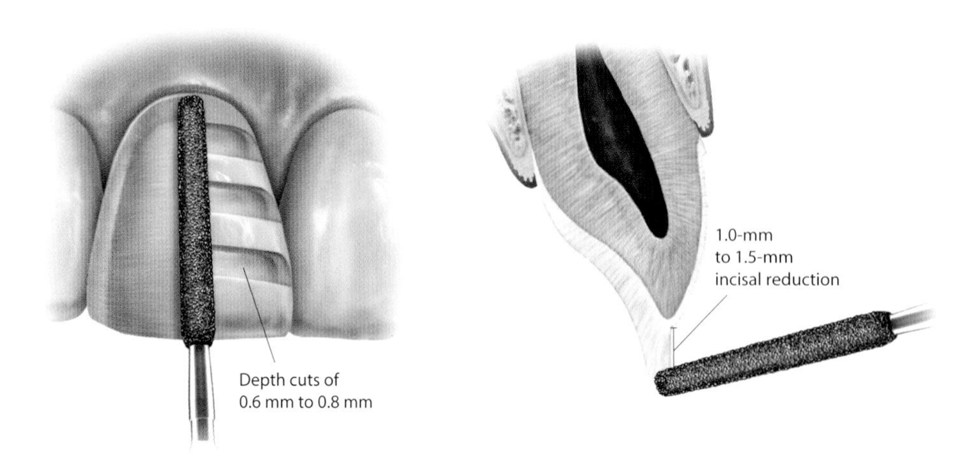

Fig. 8.11 Porcelain veneer preparation requirements.

reduction of 0.3 mm (feldspathic porcelain) to 0.6 mm (leucite and lithium disilicate material). The enamel thickness at the gingival third is 0.3–0.5 mm.

PROXIMAL REDUCTION

This may involve either stopping short of breaking the contact, or preparing through the contact area. If the contact area is to be maintained, the use of an elbow preparation, whereby the margins are extended proximally under the contact areas, may be used. This hides the margins as they extend inter-proximally. Breaking through the contact area may be required in cases with existing restorations, caries or crowding, and in cases where the dimensions of teeth are to be changed.

INCISAL REDUCTION

There is little documented clinical evidence to support one specific incisal reduction design over another. According to Calamia,[2] a tooth preparation that incorporates incisal overlap is preferable, as the veneer is stronger and provides a positive seat during cementation. This preparation design has the advantage of simple tooth preparation, and the esthetic characteristics are easier to achieve by the ceramist, as incisal translucency can be fully developed. This preparation also reduces stress concentration by distributing occlusal load over a wider surface area.[3]

ONLAYS AND INLAYS

Preparation for porcelain inlays and onlays (Fig. 8.12) requires a butt joint at the margins with rounded internal line angles. Occlusal isthmus width should be more than 1.5 mm wide, and occlusal reduction needs to be at least 1.5 mm deep.

PROVISIONALIZATION

The provision of temporary restorations is an integral element of the procedure for indirect, esthetic restorations. It is vital for periodontal and pulpal health

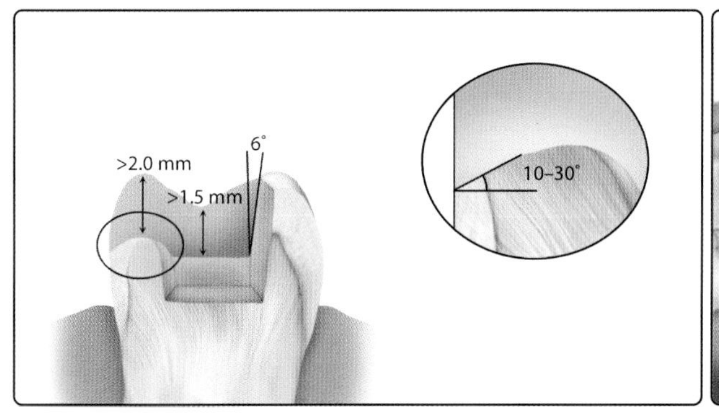

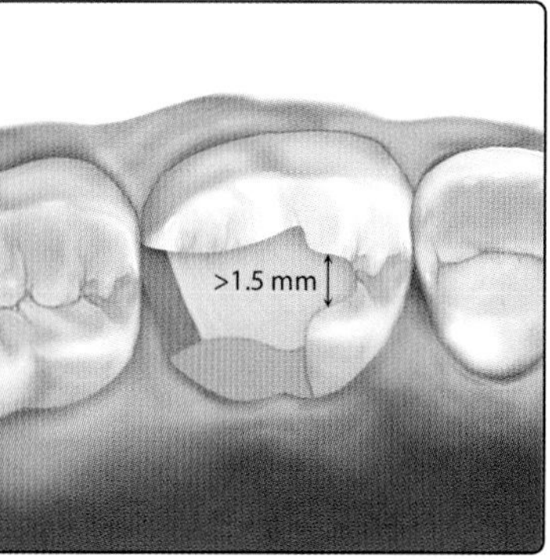

Fig. 8.12 Onlay and inlay preparation requirements.

while restorations are being constructed, and allows the clinician to demonstrate the proposed cosmetic improvements to the patient. Provisional restorations can be duplicated from a diagnostic wax-up, or constructed with a freehand chairside mock-up. This should incorporate the proposed changes that the patient, practitioner and ceramist have planned and agreed upon. These may include incisal lengthening, shade changes, and form and contour alterations. This step is essential in the planning process. It is much simpler and less costly to modify provisional restorations, according to the patient's expectations and requirements, than to remake completed restorations.

A delayed approach in the assessment of provisional restorations is recommended, so that patients are given ample opportunity to decide whether they are happy with the anticipated outcome. At the time of placing provisional restorations, the patient is often anaesthetized and cannot assess esthetics adequately. Time to allow patients to adjust to their new appearance, and to ask family and friends their opinion about their changed 'look', is invariably time well spent.

If the patient is happy with the provisional restorations, then the ceramist may construct the final restorations using the original wax-up as a blueprint. If the provisional restorations require modifications, they can be reduced or composite resin added to meet the needs of the patient. An impression of the modified provisional restorations will provide a template and serve as a communication tool for the ceramist regarding the required changes.

CEMENTATION PROTOCOLS WITH ALL-CERAMIC RESTORATIONS

The primary objective of cementation is to ensure a durable bond between the restoration and the remaining tooth tissues, and to create good marginal adaptation and seal. The cementation procedure is related to the composition and strength of the different materials. Glass-based ceramics (feldspathic and leucite- and lithium disilicate-containing ceramics) need to be bonded with resin cements to obtain a clinically acceptable strength (Table 8.5). Restorations of these materials can be etched with hydrofluoric acid, silanated and bonded to tooth structures. In contrast, glass-infiltrated and polycrystalline ceramics (e.g. alumina, zirconia) cannot be etched because of the lack of glass. Given the higher independent strength of these polycrystalline materials, restorations formed from these materials can be conventionally cemented or adhesively bonded.

Glass-based (etchable) ceramics

These materials are adhesively bonded. The ceramic is etched with hydrofluoric acid that attacks the glassy phase of the ceramic, and then rinsed thoroughly

TABLE 8.5 SUMMARY OF CEMENTATION PROTOCOLS FOR DIFFERENT CERAMICS

Type of ceramic	Cement
Feldspathic porcelain	Resin cement
Leucite- and lithium disilicate-containing ceramics	Resin cement
Alumina	1. Conventional cement – resin-modified glass–ionomer, glass–ionomer, self-adhesive resin cement or zinc phosphate 2. Surface activation and phosphate monomer-containing resin cement 3. Silicoating and resin cement
Zirconia	1. Conventional cement – resin-modified glass–ionomer, glass–ionomer, self-adhesive resin cement or zinc phosphate 2. Surface activation and phosphate monomer-containing resin cement 3. Silicoating and resin cement 4. Zirconia primer and resin cement

before silanating the surface. The acid-etch creates micro-mechanical locking, while the silane treatment allows chemical bonding. Once the surface of the ceramic is properly prepared, then the ceramic can be bonded with resin cement. Thin, translucent restorations can be bonded with light-cured resin cements, while thick or opaque restorations require the use of dual-cure resin cement.

High-strength (non-etchable) polycrystalline ceramics

These materials do not have a glassy phase and therefore cannot be etched with acid to create a roughened surface. Given their higher inherent strength, they can be conventionally cemented or adhesively bonded by:

- *Conventional cementation*, involving the use of conventional luting cements such as a resin-modified glass–ionomer cement, self-adhesive cement or a glass–ionomer cement.
- *Adhesive bonding* with aluminium oxide activation and the use of a phosphate-modified cement (e.g. Panavia–Kuraray).[4,5]
- *Tribochemical surface treatment* (CoJet/Rocatec – 3M ESPE), in which silica-coated aluminum oxide is blasted on to the ceramic surface. This creates a

surface layer of small silica particles that are fused to the surface substrate. This is followed by the application of silane primer, then bonding with a conventional *bis*-GMA resin cement.[6]

- *Use of zirconia primer and resin cement*. Using a ceramic primer containing an acidic adhesive monomer such as MDP has been found to improve the bond strength of zirconia-based ceramics.[7]

COLOUR MODIFICATION WITH CEMENT

Limited colour modifications can be made to restorations at the time of cementation with the use of pigmented cements. This may include making the final restoration more opaque to mask underlying discoloured tooth tissue. The colour modification depends on the ceramic system used, its thickness, and the translucency of the ceramic. The influence of the colour of the cement is greatest with thin translucent porcelain veneers.

KEY POINT SUMMARY

Try-in cements are recommended to assess the final colour of the restoration and to display the effect to the patient prior to cementation. Begin with a clear try-in paste; if this is not white enough, use a white cement to lighten the shade. If this is still too dark, start adding increments of white opaque cements to achieve the desired value. Do not add more than 25% opaque white cement, as this will make the restoration appear artificial, as well as rendering the margin distinct and unable to blend harmoniously.

CONCLUDING REMARKS

To achieve success in esthetic dentistry, the clinician needs to possess both technical and artistic skills, as well as a comprehensive understanding of the different treatment modalities and materials available. As in other areas of dentistry, treatment planning is paramount, and must include a comprehensive history and assessment of the patient that includes informed consent to the procedures being proposed.

The advent of adhesive dentistry has allowed restorative treatment utilizing a conservative, minimally invasive and sometimes no-preparation technique. This has revolutionized dentistry, as has the continuing development of dental materials that improve both esthetic and long-term outcomes.

Subsequent books in the series provide detailed accounts of the use of materials and techniques discussed in the present chapter.

REFERENCES

1. Gurel G, Sesma N, Calamita MA, et al. Influence of enamel preservation on failure rates of porcelain laminate veneers. Int J Periodont Rest Dent 2013;33(1):31–9.

2. Calamia JR. The etched porcelain veneer technique. N Y State Dent J 1988;54:48–50.

3. Highton R, Caputo AA, Maytas JA. A photoelastic study of stress on porcelain laminate preparations. J Prosthetic Dent 1987;58:157–61.

4. Wolfart M, Lehmann F, Wolfart S, et al. Durability of the resin bond strength to zirconia ceramic after using different surface conditioning methods. Dent Mater 2007;23:45–50.

5. Blatz MB, Sadan A, Martin J, et al. In vitro evaluation of shear bond strengths of resin to densely-sintered high-purity zirconium-oxide ceramic after long-term storage and thermal cycling. J Prosthet Dent 2004;91:356–62.

6. Valandro LF, Ozcan M, Bottino MC, et al. Bond strength of a resin cement to high-alumina and zirconia-reinforced ceramics: the effect of surface conditioning. J Adhes Dent 2006;8:175–8.

7. Lehman F, Kern M. Durability of resin bonding to zirconia ceramic using different primers. J Adhes Dent 2009;6:479–83.

CHAPTER 9

Teamwork with the Dental Technologist

BILL SHARPLING AND NAIRN WILSON

INTRODUCTION

Teamwork is fundamental to successful clinical outcomes. Team working between the dental practitioner, the practice personnel and the dental technologist, who is typically in a remote location, is critical to success in the provision of indirect restorations and prostheses. Effectiveness, as with many, if not all, other measures of success, is greatly increased by individuals working as a team, not as a team of individuals working independently. Dentistry without teamwork is not in the best interests of the patient, carrying a high risk of failures and unnecessary comebacks and complaints.

Developing a team that is capable of effective teamwork can be challenging. Inclusion of dental technologists and the dental laboratory team in this process is best achieved by reciprocal visits between the practice and the laboratory, as well as 'get-togethers' to develop the necessary relationships, share a common understanding of goals and values, agree practical arrangements and, most importantly, facilitate communication. From time to time, team building must be followed with events to reinforce team spirit, refine practical arrangements and maintain the all-important relationship between the different members of the team. A strong team is an effective team; a weak team suffers limitations, including tensions between its members. For example, when things go wrong, members of a weak team tend to blame each other, often forgetting about the needs of the patient, instead of pulling together to resolve the problem quickly and effectively.

COMMON UNDERSTANDING AND COMMUNICATION

Communication – a prerequisite to effective team working – is greatly facilitated if the participants share a common understanding, including a common use of terminology. With a common understanding of the different terms used to describe occlusal relationships, for example, the dental team, including the dental technologist and the dental laboratory team, should develop an increasing confidence that the indirect restorations and prostheses they collectively produce will have the desired occlusal relationship and function. While the dental practitioner, as the leader of the dental team, is ultimately responsible for the care of the patient, each and every member of the dental team also has a duty of care. This duty of care extends to understanding the patient's needs and expectations. For the dental technologist and the dental laboratory team to fulfil their duty of care, dentist and practice personnel must ensure that they communicate what is required in the way of laboratory support, including the use of terminology that they know will be interpreted correctly. All too often, failures in the provision of indirect restorations and prostheses are met with phrases such as 'Sorry, I didn't fully understand what you wanted' or 'If you'd made that clear, the problem wouldn't have arisen.'

Common understanding, let alone good communication, in something as complex as the provision of indirect restorations and prostheses is made exceedingly difficult, if not impossible, if the practitioner has never met the dental technologist, and if their respective teams have little, if any, knowledge of each other and their ways of working. This is particularly important when treatment is intended to enhance a complex concept such as dental attractiveness.

Many would say that the ideal – possibly the only – way to develop a common understanding and effective communication between the clinical and laboratory teams is to have the dental technologist and the dental laboratory team on site, or working in some nearby location, with ample opportunity to build up an excellent rapport. This is rarely possible, however, for a wide variety of reasons. Indeed, some of the world's largest dental laboratories work principally without direct communication, notably with the increasing use of digital technologies. As a consequence, ways must be found to overcome the difficulties posed by the physical separation of the clinical and dental laboratory teams. That said, it is suggested that there is great merit in a dental practice employing the services of a local dental technologist who welcomes visits to the laboratory and is prepared to visit the practice, possibly spending time in the surgery with the dentist and the patient, assuming the local dental technologist has the necessary knowledge, skills and technologies to provide the support required. Where such arrangements are not possible, and the dentist must rely on the services of a dental technologist in some distant location, or wishes to use a centralized high-tech service, possibly even in another country, then all the more the challenge is to ensure common understanding and good communication in the best interests of the patient. In general, the greater the separation between clinical and dental technology teams, the greater the need to work on achieving good communications.

REMOTE LABORATORIES

If, for whatever reason, a dentist must or feels obliged to seek the support of a remotely located dental laboratory for dental technology services, careful consideration should be given as to the best means of minimizing the ever-present risk of communication errors. The use of modern communication technologies – including, for example, Skype and the electronic communication of images and possibly video clips, subject to the consent of the patient – can go a long way towards realizing this goal. Despite such measures, effective communication with a remote laboratory is typically challenging. Good communication is, of course, a two-way process, requiring both the dentist/practice team and the dental technologist/laboratory team to work together to overcome the communication challenge posed by their physical separation as best they can. Communication difficulties are no excuse for the provision of indirect restorations and prostheses that fail to meet the needs and expectations of the patient. Time spent on ensuring good lines of communication is typically time well spent.

PRESCRIPTIONS

A prescription – the 'lab card' – is typically the principal form of communication between the practitioner and the dental technologist. To be effective, a prescription must include all the information necessary to achieve the desired outcome. This information must be presented in such a way that the dental technologist can, first and foremost, read and fully understand it. Hard as a dentist may try, it is important to remember that diagrams and drawings included in a prescription are at best two-dimensional illustrations of the complex, three-dimensional restoration or prosthesis that the technologist is being asked to produce. Regrettably, most dental technologists work from a collection of inappropriately brief or otherwise inadequate prescriptions – 'metal crown', 'temporary denture', 'splint' and so on – that fail on all counts to convey what is required. An example of a prescription form, which the dentist and the practice team should discipline themselves to complete in full on each and every occasion that dental laboratory support is being requested, is reproduced in Figure 9.1. Good as such forms are, the information they convey is greatly enhanced by the provision of some images of, for example, the patient's smile, the preoperative appearance of the teeth or edentulous space being restored, restorations or a prosthesis being replaced, and chairside mock-ups that the patient found acceptable and the dentist considered appropriate.

The importance of making communication a two-way process cannot be overemphasized. If a prescription is less than satisfactory, the technologist should feel free to contact the practitioner and explain this, in anticipation of a common understanding being amicably reached. Changes to a prescription agreed verbally should be confirmed electronically and recorded on the 'lab card'. If in doubt over what to include in a prescription, provide more rather than less information, mindful that most colleagues have never heard their dental technologist complain about prescriptions being too detailed. In requesting what are

Indicate modifications: Mark with + to lengthen and - to shorten

(mm) 16	15	14	13	12	11	21	22	23	24	25	26	(mm)
(mm) 46	45	44	43	42	41	31	32	33	34	35	36	(mm)

Notes Copy tooth length and proportions from the provisional restorations

COLOR

A3
A3 50%
A2 50%
A2
A3 50%
A2 50%
A1
opal WHITE
A2 50%
A1 50%
blue

Shade Guide
Vita 3D Master
Ivoclar Other

Spectrophotometer
Yes No

Value
High Low

Notes

TRANSLUCENCY +++

Fig. 9.1 A prescription form.

typically costly items from a dental laboratory, it is surprising that some practitioners leave so much room for doubt in their prescriptions for restorations and prostheses. Items returned from the dental laboratory can be no better than the quality of the information sent by the dentist.

When a prescription is being completed for dental technology support services, care should be taken to write legibly with indelible ink, which will withstand transfer to the laboratory, typically in the company of damp impressions. Despite impressions being suitably packaged in plastic bags, and subsequent careful handling by the dental technologist and the dental laboratory team, it is more common than not for the prescription card to suffer some water damage. It is good practice to retain a copy of any prescription sent to the dental laboratory in the relevant patient's clinical records. Such measures can pay great dividends when communication between the clinical and laboratory teams is compromised, through, for example, a prescription being lost or irretrievably damaged in some way; this is particularly true in the event of a dispute between the dentist and the dental technologist over responsibility for an unacceptable outcome to treatment involving dental laboratory support services. In an ideal world, such disputes should not occur, as any misunderstanding should have been discussed in the design phase, enabling the practitioner and technologist to be confident of working towards the same goal – a satisfactory prosthesis or restoration and, more importantly, a satisfied patient.

The laboratory prescription form is, of course, a document containing confidential information and as such should be treated in the same way as other medical/

dental records. Dental technologists, together with all other members of the dental team, are obliged to treat the information provided on the form in confidence. It is important to remember this, particularly when sending patient information to remote locations where professional and ethical obligations and requirements may not be so robust. A simple but potentially effective measure is to limit the patient identifier to the patient's initials, possibly together with the date of birth; however, care must be taken in adopting such an approach to avoid confusion between patients.

COMMUNICATING INFORMATION ON SHADES

Communicating what is generally referred to as the 'shade' to the dental technologist can be difficult, especially when requesting the production of indirect restorations to be included in a patient's smile. Individual teeth, and even a number of adjacent teeth, invariably encompass considerable colour variation in terms of hue, chroma and value, let alone variation in translucency.

Sadly, many laboratory prescriptions include details of just one shade, which the dental technologist must assume to be the body shade, relating to the centre of the tooth. This leaves the ceramist to best-guess what colour and translucency variation to include in the completed restoration. In the provision of a prosthesis or restoration that will replace more than one tooth, the prescription of a single shade suffers limitations, in that this approach fails to recognize the variation in colour that occurs in, for example, six upper anterior teeth.

Obvious as it may seem, in prescribing the 'shade', the dental technologist first and foremost needs to know which shade guide or shade detection device has been used; not all shade guides have specified shade 'tabs' of the same hue, chroma and value. In addition to a body shade, it is typically necessary to record at least the cervical shade, together with details of the shade and translucency of the incisal third, in the case of anterior teeth. As may be indicated clinically, the shade prescription should include details of the colour characteristics of any special features required in the completed restoration. Images of the teeth or edentulous space to be restored, with and without the selected shade 'tab(s)' included, and diagrams of the colour variation and any special features required, can be most useful, if not essential, adjuncts to a written shade prescription. Examples of the way to describe shades are illustrated in Figure 9.2.

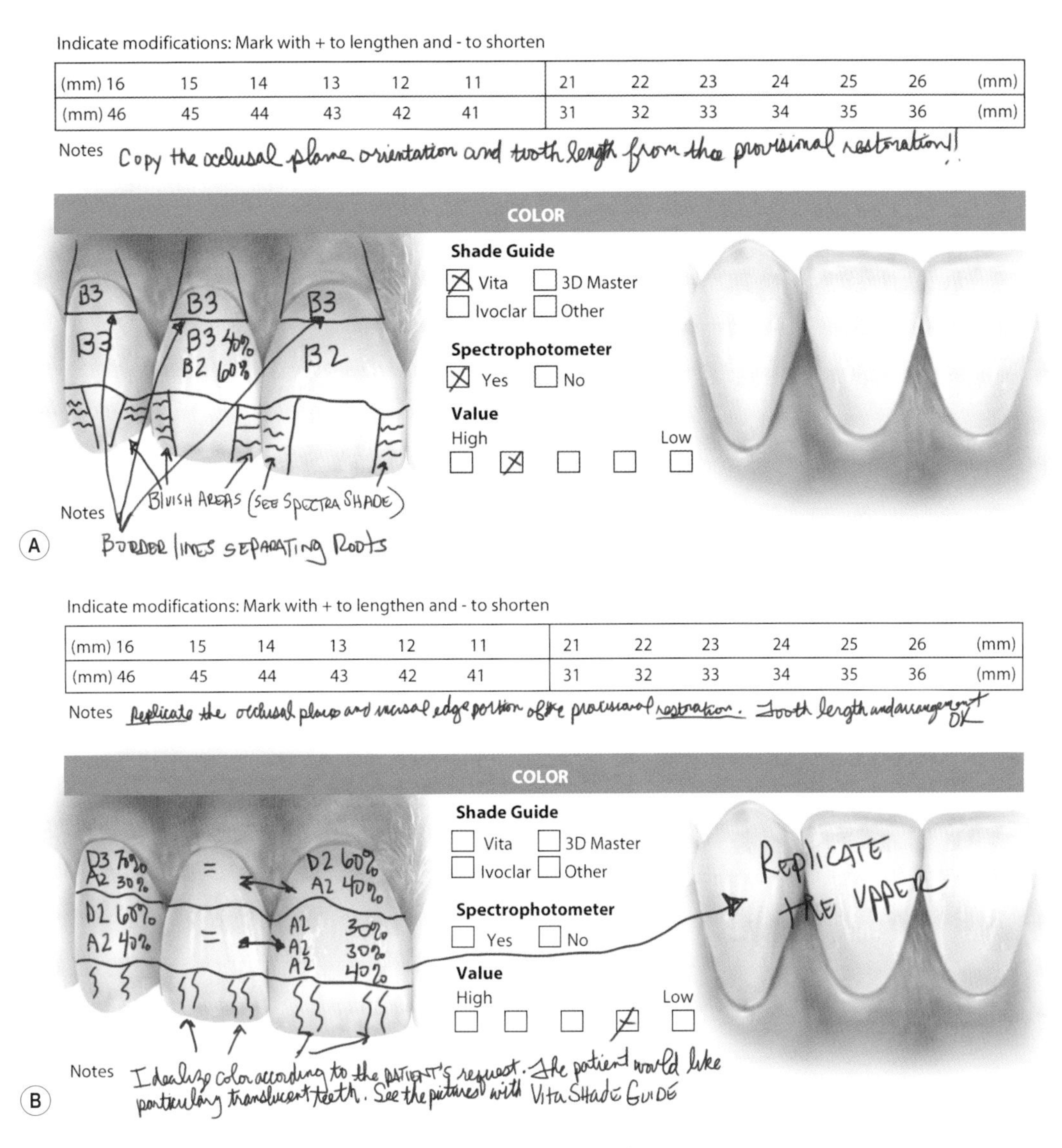
Indicate modifications: Mark with + to lengthen and - to shorten

(mm) 16	15	14	13	12	11	21	22	23	24	25	26	(mm)
(mm) 46	45	44	43	42	41	31	32	33	34	35	36	(mm)

Notes Copy the occlusal plane orientation and tooth length from the provisional restoration!

COLOR

Shade Guide
☒ Vita ☐ 3D Master
☐ Ivoclar ☐ Other

Spectrophotometer
☒ Yes ☐ No

Value
High Low
☐ ☒ ☐ ☐ ☐

Notes BLUISH AREAS (SEE SPECTRA SHADE)
BORDER LINES SEPARATING ROOTS

(A)

Indicate modifications: Mark with + to lengthen and - to shorten

(mm) 16	15	14	13	12	11	21	22	23	24	25	26	(mm)
(mm) 46	45	44	43	42	41	31	32	33	34	35	36	(mm)

Notes Replicate the occlusal plane and incisal edge portion of the provisional restoration. Tooth length and arrangement OK

COLOR

Shade Guide
☐ Vita ☐ 3D Master
☐ Ivoclar ☐ Other

Spectrophotometer
☐ Yes ☐ No

Value
High Low
☐ ☐ ☐ ☒ ☐

Notes Idealize color according to the PATIENT'S request. The patient would like particularly translucent teeth. See the pictures with Vita SHADE GUIDE

(B)

Fig. 9.2 Examples of shade descriptions included in prescription forms.

If the indirect restorations or prostheses requested form part of a phased course of treatment, it is most helpful to include in the shade prescription details of the shades and shading effects used in restorations and prostheses already completed.

Details of devices and techniques to record shades are discussed in Chapter 7.

ANATOMICAL DETAILS

In addition to information on the required shading of restorations, a note of anatomical details can be of great assistance to the dental technologist in producing a good esthetic outcome; this should cover the prominence of mamelons and marginal ridges, and surface topographical features such as perikymata, rippling or other contours. The anatomy of teeth is as varied as the anatomy of other parts of the body and reproducing it is a great art.

SURFACE TEXTURE AND LUSTRE

The surface texture and, as a consequence, reflectance of the surface of a restoration or replacement tooth can have a profound influence on its esthetic acceptability. The prescription for indirect restorations or prostheses should therefore include details of the nature and quality of the surface finish required, particularly if it is to match that of an adjacent tooth. For example, should the surface have a smooth (low in texture), glossy (high in lustre) appearance, or should it include some form of irregularities (high in texture) or specific topography and look more matt (low in lustre)? If a single tooth is to be restored or replaced, surface quality information can usually be determined from the working model, assuming a high-quality impression has been provided. If, however, two or more adjacent teeth, such as the upper central incisors, are to be replaced or restored, then surface quality requirements should be communicated to the dental technologist. The wrong surface finish can spoil an otherwise attractive esthetic restoration.

Chairside adjustment of ceramic restorations is occasionally necessary. This may affect contact areas, occlusal contacts or even the textural appearance, as mentioned above. When the glazed surface of a ceramic crown has been adjusted, it is preferable to return the restoration to the laboratory for reglazing and finishing. Very modest chairside polishing of adjusted ceramic can be carried out using specifically designed kits. If, however, either the clinician or the technologist feels that adjustments to ceramic restorations may be necessary, the option of providing a ceramic restoration for try-in at a 'bisque bake' or 'pre-glaze' stage should be considered. In this way, adjustments to ceramic restorations can be carried out prior to finishing and glazing.

OCCLUSAL RELATIONSHIP

If a single restoration or replacement tooth is required, if the inter-cuspal position (ICP) is obvious, and if a conformative occlusal approach is being adopted, then relatively little, if any, information on occlusal relationship need be conveyed to the dental technologist; the exception is when the restoration or replacement tooth is to be protected in some way from damaging non-axial loading. Indeed, an occlusal registration in simple cases adopting a conformative approach may cause more harm than good. All the technologist needs to be advised of in such cases is that a conformative approach is being used and the models should be mounted in ICP, assuming there are no deflective contacts or other occlusal complications. If a sectional impression has been recorded, then, depending on the circumstances and the extent of the impression, at least some notes on occlusal relationship will be required. These details should be provided in addition to information on the form and function of the contralateral tooth or teeth, if they are not included in the impression. Such information is essential, for example, when a quadrant impression has been taken for a crown on a premolar tooth that is to contribute to premolar guide group function. Many would say that such circumstances contradict the use of a sectional impression technique.

If multiple restorations or replacement teeth are required, then some form of occlusal registration, possibly together with a facebow recording, will be needed, as discussed in Chapter 7. In providing such information, remember that it is critical for the dental technologist to know and understand the approach that has been adopted, in particular if centric relationship (CR) has been recorded and the completed restorations are to create a new ICP in CR. As a general rule, the more complex the case, the greater the need for effective, detailed communication between the practitioner and the dental technologist.

SELECTION OF MATERIALS

Assuming a practitioner and dental technologist have an agreed understanding about which materials, including dental alloys, to use as a matter of routine in various circumstances, then the laboratory prescription need contain little information on the selection of materials; the exception is when the dentist wishes to deviate from normal practice – in which case, the laboratory prescription should specify the materials the dentist wishes to be used. Otherwise, the dental technologist must assume that the practitioner is content for the dental technology team to use the materials typically applied in the laboratory, according to the nature of the case. In the provision of porcelain fused to metal crowns (PFMs), the dentist should specify the extent to which the crown is to be faced or covered with porcelain to achieve the planned treatment outcome.

The patient's notes should contain a record of the process requested and the materials prescribed – for example, non-precious, semi-precious or precious alloy; in addition, the dental laboratory should keep a note of the alloy batch numbers used, in the event of any queries. This information may be captured in a 'statement of conformity', which should be provided with all finished laboratory work, and which all dentists are now obliged to offer to patients on completion of treatment, at least in the UK.

PHOTOGRAPHS

Photographs taken clinically or provided by the patient can greatly enhance communication to the laboratory of the requirements in individual cases, as well as constituting an important element of a patient's clinical record. In identifying photographs to be sent to the laboratory, it is important to obtain patient consent and to ensure that suitable arrangements will be in place to maintain patient confidentiality. Details of how best to record photographs clinically are discussed in Chapter 7. Poor-quality images, in particular ones that fail to record colour correctly, may add nothing to the helpfulness of a laboratory prescription; indeed, they may be misleading. A good photograph may well be worth a thousand words, however, and, in the process, may make all the difference between clinical success and failure in esthetic treatments involving laboratory support. It is important to remember, however, that photographs are two-dimensional and that views from different angles may be required to convey all the information the practitioner wishes to impart to the dental technologist.

Photographs, such as the image shown in Figure 9.3, form part of the patient records and must, of course, be treated in the same way as other records and notes in terms of confidentiality.

Good prescribing takes time and effort, but with due diligence is typically rewarded with good clinical outcomes, fewer 'remakes', and good working

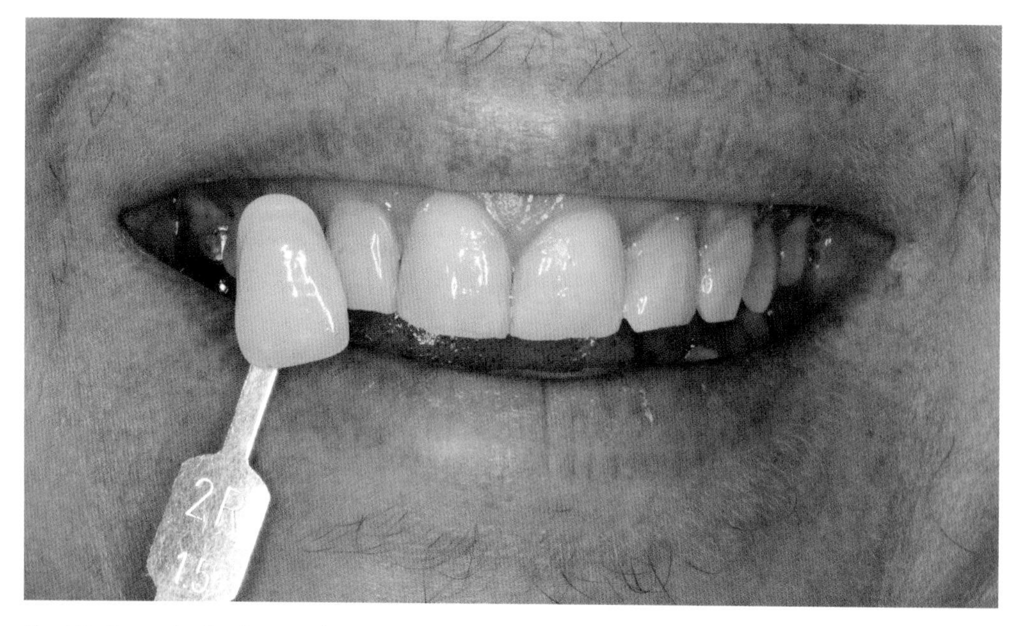

Fig. 9.3 Example of an image taken as part of shade selection. This becomes part of the patient's clinical records.

relationships between the clinical and laboratory teams. Also, the dentist must accept the judgement of the dental technologist if, for example, it becomes apparent that insufficient information has been captured by an impression when models have been cast and examined. Trust is an important aspect of the communication processes and the relationship between practitioner and dental technologist.

CLINICAL TIP

When a case goes well, take a photograph and send it to your technician with a note of thanks. Don't just communicate when there's a problem!

MOCK-UPS AND LABORATORY-MADE PROVISIONAL RECONSTRUCTIONS

In the undertaking of extensive and complex cases, and, on occasion, in the provision of even single tooth restorations or prostheses under very demanding circumstances, the use of mock-ups and laboratory-made provisional restorations can greatly facilitate communication between the dentist and the dental technologist. Traditionally, mock-ups and laboratory-made provisional restorations were principally used to communicate the form and function of restorations or replacement teeth, but they have become increasingly important in the esthetic management of the patient's dental attractiveness. A major advantage of the use of mock-ups and laboratory-made provisional restorations is the involvement of the patient, and possibly the patient's partner and family members, in the developing of the desired clinical outcome. Patients involved in this way tend to have a sense of ownership of the outcome of treatment.

As indicated above, impressions and photographs of completed mock-ups and laboratory-made provisional restorations in the mouth, possibly together with the putty indices used in tooth preparation (Fig. 9.4), can be of great assistance in ensuring effective communication with the dental technologist. They may also facilitate communication with the patient. In cases where the patient is greatly attracted by the feel and appearance of a mock-up or laboratory-made provisional restorations, the challenge for the dental technologist may be exact replication in the production of the definitive restorations or prosthesis. In the event of sending removable mock-ups or laboratory-made provisional restorations back to the laboratory to aid the production of the definitive restorations or prostheses, care must be taken to avoid colour change or distortion, caused principally by dehydration. If removed from the mouth and returned to the

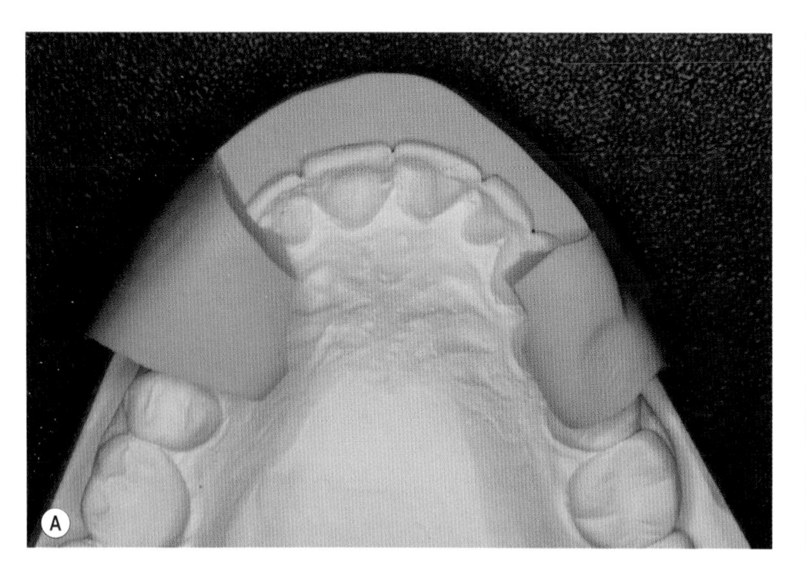

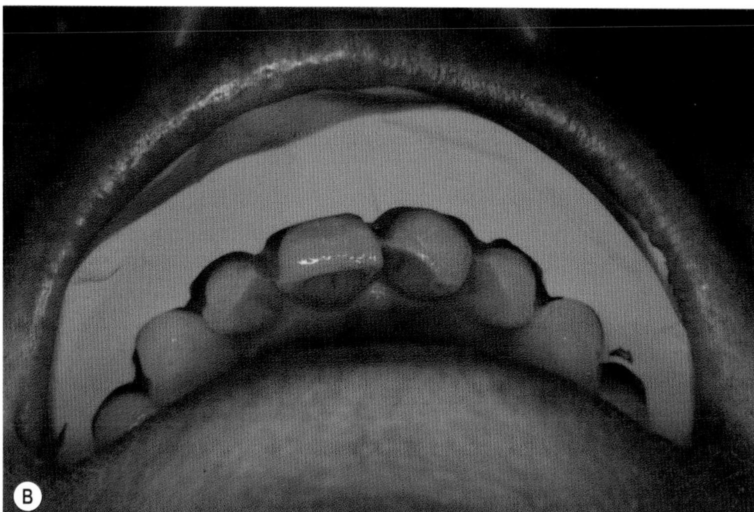

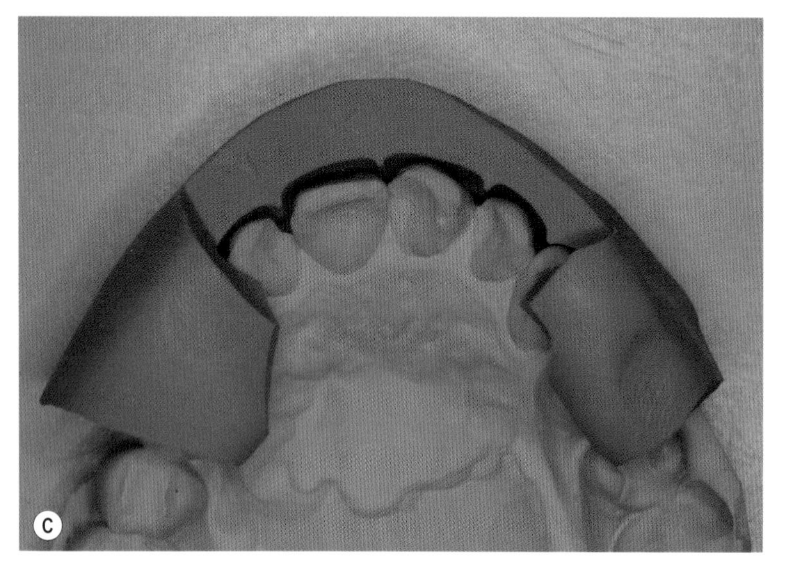

Fig. 9.4 Indices used in treatment planning and in guiding tooth preparation. A. Preoperative index of an upper anterior segment. B. Index of mock-up repositioned in the mouth to illustrate the extent of build-up required to achieve the desired esthetic outcome. C. Index illustrating the amount of tooth tissue removed during preparation. (Courtesy of Professor Brian Millar.)

laboratory, mock-ups and laboratory-made provisional restorations must be kept moist. The dental technologist must remember that the shade of the mock-up or provisional restorations may no longer be that used in the original construction, given that some shift in shade may have occurred in the mouth through, for example, staining, or possibly bleaching by toothpaste or some other oral hygiene aid.

COMPLEMENTARY INFORMATION

Information that may usefully complement a prescription for indirect restorations or prosthesis may include, for example, preoperative study casts; photographs provided by the patient, as indicated above; an impression of any mock-up provided as part of the treatment; or, better still, the mock-up itself, if removable, together with any special instructions not otherwise included in the prescription. If in doubt, include it, remembering that a completed indirect restoration or prosthesis can only be as good as the information provided by the dentist to the dental technologist.

CHAIRSIDE COMMUNICATION

Many would maintain that the gold standard in communication between a dentist and a dental technologist is to have the technologist meet the patient and work with the dentist in choosing shades and otherwise completing the laboratory prescription. This, however, is a luxury that has traditionally been available to relatively few colleagues, but it is one that has much to commend it as good practice in dental team working. It also provides an opportunity for the patient to meet the dental technologist, and, if necessary, to be told face to face, by the person who will make their restorations or prosthesis, what can or cannot be achieved in the dental laboratory. One of the great pitfalls of esthetic dentistry is when the patient develops expectations that cannot be met.

CLINICAL TIP

As part of co-decision-making, involve the patient in shade selection, particularly in a smile design case where shade-matching is not the goal, and selection of a completely new shade is the requirement. Some clinicians allow the patient to take home a shade card. It may also be worth involving other members of the dental team in shade selection, particularly dental nurses and, where possible, the ceramist.

DISPUTES

Disputes between practitioners and dental technologists are often caused by failures in communication. In the unfortunate event of a dispute developing between a dentist and a dental technologist, typically over who is at fault when a case goes wrong and a restoration or prosthesis needs to be returned to the laboratory for extensive modification or even to be remade, the priority is the satisfactory completion of the patient's treatment. Under no circumstances should patient treatment be delayed for longer than is necessary, or otherwise compromised while the practitioner and technologist sort out their dispute. Once the patient's treatment has been successfully completed, and the practitioner and the dental technologist have had opportunity to reflect on the reasons for the failure, which may well become apparent in the process of modifying or remaking the item of work, the path to resolution may become obvious. If, however, resolution is proving difficult or impossible and the costs involved justify it, consideration should be given to seeking the help of a colleague whom both sides will accept as an independent arbitrator. Being drawn into an acrimonious or even legal dispute, particularly when it involves someone with whom it would be advantageous to continue doing business, is unlikely to provide a satisfactory outcome for either of the parties. In such matters, both sides may need to remind themselves of their professional responsibility to be honest and to act with integrity in all matters. Admitting blame, even partial blame, is never easy, but it is invariably more pleasant than having to deal with the consequences of the possible alternative approaches.

The above paragraph focuses on how to act when things go wrong, but what about when everything goes well? When a well-made restoration or prosthesis is placed, the dentist can feel a great sense of pride, and this will also be shared with the dental nurse; however, as a member of the dental team, technologists should also be congratulated when they have done a particularly good job. A simple phone call, email or text message to congratulate the technologist, or to thank them for their time, effort and help, can go a long way towards cementing their position in the dental team. It may also further improve the dentist–technologist relationship, with the prospect of even better outcomes in the future.

CONCLUDING REMARKS

Much of what is written and said about communication is common sense; however, common sense does not always seem to prevail in everyday life. Communicate with others in the way you expect to be communicated with yourself, taking account of any circumstances that complicate the communication process. Building a relationship with people you need to communicate with on a regular basis, such as your dental technologist, will be time well spent.

Before signing off a prescription to a dental technologist, pause and consider:

- Does it communicate all the necessary information, together with any additional details that may help to minimize the risk of any misunderstanding or failure?
- Is the prescription not only legible but also articulate, and free of any ambiguity?
- Is it sufficient to achieve the esthetically pleasing result I am striving to obtain?

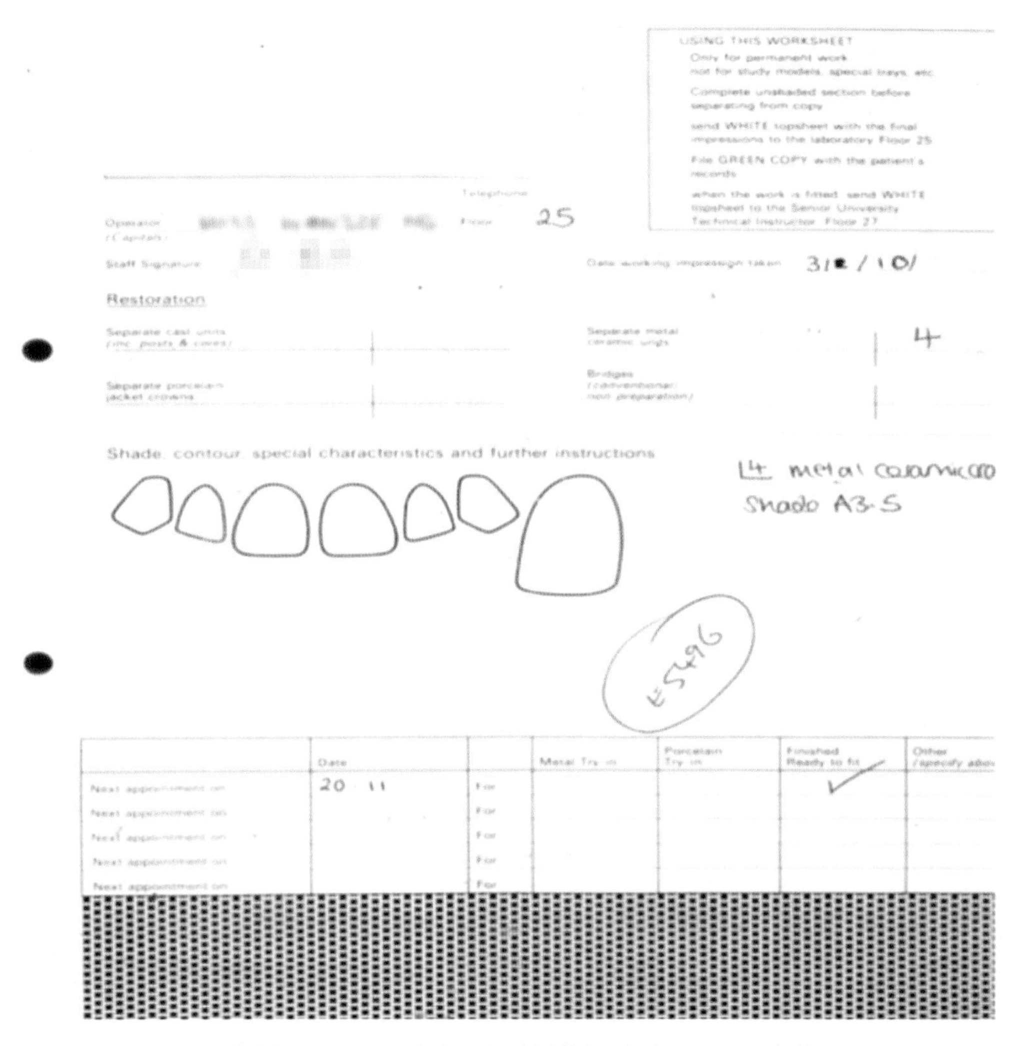

USING THIS WORKSHEET
Only for permanent work
not for study models, special trays, etc.
Complete unshaded section before separating from copy
send WHITE topsheet with the final impressions to the laboratory Floor 25
File GREEN COPY with the patient's records
when the work is fitted send WHITE topsheet to the Senior University Technical Instructor Floor 27

Telephone
Operator (Capitals) Floor 25
Staff Signature
Date working impression taken 31 / 10/

Restoration

Separate cast units (inc. posts & cores)
Separate metal ceramic units 4
Separate porcelain jacket crowns
Bridges (conventional/ non preparation)

Shade, contour, special characteristics and further instructions

L4 metal ceramic
Shade A3.5

£546

	Date		Metal Try in	Porcelain Try in	Finished Ready to fit	Other (specify above)
Next appointment on	20 11	For			✓	
Next appointment on		For				
Next appointment on		For				
Next appointment on		For				
Next appointment on		For				

Fig. 9.5 An example of a laboratory prescription that highlights the importance of effective communication between clinician and dental technologist.

- Will the laboratory work completed to this prescription satisfy the needs and expectations of the patient?

Finally, reflect on the likelihood of obtaining a good esthetic outcome based on the prescriptions in Figure 9.5.

Additional reading

Chiche GJ, Pinault A. Communication with the dental laboratory. In: Esthetics of anterior fixed prosthodontics. Chicago: Quintessence; 1994. p. 115–42.

CHAPTER 10

Maintaining Dental Attractiveness

RICHARD FOXTON

INTRODUCTION

Practitioners are professionally bound to do their utmost to ensure that any dental treatment is performed in the patient's best interests and to the best of their abilities. Esthetic dental care is no exception to this requirement. As a consequence, all esthetic dental procedures should be completed, with minimal intervention, to the satisfaction of the patient, and with a view to the best possible durability and longevity. This, however, does not ensure sustained, satisfactory performance in clinical service, as this may only be achieved with the co-operation and motivation of the patient. If the patient does not maintain a good standard of oral health and does nothing to control habits and behaviours that result in an unfavourable oral environment, then any work will be doomed to suffer early deterioration and possibly failure, irrespective of the quality of the esthetic dental care. Maintaining dental attractiveness is as much, if not more, about what patients do to maintain their dental condition on a day-to-day basis, than the actions taken by their practitioners, who, following completion of the esthetic dental care, are occasional 'visitors' in the patients' mouths.

CLINICAL TIP

Long-term maintenance and salvage options should be part of every treatment plan.

Given the above, patients wishing esthetic dental treatments must be educated, trained and motivated to maintain a high standard of oral hygiene, and to avoid behaviours and habits that may create an unfavourable oral environment, which, in turn, may compromise their dental attractiveness. To achieve this, patients may require substantial support, particularly if their esthetic concerns are, at least in part, attributable to their behaviours, habits and oral hygiene measures.

The purpose of this chapter is not to consider and discuss approaches and techniques to change the attitudes and behaviours of patients – a topic that could be the subject of a separate book – but to review the procedures practitioners may adopt to maintain dental attractiveness, subject to the patient maintaining a good standard of oral hygiene and health.

A wide range of dental procedures and materials may be used in maintaining dental esthetics. It is important for the practitioner and other members of the dental team, in particular those who provide esthetic dental care, to be competent in the selection and application of these procedures and materials. Maintenance visits, which may extend to refurbishing, repairing and possibly replacing restorations and prostheses, should be based on careful assessments and examinations.

As with the initial examination and assessment of esthetic dental care patients, as discussed in detail in Chapter 3, the examination and assessment of such patients at recall should be systematic, meticulous and detailed. If any aspect of the esthetic dental care has suffered any deterioration, let alone failed, it is not sufficient simply to identify the deterioration or failure; its causation must also be determined and addressed if the remedial treatment is to be successful, in terms of both resolving the problem and preventing recurrence.

This chapter will cover how periodontal health, restorations, including implant-supported restorations and prostheses, and procedures such as tooth bleaching should be maintained in clinical service.

Frequency of recall of esthetic dental care patients should be tailored to meet the needs and expectations of the individual. Some patients, especially those who maintain a very high standard of oral hygiene and health, may need to be recalled once a year only. Others, for various reasons, may require recall as frequently as every 3 months. The pattern of recall may vary over time. One way or another, esthetic dental care patients should, subsequent to satisfactory completion of the initial treatment, be entered into an ongoing maintenance programme. If the patient was referred for esthetic dental care, and returns to their dental practitioner for routine dental care, then the practitioner must assume responsibility to provide the necessary maintenance care, or to refer the patient back, as and when indicated clinically.

THE PATIENT'S CONCERNS

Is the patient fully aware of the potential cost and time commitment entailed by the maintenance programme?

PERIODONTAL MAINTENANCE

Whenever root surface debridement is indicated as part of esthetic dental maintenance, time should be allowed following the debridement for resolution of inflammation and healing of the periodontal tissues. This period should be around 6–8 weeks, after which time the patient should be recalled. At recall, several factors need to be assessed. These include the presence of any plaque or calculus, the condition of the gingival tissues, the presence or absence of bleeding when the pockets are probed, the depth of any pockets on probing, gingival recession, and the presence or absence of tooth mobility.[1] If thorough debridement fails to improve the periodontal status, further management may involve referral for a specialist opinion, or to the patient's medical practitioner for assessment of a possible underlying condition.

Non-surgical root surface debridement may make changes in the subgingival flora that last up to 3 months. Therefore, in cases where the medium- to long-term stability of the periodontal condition is a cause for concern, maintenance root surface debridement should be undertaken every 3 months to establish and maintain a subgingival biofilm compatible with periodontal health. Maintenance treatment should include routine examination and assessment of the status of the periodontal tissues, including radiographic examinations, as indicated clinically; an assessment of the sufficiency of the oral hygiene; and root surface debridement where residual periodontal pockets persist.[1]

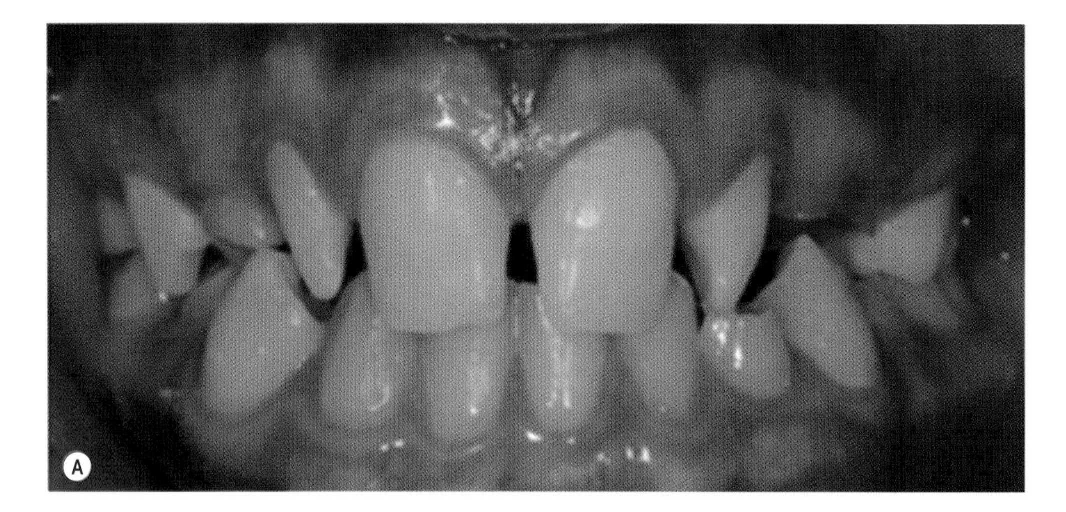

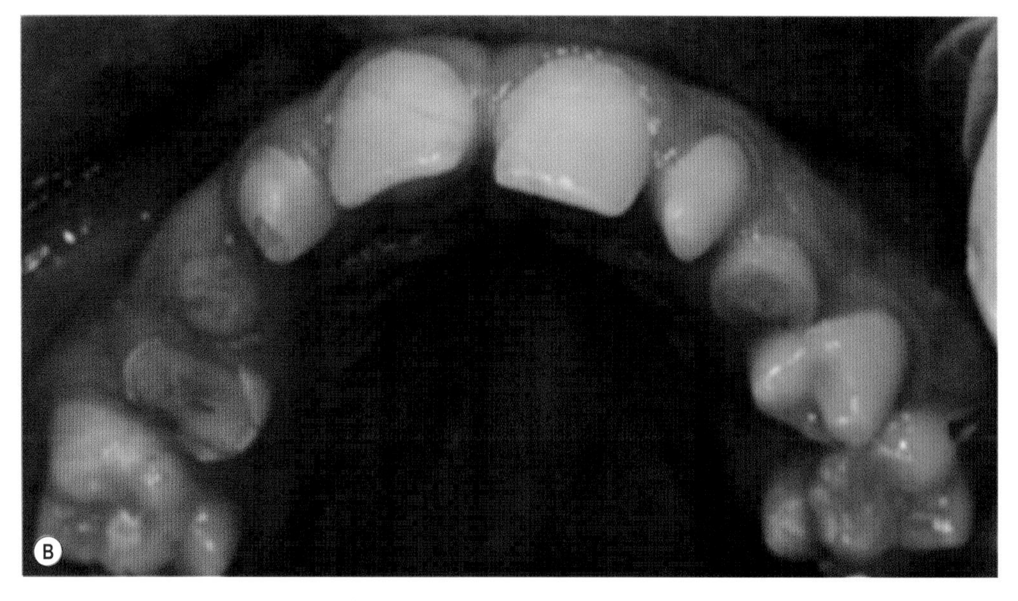

Fig. 10.1 Maintenance of oral hygiene. A and B. A 13-year-old patient exhibiting hypodontia and misshapen maxillary incisors. The maxillary incisors and retained deciduous teeth were built up with direct resin composite additions.

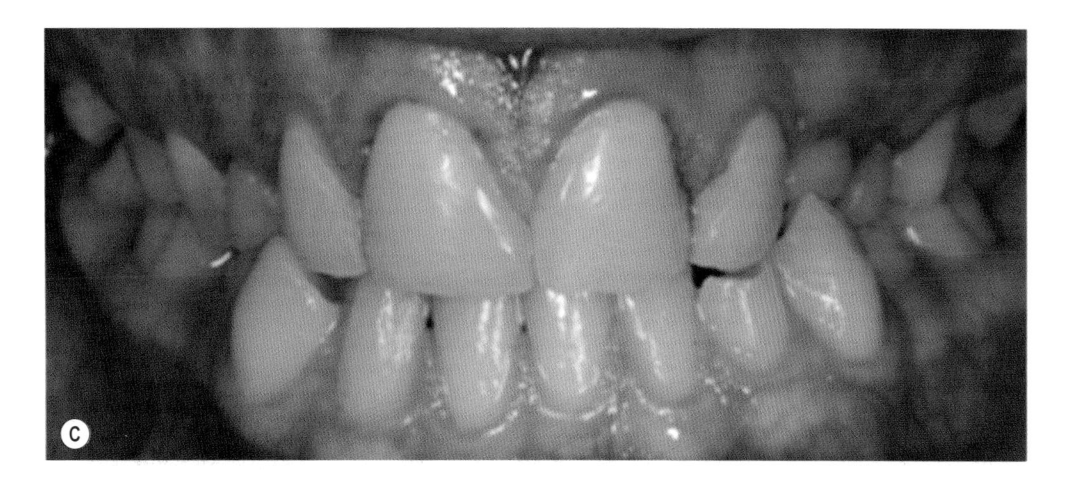

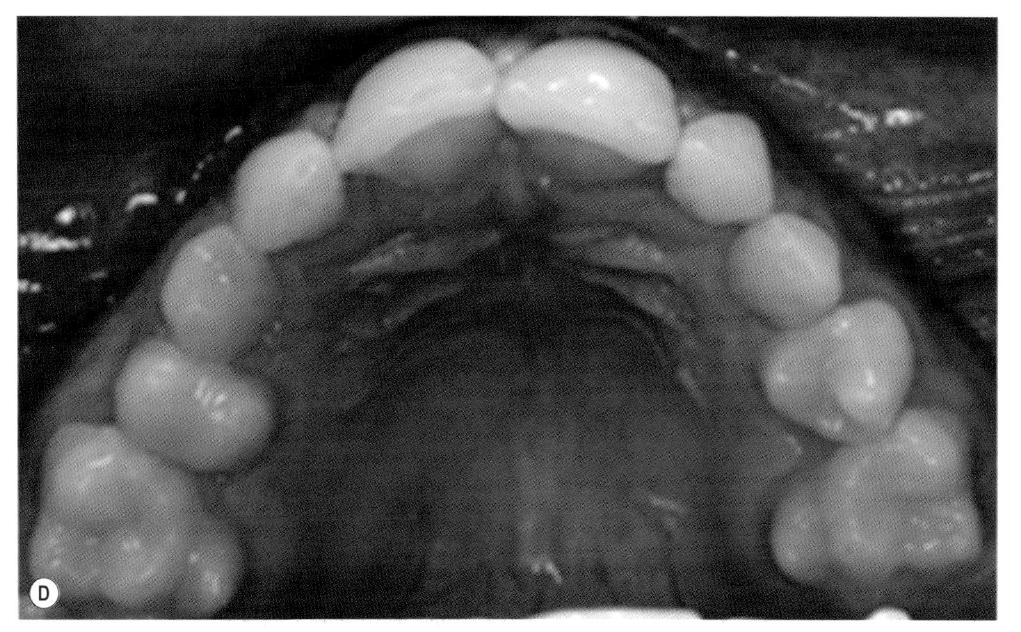

Fig. 10.1 ***Continued*** **C and D. The restorations 3 years after placement. The patient required ongoing encouragement to maintain adequate oral hygiene.**

Esthetic dental treatments may have included modifications to the anatomy and contours of teeth using adhesively bonded materials, such as resin composite (Fig. 10.1). Such modifications introduce margins between resin composite and the underlying tooth tissues, and alter the emergence profile of the tooth. At recall, such margins and altered emergence profiles should be carefully assessed as features that may be compromising oral hygiene and, in turn, periodontal health. Where there are concerns about any adverse periodontal responses to esthetically pleasing modifications to the anatomy and contours of teeth, the patient should receive detailed instruction on oral hygiene aids and procedures capable of countering the unwanted effects.

MAINTENANCE AND REPAIR OF COMPOSITE AND CERAMIC RESTORATIONS

Despite significant advances in dental biomaterial science, esthetic restorations of composite resin and porcelain suffer various forms of deterioration in clinical service; if these are allowed to progress unchecked, they may lead to premature failure, with the unnecessary loss of sound tooth tissue.

Restorations that are showing signs of failure may be managed in one of four ways[2]:

1. *No treatment (monitoring).* Monitoring is indicated if a restoration exhibits 'minor shortcomings': for example, limited, superficial staining or small imperfections in marginal adaptation that are apparent on close examination only, and do not pose any risk if left untreated.
2. *Refurbishment.* This may involve various minimal intervention procedures to correct minor shortcomings in restorations without damage to the remaining tooth tissues. Refurbishment may include the removal of limited overhangs and flash excess, refinements to contours, removal of surface discoloration, and smoothing or glazing of the surface of the restoration to eliminate or seal superficial pores and small cracks and gaps. Refurbishment techniques, which may be considered as an extension of finishing techniques for restorations, do not involve the addition of new restorative material. Refurbishment techniques that involve the application of a surface glaze should include surface preparation techniques, as described for the repair of composites (see below).
3. *Repair.* This refers to the process of correcting an unacceptable defect in an otherwise clinically acceptable restoration. Repairs typically involve some form of minimal operative intervention to remove the unacceptable defect, and the addition of restorative material to make the restoration fit for further clinical service.
4. *Replacement.* When a restoration presents with one or more defects that cannot reasonably be managed by refurbishment and repair, then restoration replacement is indicated. In all cases, restoration replacement should be undertaken in such ways as to minimize the inevitable increase in the size of the preparation, with the loss of sound tooth tissue. Detailed consideration of when to replace or repair restorations is included in the extensive review of the repair of restorations published by Hickel et al.[3]

COMPOSITE RESTORATIONS

When composite resin is placed using a direct technique, bonding between the layers of resin occurs through a process involving the oxygen-inhibited layer of unpolymerized resin on the surface of each layer of composite. When another increment of composite resin is placed and light-cured, polymerization takes place in the oxygen-inhibited layer, resulting in bonding between the two increments.[4] When the restoration is polished, or has been in service for a period of time, the unpolymerized oxygen-inhibited surface layer is lost. This makes the addition of new material to an existing restoration, as occurs in maintenance procedures, a more complicated process than the simple layering used in a composite build-up.

Indirect composite resin restorations are produced in the laboratory, or possibly at the chairside. The polymerization of indirect composites may include the application of heat to enhance the light activation of the resin. Once completed, very few free carbon double bonds are available in indirect composites for cross-linking. Therefore, as and when a repair of an indirect composite is indicated, a process needs to be followed to achieve bonding between existing and new composite.

Despite the different approaches to the provision of direct and indirect composite restorations, both types of restorations should be managed in a similar way when it comes to effecting repairs. 'Aged' composite resin, whether placed directly or formed indirectly, presents a very similar substrate from the point of view of carrying out a repair by means of the direct addition of new composite resin.

When a repair to a defective composite resin restoration is planned, consideration should be given to the cause of the defect. If the defect was caused as a result of, for example, excessive occlusal loading, then this issue should be addressed prior to carrying out the repair. If any caries is present, then this must be treated in accordance with modern concepts of caries management.

There are relatively few published data on the long-term success of repaired composite resin restorations. Laboratory studies have evaluated various surface treatments to enhance the bond between new composite resin and 'aged' composite resin. With considerable interest in this aspect of modern approaches to the maintenance of restored teeth, it is anticipated that knowledge and understanding in this area are set to increase substantially in years to come.

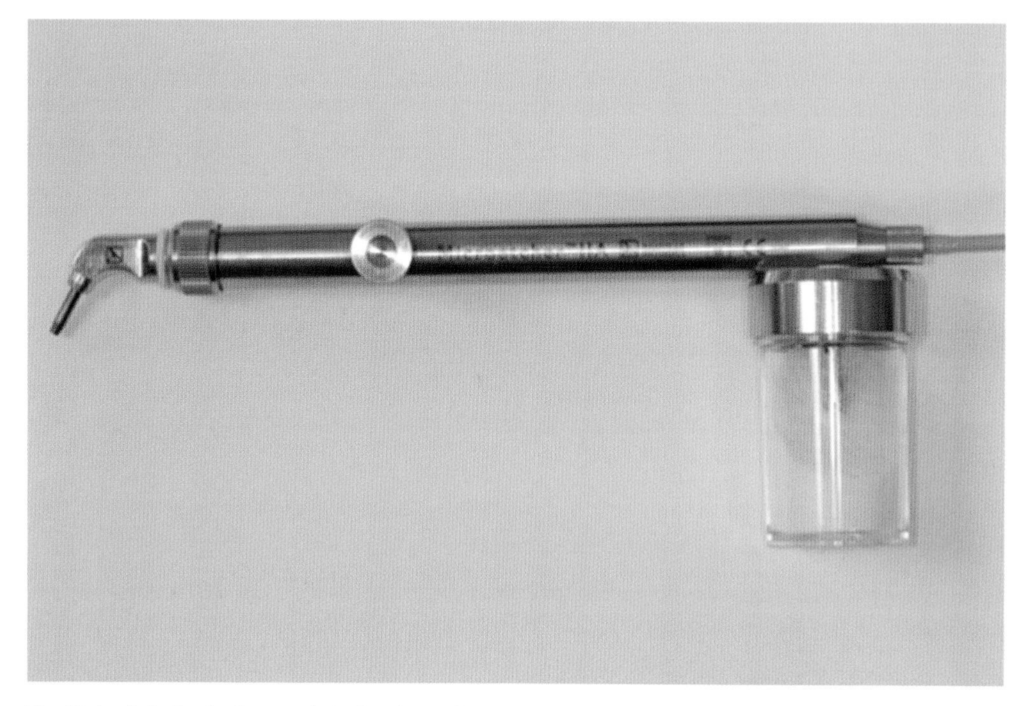

Fig. 10.2 A device for intraoral air abrasion (MicroEtcher II, Danville Engineering).

The 'aged' composite resin surface may be modified physically and/or chemically to create a micromechanical and/or chemical bond between new and existing composite resin. Composite resins essentially consist of silanated glass filler particles embedded in a resin matrix. Since it is not possible to bond chemically to the resin matrix because of the lack of free carbon double bonds, the other option is to attempt to bond chemically to the glass filler particles. Physical alteration of the composite resin surface to expose glass filler particles may be accomplished using aluminium oxide particle air abrasion (Fig. 10.2). Alternatively, silica-coated aluminium oxide particles may be used to cover the surface of the restoration with particles that are chemically reactive to a silane coupling agent and adhesive resin. The silica particles may be silanated to aid the formation of a chemical bond.

Until recently, it has been considered that the presenting composite resin surface should have around 50% of the filler particles exposed, since the composite resin is made up of around 50% by volume of glass filler particles.[4] If a silane solution is then applied to the surface, a chemical bond will be created between new composite resin and any exposed glass filler particles on the surface of the restoration. This would theoretically increase the strength of the bond of any subsequent increment of composite resin. However, it has been found, using scanning electron microscopy, that when composite resin materials contain smaller-than-average filler particles, their glass surfaces are not really exposed and therefore a silane solution applied to the surface will have no glass particles to which to bond.[4] This indicates that achieving a successful repair to composite resin may be dependent upon the type of direct resin and the size of its filler particles. Further research is clearly needed; however, based on research completed to date, it may be concluded, by way of general guidance, that[3]:

- The repair of marginal defects in composite should involve careful, minimal intervention opening and cleaning of the defect, using rotary or other means to create intact, slightly roughened surfaces in composite and adjacent tooth tissue and exclude deep undermining caries that might necessitate a substantial repair or possibly replacement of the restoration. The completed marginal defect preparation, which should be free of any sharp angular features or irregularities, should be etched with phosphoric acid and a dental adhesive should be applied, prior to filling the defect carefully with a flowable composite resin. To complete this type of procedure successfully, it is essential to have good access. If a marginal defect is located, for example, along a gingival margin, then part of the restoration may need to be removed to gain the necessary access.
- The repair of chip defects, as may occur when a marginal ridge is damaged, bulk fractures, partial loss of the restoration through wear, limited lesions of secondary caries and staining of part of the tooth restoration interface is best achieved by careful, minimal intervention preparation, etching with phosphoric acid, the application of an adhesive and placement of an appropriate composite resin restorative.

As indicated above, depending on the nature of the composite being repaired, an application of silane may also be indicated; however, more often than not, the nature of the composite being repaired is not known and the use of silane should be omitted from the procedure. If the nature of the composite to be repaired is known, the manufacturer's directions for use should be consulted to seek specific guidance as to how best to achieve a durable repair. Any such guidance should be followed meticulously.

An example of a repair to a composite restoration is shown in Figure 10.3.

CERAMIC RESTORATIONS

Ceramic restorations may be broadly classified into two groups: those that contain silicon dioxide (silica), such as feldspathic porcelains, leucite-reinforced

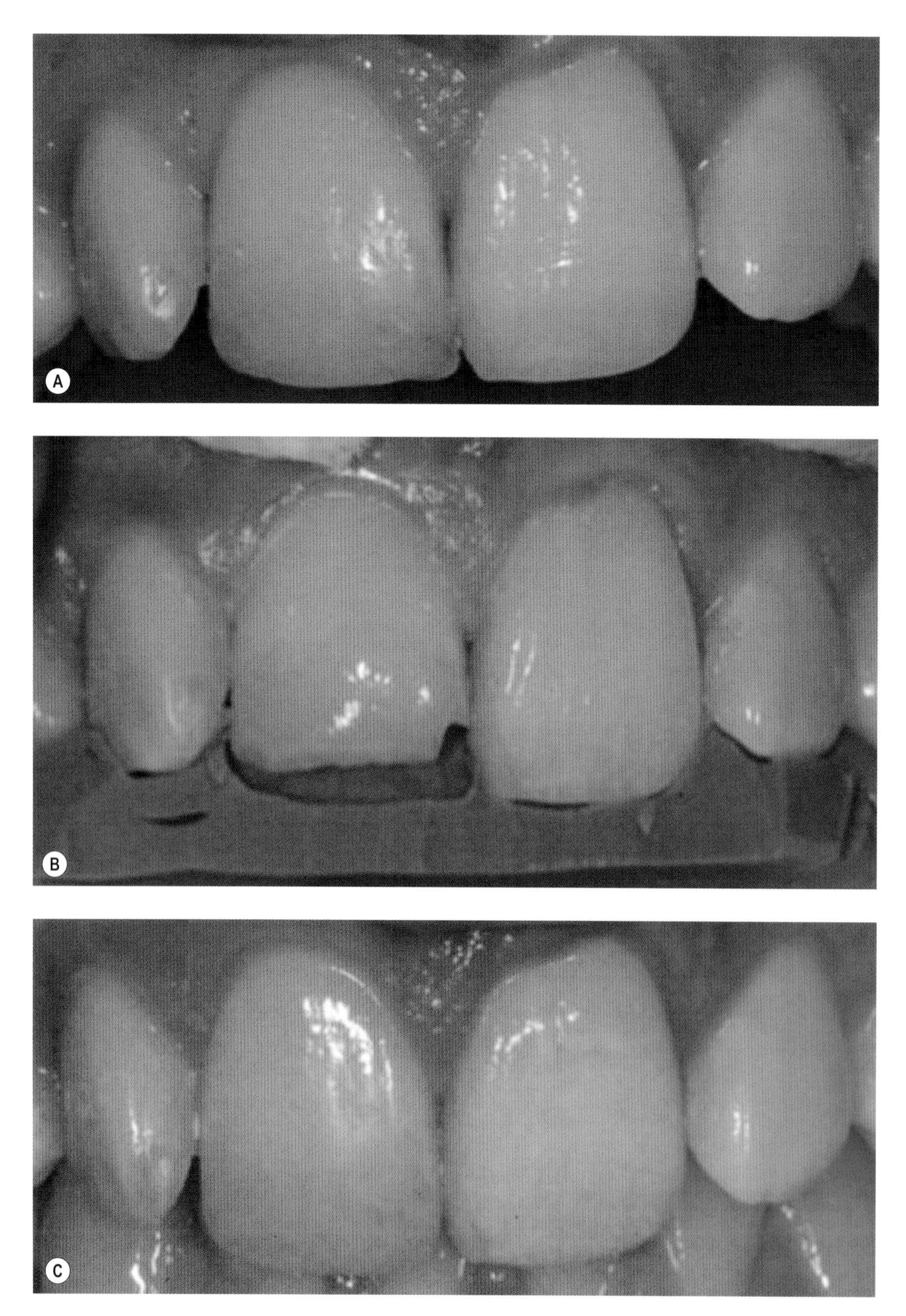

Fig. 10.3 Composite repair. A. Failing labial/incisal edge composite restoration. B. Build-up matrix applied subsequent to partial removal of failing restoration. C. Completed repair.

ceramics, and lithium disilicate ceramics; and those that do not, such as alumina and zirconia ceramic core materials. This distinction is very important when it comes to bonding composite resin to these materials, either at initial cementation of the restoration, or when attempting to repair a marginal defect or fracture.

If the restoration is made from a silicon dioxide-containing ceramic, it can be etched with hydrofluoric acid and silanated (Fig. 10.4), or air-abraded with aluminium oxide particles coated with silica to create a chemical micromechanical bond with the composite resin used to complete the repair.[5,6] The use of hydrofluoric acid in the mouth is fraught with risks of severe damage to the patient and chairside staff. If used, hydrofluoric acid must be applied with extreme care, with all the necessary precautions being followed throughout the procedure.

To simplify the silanization stage, ceramic primers are marketed as single-bottle products. However, multi-component silane coupling agents continue to be marketed as two-bottle ceramic primers, which offer the theoretical advantage that activation of the silane coupling is maximal when the two bottles are mixed at the chairside, as opposed to single-bottle ceramic primers that are maximally active immediately after manufacture.[5,6,7]

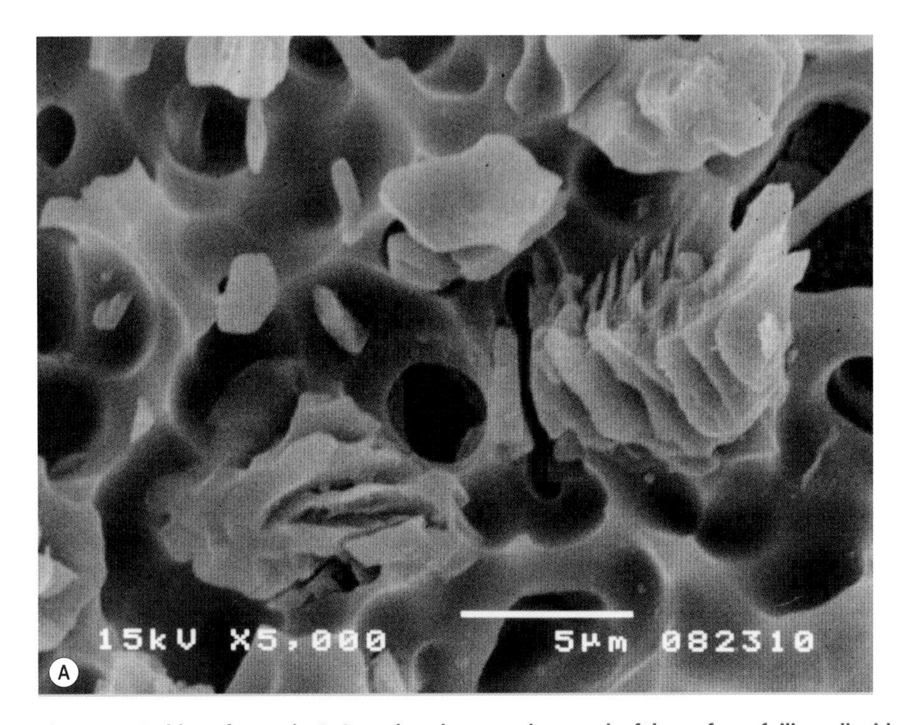

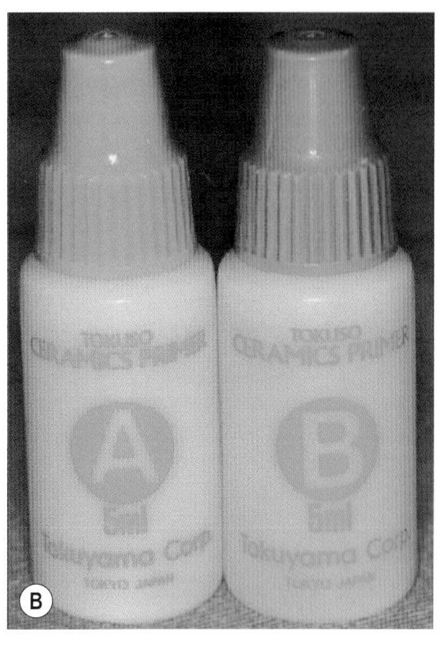

Fig. 10.4 Etching of ceramic. A. Scanning electron micrograph of the surface of silicon dioxide-containing ceramic block after etching with hydrofluoric acid. The glass phase is dissolved, creating microscopic pores, which allow micro-mechanical retention of a resin placed on the surface. B. Two-bottle ceramic primers are silane coupling agents that can be maximally activated when mixed at the chairside.

At present, it remains difficult to achieve a durable bond to zirconia or alumina ceramics. As such, attempting to repair a restoration of veneering porcelain would be very unpredictable.

In the process of repairing ceramic restorations, the removal of any bonded composite resin lute that may be present carries with it the risk of removing sound, healthy dentine because of the challenge in differentiating between the composite resin and the underlying tooth structure. Laboratory research has indicated that recently developed bioactive glasses, such as Bioglass® (45S5), may effectively remove resin, whilst being conservative of the underlying tooth structure (Fig. 10.5).

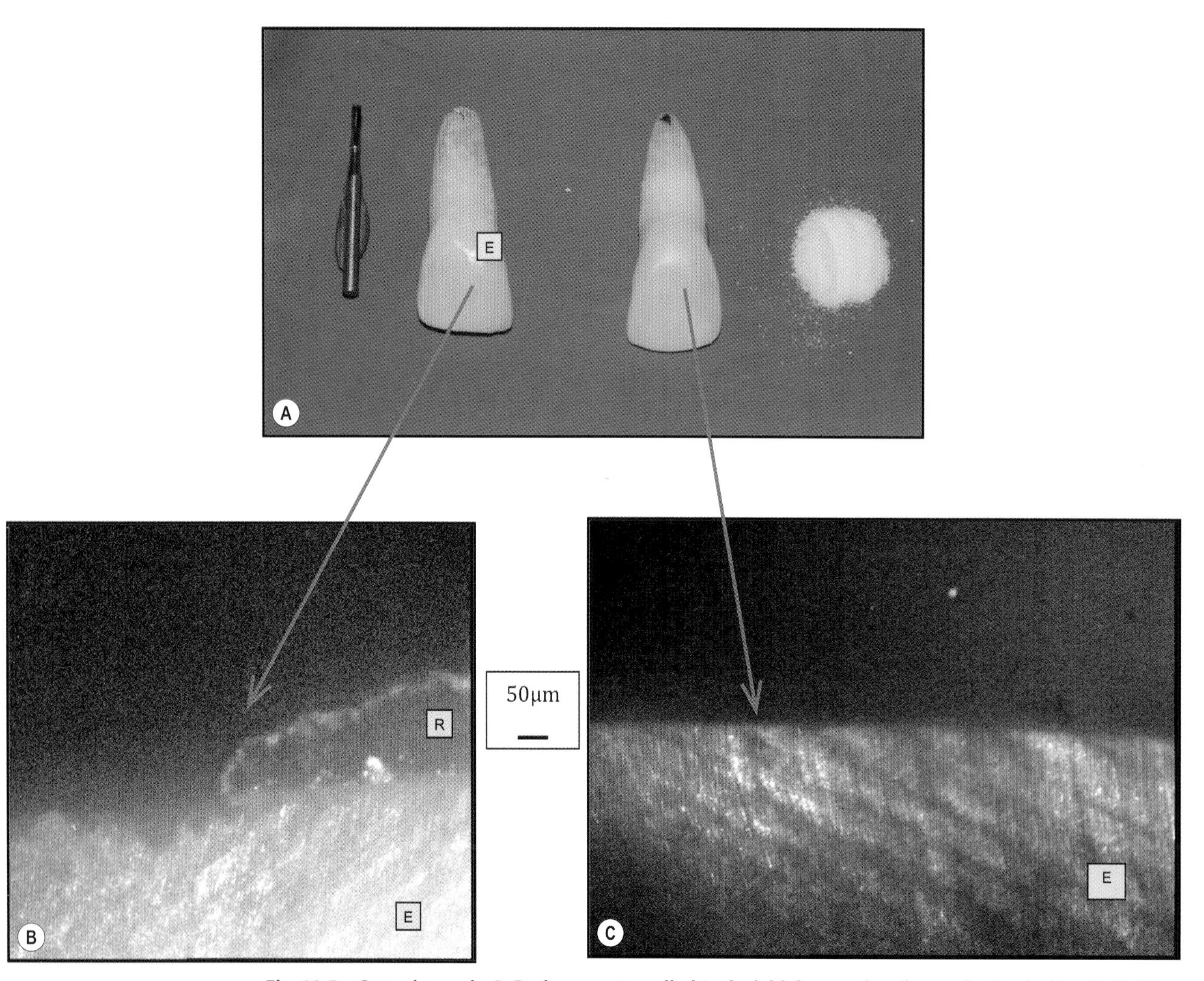

Fig. 10.5 Ceramic repair. A. Resin cement applied to the labial enamel surfaces of extracted teeth. B. After visible removal of the resin cement, laser scanning microscopy revealed that the tungsten carbide bur had removed enamel as well as the resin cement. C. After visible removal of resin cement with Bioglass® (45S5), the resin cement is removed without interfering with the underlying enamel.

Small additions of porcelain or any other ceramic material cannot be bonded to a fractured ceramic restoration in the mouth. Repair of small ceramic fractures must be carried out using composite resin. Because ceramic materials are quite different from resin composites, chemically and esthetically, the opportunities for achieving a successful, esthetically pleasing, long-lasting repair to a ceramic restoration are relatively limited. Moreover, when damage occurs to a ceramic restoration in an area of high occlusal loading, the bond between a composite repair and ceramic may not be sufficient to withstand the loads applied to it in clinical service. That said, repairs to ceramic restorations can be a reliable, low-cost means to extend the clinical serviceability of expensive, possibly difficult-to-replace restorations. If for no other purpose, a repair to a ceramic restoration may serve as a temporary means to restore the appearance of the restoration until such time that a replacement restoration can be provided.

PORCELAIN FUSED TO METAL CROWNS

Repairs to porcelain fused to metal (PFM) crowns are made using similar techniques to those employed for repairs to ceramic restorations, when the damage is contained within the porcelain. If the damage to the crown has exposed metal, then the metallic surface should be air-abraded with aluminium oxide particles coated with silica, prior to masking the metal with an opaque resin composite. Once the metal has been masked, the restoration may be repaired in a similar manner to a ceramic restoration. As with ceramic restorations, a repair to a PFM crown may be best viewed as a short- to medium-term temporary measure until such time as a new restoration can be provided. In older patients for whom the replacement of a damaged PFM may not be in their best interest, a repair may be maintained by refurbishment and new additions, as may be indicated clinically.

TOOTH BLEACHING

Tooth bleaching, as discussed in an earlier chapter, may be accomplished using at-home or in-office techniques. A randomized clinical trial compared the whitening results of an at-home technique using 10% carbamide peroxide and an in-office technique using 38% hydrogen peroxide. Both these techniques were shown to produce satisfactory and long-lasting bleaching results at the 9-month recall visit.[8] At home, nightguard vital bleaching using a 10% carbamide peroxide solution in a custom tray has been shown to be safe and effective over a period of 10 years.[9] Colour stability was found to last 108–144 months post-whitening. On the other hand, a double-blind randomized clinical trial of two at-home carbamide peroxide tooth-bleaching agents found that there was a tooth shade relapse at a 2-year follow-up.[10] Top-up bleaching can be carried out when tooth shade relapse has occurred. The procedure for top-up bleaching is the same as for initial bleaching but may not take as long to complete, given that the shade relapse may be relatively limited.

A clinical case in which a single dental implant was placed to replace an avulsed upper right central incisor is illustrated in Figure 10.6. The adjacent upper left central incisor was bleached using 'home bleaching' with 15% carbamide peroxide gel prior to restoring the dental implant. The bleaching was continued to give a slightly 'whiter' shade than selected for the implant-retained crown in anticipation of some shade relapse.

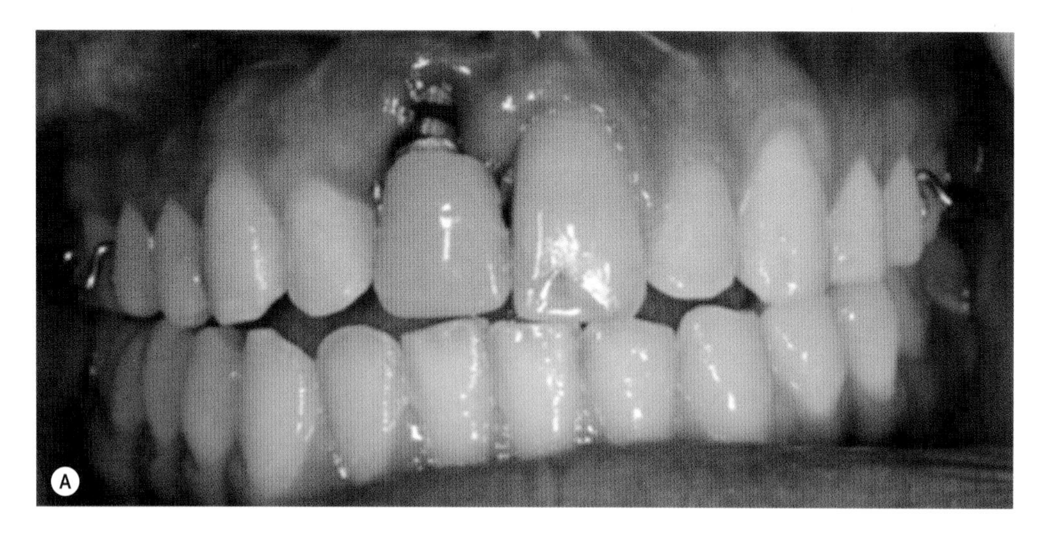

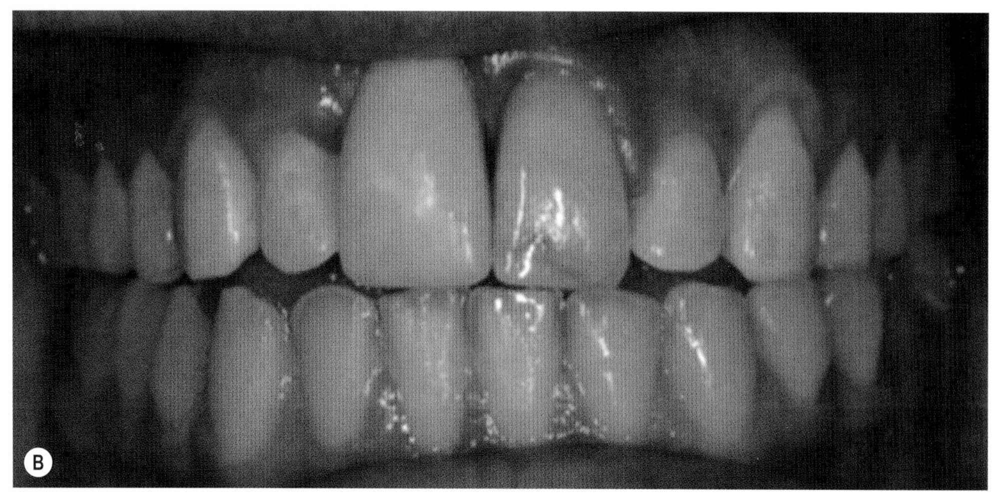

Fig. 10.6 Bleaching in implant dentistry. A. A dental implant has been placed in the upper right central incisor space and the darkened upper left central incisor has been root-treated. The upper left central incisor was lost because of trauma. Additional loss of labial bone resulted in the implant being placed buccally. B. A provisional composite resin screw-retained crown has been placed to allow healing of the gingival tissue around the dental implant.

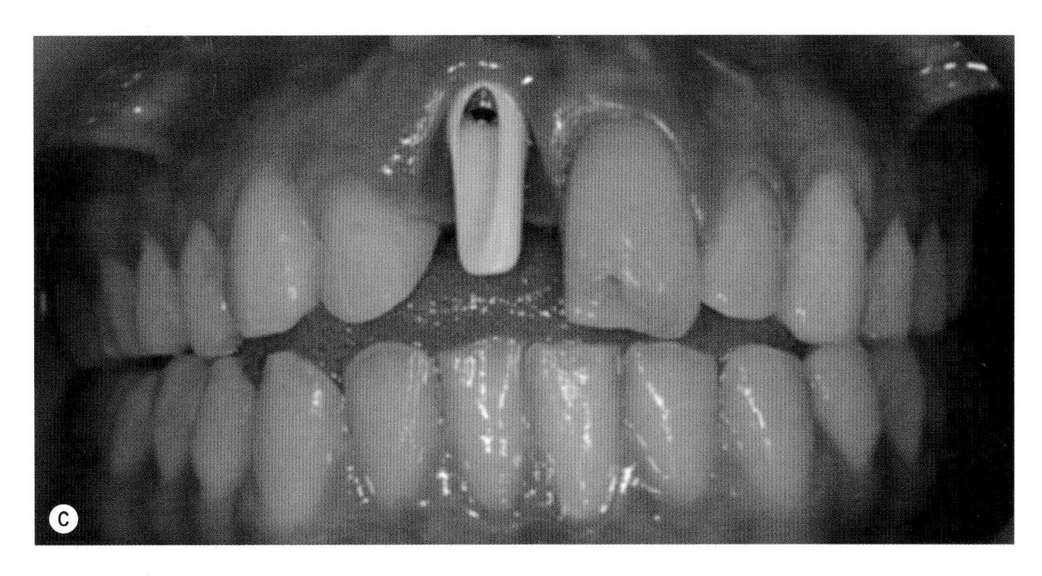

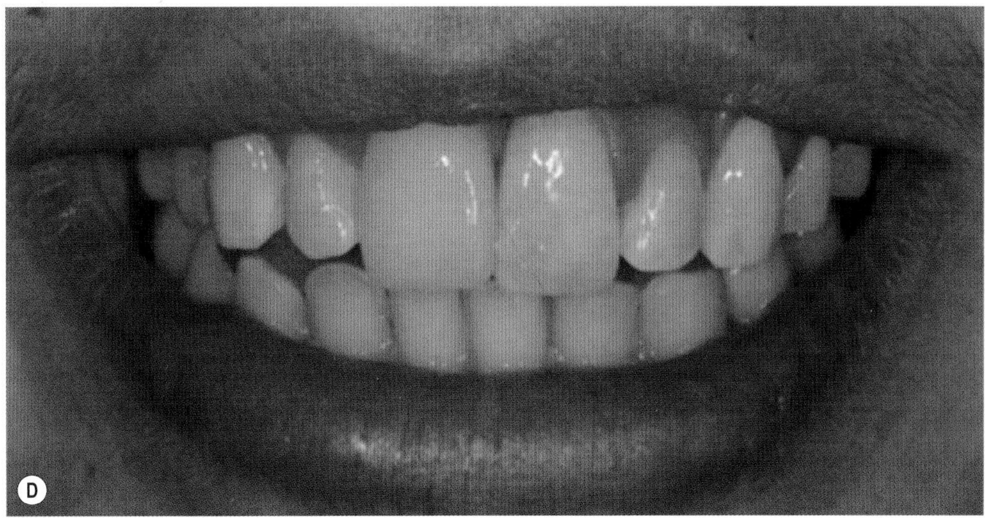

Fig. 10.6 ***Continued*** **C. A zirconia abutment was placed in the implant following bleaching of the upper left central incisor. D. The dental implant was restored with a crown cemented on the zirconia abutment and the discoloured composite resin restoration in the upper left central incisor repaired. The gingival margins of both the implant-retained crown and upper left central incisor are not visible when the patient smiles.**

DENTAL IMPLANTS

Dental implants require maintenance which may require regular visits to a specialist and can be expensive, although less costly than implant failure to the patient or a legal challenge to the dentist who placed the implants or the general practitioner landed with reviewing them. All patients with implant-retained restorations or prostheses should be recalled at least annually. Single-unit crowns may become loose or displaced if provisional cement has been used. Fixed prostheses should be monitored for signs of wear and the screws used to retain the prosthesis or the abutments should have their torque checked.[11] It is important for the patient to maintain good oral hygiene; otherwise the surrounding soft tissues may become inflamed. Long-cone periapical radiographs should be taken of the fixtures on an annual basis, at least for the first few years, to monitor the marginal bone levels.[11] If there is inflammation of the surrounding tissues and loss of the marginal bone, a diagnosis of peri-implantitis may be made. In such cases, intervention, up to and including surgical treatment, may be required to remove the inflamed and damaged tissue and disinfect the implant surface.[11]

KEY POINT SUMMARY

It's not just other dentists' work that fails! So be honest when you answer your patient's questions.

- *Don't* oversell the longevity.
- *Do* discuss failure and future options.

CONCLUDING REMARKS

In esthetic dentistry, maintenance care is important to long-term clinical success. Esthetic restorations and prostheses, in a similar manner to all other forms of restorations and prostheses, should be monitored and refurbished or repaired to delay, if not prevent, replacement. The need for ongoing maintenance of esthetic restorations and prostheses must be explained to and accepted by the patient prior to embarking on initial provision. Typically, once an esthetic dental care patient, always an esthetic dental care patient, but hopefully a patient who can be managed on an ongoing basis by minimal intervention approaches and procedures.

REFERENCES

1. Eley BM, Soory M, Manson JD. Periodontics. 6th ed. London: Churchill Livingstone/Elsevier; 2010. p. 221–5.
2. Hickel R, Roulet JF, Bayne S, et al. Recommendations for conducting controlled clinical studies of dental restorative materials. Clin Oral Investig 2007;11:5–33.
3. Hickel R, Bushaver K, Ilie N. Repair of restorations: criteria for decision making and clinical recommendations. Dent Mater 2013;29:28–50.
4. Akimoto N, Sakamoto T, Kubota Y, et al. A novel composite-to-composite adhesive bond mechanism. Dent Mater J 2011;30:523–7.
5. Matsumura H, Kato H, Atsuta M. Shear bond strength to feldspathic porcelain of two luting cements in combination with three surface treatments. J Prosthet Dent 1997;78: 511–17.

6. Aida M, Hayakawa T, Mizukawa K. Adhesion of composite to porcelain with various surface conditions. J Prosthet Dent 1995;73:464–70.

7. Franses LS. MClinDent Thesis. King's College London Dental Institute, King's College London; 2006.

8. Giachetti L, Bertini F, Bambi C, et al. A randomized clinical trial comparing at-home and in-office tooth whitening techniques: a nine-month follow-up. J Am Dent Assoc 2010;141: 1357–64.

9. Ritter AV, Leonard RH Jr, St Georges AJ, et al. Safety and stability of nightguard vital bleaching: 9 to 12 years post-treatment. J Esthet Restor Dent 2002;14:275–85.

10. Meireles SS, Santos IS, Bona AD, et al. A double-blind randomized clinical trial of two carbamide peroxide tooth bleaching agents: 2-year follow-up. J Dent 2010;38:956–63.

11. Palmer RM, Smith BJ, Howe LC, et al. Implants in clinical dentistry. Abingdon: Taylor & Francis; 2002. p. 238–48.

INDEX

Page numbers followed by 'f' indicate figures, 't' indicate tables, and 'b' indicate boxes.